About the A

ARTHUR C. K

(Robinson, 1

based on an unprecedented and extensive survey of

1,000 people in the USA with oste   The

result was described i   nt

book'

T   exercise was the most powerful   for

many forms of arthritis led to a follow-up book, *Arthritis: What Exercises* Really *Work*, which was published in the UK in 1996. The two books were issued in a combined edition, *Arthritis: The Complete Guide to Relief* (Robinson, 1998).

Arthur C. Klein is a member of the American Society of Journalists and Authors, and the American Medical Writers Association.

The Daily Telegraph

BACK PAIN

What Really Works

Arthur C. Klein

ROBINSON
London

For Zoë Rachel Klein

Constable & Robinson Ltd
3 The Lanchesters
162 Fulham Palace Road
London W6 9ER
www.constablerobinson.com

This revised edition published in the UK by Robinson,
an imprint of Constable & Robinson Ltd 2006

A combined edition first published in the UK by Robinson Publishing Ltd 1999.
Backache Relief first published in the USA by St Martin's Press 1985.
Backache: What Exercises Really Work first published in the UK by Robinson
Publishing Ltd 1996; first published in the USA by St Martin's Press 1994.

Exercise illustrations by Lauren Jarrett and prelim illustrations by Stephen Dew.

A copy of the British Library Cataloguing in Publication data
is available from the British Library

ISBN 13: 978-1-84529-098-6
ISBN 10: 1-84529-098-4

Printed and bound in the EU

1 3 5 7 9 10 8 6 4 2

Contents

x CONTENTS

Acknowledgements

Thanks to Donna Danyluk, Millie Mascia, Page McBrier, and especially Evelyn Poitras for their help with the research on which this book is based and the preparation of the manuscript;

To my literary agent, Max Gartenberg, who helped define the scope and structure of the book;

To Miriam Fisher, my first survey participant, for her many contributions to the background research;

To Frank Anello for his support and inspiration;

And to Jonathan B. Segal of Times Books for his advice, encouragement and enthusiasm.

The publishers wish to express their thanks to BackCare (registered as the National Back Pain Association), an independent national charity, for their help in conducting the UK survey.

Introduction

For virtually everyone, the chances that at some time in their lives 'something will go wrong' with their backs are considerable. There are, after all, more muscles, joints, bones, nerves and ligaments running up and down the vertebrae in close proximity to each other than in any other part of the body. The subtle complexity of the interaction of these spinal structures, as back pain sufferers know only too well, can make it difficult for even the best-trained doctors with the most sophisticated diagnostic techniques to determine precisely what is amiss.

Tens of thousands of people are laid low with back pain every year. For some, the lucky ones, it resolves within a few weeks with a judicious combination of exercises supplemented by painkillers and anti-inflammatory drugs. But what of the rest? There are, as Arthur Klein points out, a myriad of different specialists involved in the treatment of back pain, each with their own opinion as to the likely explanation and the best way of putting it right. Amidst this babble of competing views, the back pain sufferer can understandably find it difficult to know where to turn or how to evaluate their claims of efficacy. One vital source of information, much neglected but of great importance, is the judgement of the real experts, back pain sufferers themselves.

It was a most ingenious idea to invite the jury, nearly 500 American back pain sufferers, to deliver their verdict based on their own personal experience of the relative efficacy of the various treatments on offer. For this second UK edition, the results of the US survey have been extended and updated with another larger-scale survey conducted online in the UK in 2004. This survey gleaned responses from 2,240 back pain sufferers.

There are, of course, several different types of back pain, even though in any individual the precise pathology that gives rise to their symptoms may not be easy to pin down. These subdivide into a few main groups – such as slipped (or ruptured) disc, arthritis, sciatica and spondylosis – and participants in the surveys have been invited to assess which of the several options, including physiotherapy, cortisone injections or an operation, proved most effective and in what situation.

The overall impression is of 'horses for courses' where the efficacy of the various approaches varies widely. However, most participants agree on the importance of self-help measures and staying as active as possible, with many getting great relief from yoga and from carefully designed exercise programmes.

There are obvious limitations to this personal and anecdotal assessment of therapy but this is far outweighed by its virtues. First, it conveys very well the scope of possible treatments, both orthodox and otherwise, along with their drawbacks. Further, it emphasizes how, for many of those with chronic back pain the best solution lies in going beyond expert opinion to take control of their condition by deploying judicious forms of self-treatment. Much the most important of these are the exercises deemed safe and effective by specialists at Cornell University in New York that increase the suppleness of the spinal column and strengthen the muscles that sustain it. These are described in detail in the second half of this book.

Like all family doctors, I see at least a couple of patients with back pain every week and am delighted that in addition to other appropriate advice and specialist referral I can now recommend a book that offers the best hope of long-term relief of their symptoms for many of them.

Dr James Le Fanu

Author's Preface

This updated edition provides important new information about diagnosing and treating back pain, and answers the major questions on back pain sufferers' minds. For example, what steps can you take right now to stop pain? Which kinds of healthcare practitioners are most likely to help you . . . or waste your time . . . or make you worse? Which new treatments should you know about? What are the best exercises for your back? Which methods work best for specific kinds of back pain? Are there unorthodox healing approaches that get proven results?

Back Pain: What Really Works brings you solutions based on surveys of the ultimate experts on back pain – sufferers themselves. These are the individuals who have found ways out of seemingly incurable back pain. They are the people who have been through it all, heard it all, tried it all, and yet managed to emerge on the other side with life-changing answers.

I am one of these people, although, ironically, there was a time in my own life when I would have looked down my nose at anyone who couldn't manage back pain.

Low back pain ran in my family and I had my first acute episode of muscle spasms at 18. For more than 20 years, I held back pain at bay. I bought a bed board and a firm mattress. I found a good 'writer's chair' – one that supported my lower back. I worked out three times a week at a gym. I did daily stretching and strengthening exercises for my back. I swam. I ran six miles a day. Incapacitating back pain? Lost work days? Ha! No way. Not me. That was for other people.

Then one day my right Achilles tendon swelled up and my ankle all but locked in place. I had to walk with crutches. I got to the gym pool every day, but, generally, I had to sit more and exercise less. My legs, hips and buttocks began to spasm day and night. The backs of my thighs ached intensely. Still, I felt relatively fortunate. I had a diagnosis for my ankle problem. I was sure I could find a treatment for it. I eagerly envisioned the day when I could walk normally again and get my back into better shape.

That didn't happen for a while. One evening, after dinner at a restaurant with my wife, I felt a horrid vice-like aching in my back and legs. The tightening soon became unendurable and I lowered myself to the floor before I fell. It was hours before I could crawl to my bed.

A year later, I still wasn't on top of the world, in spite of having seen an internist, two orthopaedists [orthopaedic surgeons], a sports podiatrist, a neurologist, a Chinese herbal specialist, a doctor of physical medicine, an acupuncturist, a chiropractor and a physical therapist [physiotherapist].

Eventually, I found the help I needed. Had I known then what I know now, however, I would have saved myself an awful lot of anguish, including the almost unbearable emotional pain of not being able to pick up, hold and cuddle my newborn daughter.

I don't mention all this because the answers I found for myself will solve your problems. I needed ankle surgery and treatment of a neuromuscular disorder to correct the underlying cause of my back pain.

I mention my own experiences because they motivated me to carry out the research for this book. I simply couldn't get the same answer twice about back pain. And, many times, I couldn't get any answers. Small wonder. Owing to the thinness of research in the field, even back practitioners themselves often don't know how well or poorly most treatments work. The common cold is taken more seriously. However, I believe that the research in this book will help change that. For certain, I expect, hope and pray that this book will be the start of the end of your back misery.

Arthur C. Klein
January 1999

About Your Back

Before you find out about back pain relief, here is a brief summary of the main 'moving parts' that make up your back and why they can sometimes be vulnerable to stress or injury. Firstly, you may have noticed that your spine is not straight but slightly curved (in an S-shape).

Not everyone's back is exactly the same shape, but we all have a slight hollow in the base of the neck and in the small of the back (lumbar region). You should try to maintain this shape as much as possible, especially when carrying out day-to-day activities.

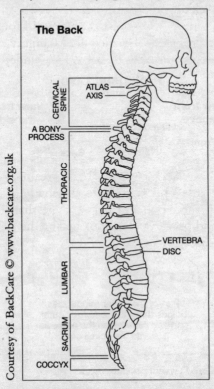

The Back

CERVICAL SPINE

ATLAS
AXIS

A BONY PROCESS

THORACIC

VERTEBRA
DISC

LUMBAR

SACRUM

COCCYX

Courtesy of BackCare © www.backcare.org.uk

The spine is made up of thirty-three small bones called verte-brae, with discs that act as 'shock absorbers' and enable the spine to be fairly flexible. The inside (nucleus) of each disc is made up of a soft jelly-like substance. This is contained within a thick, stretchy, fibrous outer layer (annulus). When people talk about a 'slipped' or herniated disc, it is important to realize that discs don't actually slip – there is nowhere for them to go! Instead, the annulus develops a crack and either it or the nucleus then puts pressure on the surrounding nerves. This results in pain and sometimes 'pins and needles' feelings or sensations of weakness.

The spine also protects the spinal cord, which contains the nerves that come from the brain. Nerves come out from between the vertebrae to send messages to various parts of the body, as well as receiving messages. Each nerve supplies both muscles and joints and therefore has more than one role.

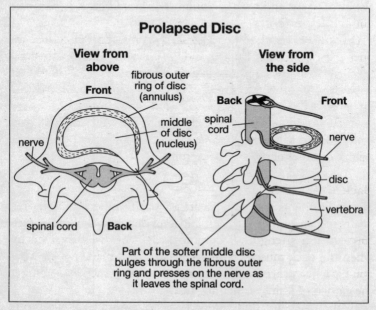

Prolapsed Disc

View from above

fibrous outer ring of disc (annulus)

Front

middle of disc (nucleus)

nerve

spinal cord   **Back**

View from the side

Back   **Front**

spinal cord

nerve

disc

vertebra

Part of the softer middle disc bulges through the fibrous outer ring and presses on the nerve as it leaves the spinal cord.

Prolapsed Discs ('Slipped Discs')

When you have a prolapsed disc, the bulging disc may press on a nerve coming from the spinal cord. There may also be some inflammation around the damaged disc. The most common discs to prolapse are at the base of the spine.

Nerve Root Pain and Sciatica

Nerve root pain occurs because a nerve coming from the spinal cord is pressed on ('trapped') by a prolapsed disc, or is irritated by the inflammation around the injured disc. Although the problem is in your back, you are also likely to feel pain right down your leg. This leg pain can be more intense than back pain. With a slipped disc, the sciatic nerve is the most commonly affected nerve. (The term 'sciatica' means nerve root pain of the sciatic nerve.) The sciatic nerves are made up of several nerves that come out of the spinal cord in the lower back. There are two sciatic nerves – one for each leg – and each sciatic nerve runs deep inside the buttock and down the back of the leg.

The irritation or pressure on the nerve next to the spine may also cause 'pins and needles', numbness or weakness in part of a buttock, leg or foot.

(In a few cases, the nerves pressed on by a prolapsed disc are ones that control the bladder and/or bowel. If this occurs it is a medical emergency and needs urgent treatment. You should tell your doctor immediately if you have any sudden problem with incontinence of urine or faeces, or if you cannot pass urine, especially if these symptoms develop at the same time as back pain, numbness in the inner 'saddle area' of your bottom and thighs, or other nerve root symptoms.)

Back Muscle Problems

Strong ligaments and muscles are attached to the vertebrae. The ligaments and other surrounding muscles give the spine extra support and strength. A common form of back pain occurs when the back muscles go into spasm. This may happen when you have been carrying out strenuous activity, such as digging in the garden or lifting something heavy.

If the pain dies down and there are no unusual symptoms (e.g. numbness, 'pins and needles' or pain down the leg), it may be caused by muscle spasm. However, if the pain lasts more than 48 hours and increases (rather than decreases), you should contact your doctor.

The lower (lumbar) region of the back is the most vulnerable area of the spine, because it bears the entire weight of the upper body. It is also the point where your mobile spine meets a fused bony ring (your pelvis), and so takes a great deal of stress and strain. Your spine is strong however. It's a clever piece of engineering that is designed to be used and is important *not* to be frightened of moving it.

A Note on Healthcare and Drugs in the UK

While the kinds of practitioners and treatments described in this book are very similar in both the UK and USA, the structure of healthcare in the two countries is very different. Access to free healthcare for individuals in the UK is provided through the National Health Service (NHS), and your first port of call as a person with back pain should always be your GP. He or she will then refer you to your local hospital or other specialist practice for the appropriate consultancy and treatment. Since the introduction of the 'internal market' in the NHS, the facilities your doctor will be able to offer you and the details of the necessary arrangements may vary from one practice and health authority to another, but in all cases it is usual to obtain a referral from your GP before you see a specialist.

Your GP may also be willing to refer you to a chiropractor, osteopath or acupuncturist if you wish; alternatively, you may consult any of these practitioners privately, in which case of course you will have to bear the full cost.

One or two differences in terminology should be noted. Physiatry in the USA has much in common with physiotherapy as practised in the UK, although there are some differences. Access to physiotherapy is via referral from your GP or hospital consultant, unless you wish to consult a private physiotherapist. Some GP practices employ their own physiotherapist. Podiatry is more usually known as chiropody. Osteopaths in the USA are classified as medical doctors and may prescribe drugs, whereas their counterparts in the UK are classified as non-medical practitioners and therefore may not issue prescription-only drugs. A minority of GPs may practice osteopathy in the UK.

Many of the drugs mentioned in this book are known under different brand names in the UK and the USA. A few are not available in the UK, and in addition new drugs, not mentioned here, have become available since this book was first written. The following list covers the different names under which the principal drugs mentioned in the text are known in the two countries:

Drug name in USA	Drug name in UK
Acetaminophen	Paracetamol, Panadol
Ascriptin	Aspirin
Ben-Gay	Deep Heat
Chymopapain	Not widely available in UK
Clinoril	Available in UK
Darvocet	Paracetamol
Darvon	Paracetamol
Demerol	Morphine
DMSO	Not widely available in UK
Equagesic	Available in UK
Indocin	Indomethacin
Mobisyl	Deep Heat
Motrin	Available in UK
Naprosyn	Naproxen
Pantopaque	Not available in UK
Parafon Forte	Not available in UK
Percodan	Oxycodone (available in UK as suppository)
Robaxin	Available in UK
Salon Pas	Paracetamol
Soma	Carisoma (not available in UK)
Tylenol	Tylex (prescription only)
Valium	Available in UK

A Note on Safety

Many of the exercises in this book involve getting on to the floor. To help you get down to this position, we advise you to: get down on to your hands and knees; then roll on to one side by first lowering your bottom, then your shoulders, to the floor. You can then roll on to your back. Keep your knees bent all the time. To get back up, bend your knees and roll on to one side, then on to your hands and knees. Make sure that you have a solid chair or low table nearby. Get up on to one knee, then press down with your hand on the chair or low table to support yourself as you rise to a standing position.

Part 1
Back Pain: What Really Works

Section 1
An Introduction

It is unlikely that medical advances alone can solve this terrible problem. The back pain epidemic does not revolve solely around medical issues.

Mark L. Schoene, 2004 Editor, The Backletter, in the foreword to
The Back Pain Revolution by Gordon Waddell CBE DSc FRCS,
Orthopaedic Surgeon, Glasgow

I believe that back sufferers could help one another a lot by sharing their experiences.

A survey participant

Chapter 1
Relief Is in Sight

Back pain affects over one-third of the UK's adult population. To add to their woes, British back pain sufferers also endure the frustration of having to work out for themselves which of the many kinds of practitioners, all of whom claim high degrees of success, can help them — and which of the numerous, highly touted treatments and self-help approaches may offer relief.

Suppose you have recurring and incapacitating muscle spasms with accompanying low back pain. Do you simply start making the rounds and hope for the best? Is self-treatment the best answer? Do you listen to your neighbour when she suggests acupuncture? If the meter reader was helped by trigger point injections, does that mean they will work for you? Is your mother-in-law right about the value of manipulation? Which kinds of exercises help most? Does gravity inversion help at all? Are biofeedback and yoga effective?

What about medical doctors versus other practitioners? Do doctors know best? If so, which kinds of doctors? The orthopaedic surgeon, the musculoskeletal physician, the sports medicine specialist, the pain consultant, the neurologist, the rheumatologist, the acupuncturist? Will your general practitioner do just as well?

How about the sometimes maligned but increasingly popular complementary health practitioners like chiropractors, holistic massage therapists, Alexander teachers, kinesiologists, Rolfers, posture therapists and yoga instructors? What do their track records look like for various back problems? And why do a majority of back sufferers eventually get around to seeing one or more of them?

The questions are almost endless. Answers, at least unbiased and documented ones, scarcely exist. More research urgently needs to be done on back ailments. According to the *European Guidelines for the Management of Acute Nonspecific Low Back Pain in*

Primary Care, published in 2004, 'Pain is not attributable to pathology or neurological encroachment in about 85 per cent of people . . . Risk factors are poorly understood.'

Back Pain: What Really Works was written to fill this void – to provide answers that can save you literally months and years of needless pain and incapacitation. No matter how long you've suffered back pain, no matter how many practitioners, treatments, and self-help approaches you've tried, you'll find answers here that will help you.

Back Pain: What Really Works is the only resource that actually documents the effectiveness (or otherwise) of more than 100 different practitioners, treatments and self-help therapies. The original book's findings were based on an extensive survey that took two years to complete – correspondence and interviews with nearly 500 back sufferers from every state in the USA. This second UK edition has been updated with the results of a web-based survey conducted in the United Kingdom in 2004. A total of 2,240 back pain sufferers responded to the survey questions and provided new insights into the conventional and complementary treatments they found helpful.

These people have a great deal to offer you. They understand the time- and money-saving truths about a fragmented area of healthcare. They know when self-care should include professional care – and when you're better off treating yourself. They can tell you what works and what doesn't in treating the following kinds of back pain: low back syndrome, sciatica, herniated discs, osteoarthritis-based back pain, neck pain, scoliosis and spondylolisthesis. They know because, collectively, they have tried everything.

They can also help you steer clear of unhelpful or harmful practitioners and treatments that account for a significant chunk of the roughly £1,632 million spent every year in the UK on back care. They can tell you which commonly used complementary therapies may be injurious. And non-medical practitioners are not the only villains. Practitioner-related injuries occur throughout the field of back care.

Here are some specific ways in which you will benefit from the unique information in this guide:

- You will discover how to put together an individualized back exercise programme.
- You will learn who is considered by survey participants to be more effective, the orthopaedic surgeon or the chiropractor.
- You will receive documented results about the use of new or controversial techniques such as anti-gravity devices, sclerotherapy, acupuncture, nerve blocks, nutritional supplements and many others.
- You will find out why a hospital accident and emergency department can be a dangerous place to go when you have a back problem.
- You will learn the twenty-five most popular and proven-effective tips from back sufferers all over the country as well as suggestions on safely carrying out twenty-five common activities, from making love to raking leaves and shovelling snow.
- You will receive information about 'home remedies', from liniments to hot soaks to facts and figures about the illegal substances DMSO (an industrial solvent called dimethyl sulfoxide) and marijuana.
- You will learn to identify, and avoid, the many widely prescribed back treatments that have no more value than a placebo.
- And women readers will discover why it is often a mistake to mention back pain to an obstetrician.

The numbers tell the story. More than 17 million British people have back pain at some point in their lives. And this figure continues to grow, despite the burgeoning number of books and magazine articles on the subject.

The myths also tell the story. The most widely seen practitioners – orthopaedic surgeons and chiropractors – may not be the most effective (although this book tells you how to select members of both professions who are highly successful). The most helpful practitioners are seldom heard about, and many are not even thought of as back practitioners. A majority of routinely administered treatments are almost worthless, while less expensive, less publicized and more beneficial approaches are seldom brought to the public's attention.

All in all, and certainly through no fault of their own, back sufferers are misinformed and uninformed. Hence, we have the unmerry-go-round effect in which many long-term back sufferers have seen five practitioners and have incurred untold expense and pain for twelve years before getting the problem under control. *Back Pain: What Really Works* gives you the information you need to minimize or eliminate pain – not just in the short run, but for a lifetime. In effect, it puts you in touch with hundreds of people with back pain similar to yours – people who have 'been through it all,' but, more important, people who have put their problems behind them.

Most of the information in this book takes the form of immediately usable, pain-preventing advice. The remaining information is subtler but no less valuable. It includes knowing what questions to ask; being knowledgeable enough not to be taken in by meaningless or irrelevant diagnoses; understanding the odds that certain therapies have of working; knowing if you are on a dead-end course, and if so, what to do about it; taking comfort that you are not the only person who has a chronic back problem; realizing that a 30-minute daily regime of back exercises does not prevent or solve everyone's problems – but that there are alternatives.

This book is filled with real people who had or still have problems like yours, who made the rounds without the benefit of guidelines. The average participant in the US survey was given half a dozen different kinds of treatments and relieved of untold amounts of time and money in the process.

It doesn't have to be that way for you. This book lets back pain sufferers speak for themselves, and to each other, to help one another.

Chapter 2
These People Can Help You

At the age of 45 Tony was a superb physical specimen. He ran 16 km (10 miles) every day. His abdominal muscles were so highly developed that fifty bent-knee sit-ups felt like child's play. He was also remarkably supple. The yoga Plough was a comfortable exercise for him. So was bending over with his legs straight and touching his palms to the floor.

This was Tony's physical condition when he first experienced back pain – 'twisting his back', as he put it – while playing basketball with his 16-year-old son.

More than four years passed before Tony found a way to treat and solve increasingly incapacitating muscle spasms. For four years, he somehow coped well enough with the pain to make a living as a top executive for a computer company. He saw some of the most illustrious back specialists in the USA, including an orthopaedic surgeon for a professional football team, the chief neurologist of a major rehabilitation centre, and a doctor of physical medicine who is a well-known author. He tried a wide array of treatments, from trigger point injections to biofeedback, from manipulation to acupuncture to a prescribed exercise programme.

Tony finally did find a solution. But the trial-and-error course he had to trace through a maze of practitioners and therapies cost him dearly in money, time and suffering.

It doesn't have to be that way.

For thirteen years Teresa worked as a teacher, spending most days on her feet, stooping to look at children's work, bending to help tie shoelaces, and stretching to write on the blackboard.

Throughout these years, although she never did any kind of regular exercise, Teresa was free of back pain – until she painted her house during a summer holiday. Then she felt aching in her legs, and a week later, she recalled, 'I couldn't move, couldn't get dressed or get to the bathroom, and I was admitted to the hospital.' The orthopaedic surgeon in charge of her case pre-scribed muscle relaxants, painkillers and traction. By the end of the summer, Teresa had improved enough to return to work.

A few months later, though, the pain returned. This time it was even worse. 'It was decision time,' Teresa said. 'My family doctor was finished with me. Should I try another orthopaedic surgeon, an osteopath, a chiropractor, a neurosurgeon? My husband and I discussed it at length and we decided to try a chiropractor.'

After fifteen months of chiropractic care, Teresa was hanging on, but just barely. Something else had to be done. 'It looked like I was going to be tied to this chiropractor for life . . . never mind the monthly expense. I really couldn't figure out where to turn.'

Eventually Teresa stumbled on an alternative plan that worked. But the misery she suffered probably could have been avoided if the information she needed had been available.

Ann could always put up with the minor low back pain she felt for a few days every month before her period. But the pain flared up during her first pregnancy and then continued to grow con-siderably worse.

'That's the price we pay for walking upright,' a gynaecologist told her, adding, 'No one ever died of low back pain.' He also told her that she would be fine once she had given birth.

When Ann's pain worsened during her child's infancy, she went to an orthopaedic surgeon. He found nothing wrong and suggested exercises including sit-ups. The pain increased until she had to rule out exercise of any kind.

As her child became heavier, Ann suffered every time she picked him up. About every three months she had an episode of back spasms that made it impossible for her to get out of bed without her husband's help. Five years and numerous practition-ers later, Ann finally managed to get her problem under control.

'But my back problem should never have got out of control in the first place,' Ann concluded. 'I listened to the usual medical advice and wound up with the usual outcome – more back pain. Back sufferers deserve to know some hard facts and truths. And this kind of "consumer guide" information simply hasn't been available.'

Bob is the kind of back sufferer no back specialist likes to talk about. He has been examined and treated by orthopaedic surgeons and chiropractors, osteopaths and naturopaths, and other conventional and alternative healthcare practitioners. He doesn't know what is wrong with his back. No two of his twelve diagnoses are the same – and none makes sense to him. He has read widely about back pain, been everywhere, tried everything.

There are at least 1.5 million – and maybe as many as 5 million – severely disabled back sufferers like Bob in the USA.

'Some doctors who know about the chronicity of my problem,' Bob said, 'won't even allow me to make an appointment to see them. If they do agree to examine me, they're all but itching to get me out the door. It is assumed that I have workers' compensation or some other kind of insurance, which I don't, or that I am a neurotic who enjoys the attention. Actually I live alone and nobody pays me any attention unless I'm up and about. Some obviously think I'm a malingerer, even though I worked from age 14 to 40. It's just been the past five years that I've not been able to be on my feet long enough to hold down a job. I am living off my savings, which are about depleted.'

After filling out his survey questionnaire, Bob wrote in a post-script, 'I hope that your book won't leave out people like me. I hope it won't be another simplistic *Six Minutes a Day to Relief*, full of "guaranteed safe" exercises I can't even do.'

In my own postscript, I am happy to add that Bob has started to find a way out of his prolonged nightmare of disability. His prognosis for normal functioning is good.

Teresa, Tony, Ann and Bob – and the 488 other people in the US survey and 2,240 people in the UK survey – give you informa-tion, insights and practical advice that have never before been available, and that often run counter to so-called common wisdom.

The experts have had their say about relieving back pain. Now listen to the people who know which prescriptions work.

Section 2
Back Practitioners

Health practitioners use many different methods to treat back pain and the road to recovery is very individual. What works for you may not work for the next person and it is a question of working out for yourself — with the help of medical professionals — what suits you best.

Sarah Rastrick, writing in *Arthritis News*, August/September 2003

The goal of every back sufferer should be self-care. The question is who can best help us to reach that goal.

A survey participant

Chapter 3
Medically Qualified Practitioners

General and Family Practitioners • Orthopaedic Surgeons • Spinal Orthopaedic Surgeons • Pain Clinic Doctors • Neurosurgeons • Rheumatologists • Neurologists • Musculoskeletal Physicians • Accident and Emergency Department Doctors • Sports Medicine Specialists • Obstetricians • Gynaecologists

Many unexpected facts and helpful insights about medically qualified practitioners that emerged from the US and UK surveys can help you pursue the proper treatment for your back now and help you care for it yourself in the long run. Here are some highlights that will be explored further in this chapter:

• Doctors who catch your attention in the mass media are not necessarily representative of their colleagues. For example, the orthopaedic surgeon who talks about his new book on a radio programme may indicate a great interest in working with most back sufferers – not just the few who require surgery – but this interest is atypical. And unless you learn how to select the right kind of doctor, the search can take years of hit-and-miss appointments.

• Despite the positive attitude of the American Medical Association towards back exercise, and the advice about exercise published in its own consumer back book, the US survey found that only 15 per cent of doctors prescribed (or even mentioned) exercise. More positively, in a 1996 UK BackCare Association survey, 58 per cent of GPs said they gave specific back exercises and 66 per cent reported recommending general fitness to people with acute lower back pain. By knowing which kinds of doctors to see, you can practically guarantee yourself a beneficial exercise regime if a self-help programme isn't helping you maximize your progress.

- Prominent back specialists have popularized the idea that stress contributes to back pain. Yet only 29 per cent of the US doctors mentioned stress to their back patients.
- Even if you decide not to see a medical doctor for treatment, you still should have a thorough medical examination to rule out illness, disease, neurological impairment or structural abnormality as a cause of your back problem. Gordon, from Scotland, had this to say: 'If your back pain is caused by injury, insist on . . . an early, accurate diagnosis. Do not be fobbed off with a packet of painkillers.'

The following doctors are listed according to frequency seen by UK survey respondents, not according to their effectiveness in helping back patients.

Note: In a few cases, where figures have been rounded to the nearest whole number, survey percentage results will not total 100.

General Practitioners (GPs, Family Practitioners)

General practitioners are the starting point for almost everyone with back pain. But many back sufferers quickly move on to other kinds of practitioners. Among US respondents, there was a general feeling that GPs relied too much on prescribing painkillers. Meanwhile, some UK respondents were concerned that their GPs couldn't distinguish between an injury and a degenerative condition. On the other hand, general practitioners know their patients better than specialists do. With this advantage, and with appropriate interest and skill, they can sometimes do more than any other type of doctor to eliminate back problems or prevent them from happening in the first place. Many medical schools now train their students to be 'compassionate healers' by emphasizing the promotion of health and prevention of degenerative ailments, including back pain.

If your family doctor is determined to help you all the way through a back problem, count your blessings. Running around to see this or that specialist just because 'common wisdom' says that you should, will often cause you needless trouble.

One young woman, a recreational counsellor, was making slow progress under the care of her general practitioner, whom she described as 'very gentle, thorough, concerned about lifestyle, habits, exercise and activity.' The GP diagnosed the patient's problem as spinal stenosis (a narrowing of the spine, which puts pressure on nerve roots). This diagnosis was confirmed at the doctor's request by an orthopaedic colleague. Fine so far. But the young woman was berated repeatedly by well-meaning friends for taking the word of 'just a GP', so she went to an orthopaedic surgeon privately, paid a handsome fee, and got nothing more for her efforts than 'a rushed examination and a sheet of do's and don'ts'.

In contrast, her GP provided 'a relaxed and inquiring examination, and concern for long-run progress.' Also, as the patient explained, 'My GP treated acute pain with drugs to relax muscle spasms and reduce inflammation. Then the doctor provided me with an extensive exercise programme, with notes and suggestions for exercise to start with and a progression to build into as pain subsided and strength increased. She also provided pointers about posture and a good mattress.'

	US survey	UK survey
Number of people treated	266	1,150
Responses	%	%
Provided dramatic long-term help*	8	9
Provided moderate long-term help*	12	14
Provided temporary help	14	41
Ineffective	54	31
Made patient feel worse	12	5

* Includes help that eveually came from appropriate referrals.

What to Do If Your General Practitioner Makes a Referral

If a specialist is needed, a competent general practitioner will make a referral. For example, 5 per cent of the general practitioners in the US survey referred their patients to a physiotherapist and achieved outstanding results. These doctors wanted to stay involved, to be ultimately responsible for their patients' care, and appreciated the value of having someone work closely with the patients in a comprehensive rehabilitation programme.

But what happens when you're referred to another medical doctor, such as an orthopaedic surgeon, neurologist or neurosurgeon? Should you simply accept the referral? Or should you try to discuss it with your doctor?

Most people in the US survey found that a few key questions were essential:

1. What will be the next step if the diagnostic procedure conducted by the specialist does not reveal a tangible reason for my problem?
2. Will you or the specialist still try to help me even if there is no disease or serious malformation?
3. What will be done about my soft-tissue (muscular) problems? (Even if you are a candidate for surgery, your musculature will still need post-operative rehabilitation.)

If the answers to any of these questions is unsatisfactory to you, you may be better off finding a good back practitioner on your own. In the UK, this may mean seeking private treatment. If this seems a daunting prospect however, asking for a second opinion from another NHS doctor may be the solution. If you learn that your general practitioner will act as coordinator for all forms of treatment involving your back, you can relax. Having a GP pave the way for you with other healthcare practitioners often guarantees a more positive reception, especially if you are a chronic back sufferer. As a retired teacher suffering through years of sciatica pain remarked, 'My GP's involvement with my problem has made a big difference. Even when nothing significant can be done for my pain, he confers with other doctors and talks with me about ways to lower the stress from my pain.'

Orthopaedic Surgeons

Orthopaedic surgeons tend to ask the question: is this person likely to benefit from surgery? If not they are unlikely to keep you on their books, and may refer you on for conservative treatment, such as physiotherapy. Orthopaedic surgeons are specialists at diagnosing and treating injuries and diseases of bones and muscles, as well as joints, tendons and ligaments. Hence, you would expect them to provide at least some relief for back sufferers or, at least, to refer patients to someone who could help.

However, as with many other professionals, the experiences of our survey participants were variable.

According to many respondents, effective orthopaedic surgeons spend more time listening than examining. If you sense a lack of interest during your initial consultation, the orthopaedic surgeon is unlikely to help you. Survey participants who found orthopaedic surgeons uninterested and difficult to talk to were usually disappointed in the treatment they received.

A construction worker with low back pain said, 'My orthopaedic surgeon seemed not to even care about my problem,' while a young housewife felt that her orthopaedic surgeon wasn't prepared to spend time trying to find out what the problem was.

Orthopaedic surgeons may make terrific surgeons. But unless you need surgery, and the chances are at least 95 per cent that you don't, you will probably find other practitioners more helpful. Back patients are emphatic about this point. 'Two orthopaedic surgeons showed little interest when no surgery was indicated,' reported a teacher. And a photographer who was ultimately helped by acupuncture and biofeedback said, 'My X-rays yielded no sign of injury. Therefore, from the viewpoint of the orthopaedic surgeon, there was no injury.' Meanwhile, Alison, from the UK, said: 'Don't let medical practitioners, such as orthopaedic surgeons, get you down. I had several years of being told that I should not be suffering so much pain, which I construed as meaning that they felt I was "putting it on".'

In contrast, some survey participants had much more positive experiences with orthopaedic surgeons. For example, the owner of a sporting-goods shop said: 'I had muscle strain in the low back and my family doctor sent me to an orthopaedic surgeon who said, "You don't need surgery; it's just the price you pay for walking upright!" Well, I wasn't walking upright. I was bent over from the pain. So I called orthopaedic surgeons in the Yellow Pages and asked the receptionists if the doctor treated a lot of back patients who didn't require surgery. Three seemed put off by my question. The fourth was very positive, gave me an appointment, and that was the beginning of the end of my back problem.'

Orthopaedic surgeons willing to deal with soft-tissue problems (often by referring the patient to a physiotherapist) are most helpful to back sufferers. Soft-tissue problems are what most back sufferers have. They usually involve a strain (torn fibres caused by overstretching), spasms or inflammation of back muscles – or all of the above. Soft-tissue problems can also involve damage to ligaments, tendons or connective tissue. Although helpful orthopaedic surgeons use a variety of procedures, they all have certain approaches and attitudes in common.

For starters, the effective orthopaedic surgeon realizes that prescription drugs will probably play a fairly minor role in your recovery. He may prescribe pills, but he keeps the role of drugs in perspective and does not end your treatment with them.

Also, the effective orthopaedic surgeon will insist that you keep in touch with him (or a physiotherapist) on a regular basis until you're fully recovered. He knows that personal interaction is the only way to keep tabs on how you feel and what new steps you're ready to take.

	US survey	UK survey
Number of people treated	429	413
Responses	%	%
Provided dramatic long-term help	13	16
Provided moderate long-term help	10	15
Provided temporary help	9	30
Ineffective	61	29
Made patient feel worse	7	10

Spinal Orthopaedic Surgeons

Spinal orthopaedic surgeons did not feature in the US survey but got a good rating in the UK survey, providing dramatic or moderate long-term relief for 45 per cent of patients. Spinal orthopaedic surgeons specialize in spinal surgery (whereas many orthopaedic surgeons specialize in hand surgery or knee operations.)

Number of people treated in the UK survey	204
Provided dramatic long-term help	24%
Provided moderate long-term help	21%
Provided temporary help	23%
Ineffective	21%
Made patient feel worse	11%

Pain Clinic Doctors

Pain management clinics are specialized clinics for the treatment of all forms of chronic pain. Pain clinics take a multidisciplinary approach to the treatment of pain and various options may be considered, including nerve blocks, analgesics and psychological therapy. You will need to be referred by your GP. Your pain will be assessed and a treatment plan discussed with you; the plan will be sent to your general practitioner or to your referring consultant.

The aim of pain clinics is to reduce your level of pain, to restore your functioning and to improve your sense of well-being. Pain clinics did not feature in the US survey. However, according to UK survey participants, pain clinic doctors offer reasonably effective treatment, with 67 per cent of patients receiving temporary relief or better.

Number of people treated in the UK survey	342
Provided dramatic long-term help	15%
Provided moderate long-term help	14%
Provided temporary relief	38%
Ineffective	22%
Made patient feel worse	11%

Neurosurgeons

Neurosurgeons specialize in operations involving the nervous system. They hardly ever treat backs in general; they treat them surgically. They also prescribe medication, including painkillers and antidepressants (which have been shown to have beneficial effects on pain originating in the nerves).

There seems to be a considerable difference between the US and UK survey findings in relation to neurosurgeons. A number of US survey participants felt that neurosurgeons tended to over-prescribe medication. But what neurosurgeons can provide, 13 per cent of the time in the US and 33 per cent of the time in the UK, is the skill to achieve extraordinary results with some patients in severe pain.

Consider the testimony of this Indiana truck driver: 'I saw a GP and a chiropractor for three years. They never relieved my pain from osteoarthritis, bone spurs and a ruptured disc, and I never received a referral until I was totally incapacitated. The neurosurgeon was my salvation. His corrective surgery to remove a large bone spur and a disc provided me with the first relief from years of agonizing and sometimes paralysing pain.' The patient was able to resume his truck driving and loading activities after a few months of instruction and care from a physiotherapist recommended by the neurosurgeon.

More typical of US participants is the comment of a research sociologist who had a disc removed by a neurosurgeon: 'Back surgery worked well for my acute pain. However, the neurosurgeon was not helpful for anything except surgery. He did not mention stress, exercise or anything else for that matter.' This patient's greatest progress came through a physical fitness instructor at a local health spa, but the surgery did relieve her pain enough for her to take up the exercise.

Perhaps only 1 per cent of all back sufferers need surgery. But if you see a surgeon and are advised to have an operation, participants in the US survey suggest the following:

1. Try to get additional opinions from at least one other surgeon and one practitioner who is not a surgeon, even though this can be difficult in the UK healthcare system. Explore the potential benefits of physiotherapy and exercise as well as chymopapain (see Chapter 5) if you have a ruptured disc.
2. Ask about your chances of success. Specific figures should be available at every hospital.
3. Ask about post-operative care. According to one US neurosurgeon, 'Successful surgery is only 10 per cent of the process of making you well.' If your surgeon isn't interested in the remaining 90 per cent of treatment needed to restore you to full activity, consider changing doctors (though this may not be easy in the UK, where there are relatively few surgeons available).

	US survey	UK survey
Number of people treated	53	166
Responses	%	%
Provided dramatic long-term help	13	33
Provided moderate long-term help	13	14
Provided temporary help	8	19
Ineffective	51	23
Made patient feel worse	15	10

Rheumatologists

Rheumatologists are medical doctors who specialize in diagnosing and treating the more than a hundred forms of arthritis and related diseases. Certainly, if you have reason to believe that arthritis plays a role in your back condition, you should consult this specialist. But people with chronic and serious back problems not primarily due to arthritis can also benefit from a rheumatologist's care. They frequently find this specialist both interested and experienced in working with long-term, soft-tissue problems. In both surveys, around 60 per cent of patients got some degree of relief from their back pain as a result of seeing a rheumatologist.

The following comments are typical of those from US survey respondents:

'I was lucky that the rheumatologist I consulted recognized my problem and believed as I do in moderate treatment,' said an editorial researcher, who received non-prescription pills for pain and inflammation. He also got good advice about changing his work routine and sticking to a sensible exercise plan.

'So far, the rheumatologist has proved the most useful of all doctors,' reported a speech therapist who had been assured by her family doctor that her pain would vanish on its own. When she could no longer sit without severe pain, she sought help from a specialist. 'The rheumatologist was very supportive about my joining a YMCA exercise programme. He also talked constructively about stress, not as a single cause, but as a contributing factor to back pain.'

	US survey	UK survey
Number of people treated	15*	128
Responses	%	%
Provided dramatic long-term help	7	18
Provided moderate long-term help	33	12
Provided temporary help	20	28
Ineffective	40	30
Made patient feel worse	0	12

* Forty-six people were cited in the US survey data, but only those who had osteoarthritis were included in the statistics for the final report. Other forms of arthritis, although they do cause back problems, are beyond the scope of this project.

Neurologists

Neurologists are consulted by patients who have complex back problems involving the nervous system. These patients may suffer a high degree of pain and disability and the neurologist therefore tends to prescribe more medication than other practitioners. Low-dose antidepressants may sometimes be prescribed, as they have been found to be helpful in treating neuropathic pain. UK survey participants responded much more positively than US participants to these practitioners. In the UK survey, 41 per cent of respondents gained some form of relief, as opposed to only 8 per cent in the US survey.

	US survey	UK survey
Number of people treated	44	104
Responses	%	%
Provided dramatic long-term help	2	9
Provided moderate long-term help	2	11
Provided temporary help	4	21
Ineffective	76	44
Made patient feel worse	16	15

Musculoskeletal Physicians

Musculoskeletal medicine is an emerging discipline and several hospitals in the UK now have musculoskeletal departments. Musculoskeletal physicians are orthodox medical doctors who have done lengthy additional training in the specific diagnosis and treatment of conditions of the spine, muscles and joints. Their treatment may consist of manipulation and exercises but they are also able to perform injections, such as prolotherapy and epidurals and the more invasive techniques such as discography and intra-discal electrothermal therapy (IDET) under X-ray guidance. No US or UK survey data is available at present for these practitioners.

Other Medical Doctors

Reports of other medical doctors seen by survey participants were too few to yield significant statistics. Nevertheless, some comments are included here because they offer valuable firsthand experience.

Accident and Emergency Department Doctors

Stay out of accident and emergency departments if at all possible. Of the nine patients in the US survey who were treated in emergency units, none received even temporary relief. All found that their pain grew worse during the wait for examination and treatment (the average wait was two hours). Two of the patients ended up back in hospital within a few days of leaving the accident and emergency department because of vertebrae fractures that had been overlooked.

Of course, if you are in an accident and sustain a serious injury, you have no alternative but to seek emergency care. On the other hand, if you reach for a tissue and your back 'goes out', resulting in severe pain, you probably do have a choice, including trying to convince a doctor to see you at home. Making a trip anywhere is likely to increase your pain.

Sports Medicine Specialists

Sports medicine is a relatively new and under-populated branch of medicine. Only five sports medicine doctors treated participants in the US survey. (Another ten survey participants tried unsuccessfully to make appointments with sports medicine doctors, many of whom were physicians for professional sports teams and unable to see 'ordinary' back sufferers within a month of their call.) Of the five, four helped their patients achieve dramatic long-term help; the other provided moderate long-term help. The physical-medicine orientation of these doctors makes them a good choice for a wide range of back problems.

A Kentucky journalist who had suffered debilitating back pain for six years before he saw one of these practitioners said: 'Stretching exercises prepared specifically for me by a sports medicine specialist solved my problem in the long run. Since I started my programme, except for two occasions when I was lax in performing my required exercises, I have had little pain and no major problems.'

In the UK survey, 78 per cent of respondents who consulted sports medicine professionals gained some degree of relief from pain.

Number of people treated in the UK survey	84
Provided dramatic long-term help	18%
Provided moderate long-term help	12%
Provided temporary help	48%
Ineffective	17%
Made patient feel worse	5%

Obstetricians/Gynaecologists

These practitioners specialize in treating problems related to pregnancy, childbirth and women's reproductive health.

'I explained the problem of my back pain to my gynaecologist,' a US librarian said. 'But he has never referred me to a back specialist or done anything about it. He said it was common for women to have back pain, especially when they reach my age.' This patient is 32 years old and performs her job in spite of almost intolerable pain.

According to US survey participants, unless you are certain that your back pain has a gynaecological basis, you probably shouldn't expect much help from obstetricians and gynaecologists. However, obstetricians got a better rating in the UK survey, providing some degree of relief for over half the patients who consulted them.

Number of people treated in the UK survey	37
Provided dramatic long-term help	19%
Provided moderate long-term help	2%
Provided temporary relief	35%
Ineffective	22%
Made patient feel worse	22%

Chapter 4
Non-Medically Qualified Practitioners

Physiotherapists • Chiropractors • Osteopaths • Acupuncturists • Massage therapists • Physical fitness instructors • Nurses • Reflexologists • Pharmacists • Psychotherapists • Occupational therapists • Alexander teachers • Aromatherapists • Yoga instructors • Homeopaths • Faith healers • Chiropodists/Podiatrists • Nutritionists • Herbalists • Tai Chi instructors • Kinesiologists • Shiastsu or acupressure massage therapists • Hypnotherapists • Naturopaths • Dance instructors • Rolfers • Feldenkrais therapists • Biofeedback instructors

Many back sufferers get the help they need from the non-physician practitioners described and rated in this chapter. Some of the practitioners, like chiropractors and massage therapists, are well known, but there is little documentation about their relative effectiveness or ineffectiveness. Others, like Tai Chi instructors and Feldenkrais therapists, are unknown to many back sufferers. Still others, like physiotherapists, usually need a doctor's authorization to treat you. And a few, like chiropodists, who seem far removed from back care, can be surprisingly helpful with certain back problems. Collectively, these practitioners are enormously popular. Twenty-eight kinds of practitioners are evaluated in this chapter. But as you'll see, only about one-third of them can benefit most back sufferers in a major way. The rest are included because knowing the truth about them enables you to avoid wasting your time and money as so many other back pain sufferers have. It also gives you greater peace of mind when well-meaning friends ask you whether you have seen this or that kind of healthcare specialist.

The practitioners in this chapter are listed according to frequency seen, not according to their effectiveness in helping back patients.

Evaluating Complementary and Alternative Health Practitioners

In recent years, there has been much controversy concerning complementary and alternative medicine. In November 2000, in the UK, the House of Lords Select Committee on Science and Technology published a report on complementary and alternative medicine (CAM).

The Committee concluded that most therapies were relatively safe. However, they were concerned that a vital medical diagnosis and treatment could be missed if patients chose to see only a CAM practitioner, who might not have the training to recognize symptoms that should be taken to a doctor immediately.

The Committee also found that there was very little research into whether the therapies worked, training was often inadequate, and too many therapies were unregulated in any way.

They divided complementary and alternative therapies into three groups:

Group One: This covered the 'big five' – acupuncture, chiropractic, osteopathy, herbal medicine and homeopathy – which had the best professional organizations and training standards. Chiropractic and osteopathy are now statutorily regulated, which means it is illegal for anyone to practise without being registered with the professional body. Herbalists and acupuncturists were well on the way to being regulated by the end of 2005.

Group Two: This included those therapies that – although supporting evidence was lacking – were considered harmless enough to complement conventional medicine. These include Alexander Technique, aromatherapy, massage therapy, hypnotherapy, reflexology, shiatsu, healing, nutritional medicine and yoga. The Select Committee felt that voluntary self-regulation under one professional body for each therapy in Group Two should be sufficient, although it could not prevent somebody practising as an 'aromatherapist', for example. Each body would:

- maintain a register of individual members or member organizations
- set educational standards and accredit training establishments
- provide codes of conduct, ethics and practice

- organize a complaints mechanism and disciplinary procedure accessible to the public
- require members to take out adequate professional indemnity insurance

Group Three: This category, which was the most controversial, covered those therapies that the Committee considered scientifically unproven and unregulated, such as naturopathy and kinesiology. There is still much debate about which practices should be included in each of these groups.

Tips on Getting the Best from CAM Practitioners

Many people are keen to try CAM therapies. Here are some tips that should help you take advantage of them in an informed, safe way:

1. Start by talking to your GP, and then perhaps your local complementary medicine centre, in order to find out which therapy is suitable for your particular health problem. It's also a good idea to get personal recommendations.
2. Copies of the regulations governing individual therapies are available from organizations such as the Research Council for Complementary and Alternative Medicine (see Useful Addresses, p. 463). Individual associations can also provide information about therapists in your local area.
3. Most CAM practitioners charge between £25 and £45 per session. Always check on the total cost of your treatment before you start. Many private medical insurers now cover the better-known complementary therapies and some therapies are available on the NHS.
4. When going to a new therapist, you should be given time to discuss your health problem before starting treatment. If you don't feel comfortable with a therapist, trust your instincts and walk away.
5. Find out what qualifications your practitioner has. It's also a good idea to ask how long they have been practising and what experience they have in treating your particular problem.
6. Check that your practitioner is covered by professional indemnity insurance in case something goes wrong. (Most of

them get this cover when they register with their professional body.)

7. Always discuss any complementary therapies you are having with your GP, especially if you are taking any homeopathic or herbal remedies. Most doses of herbal medicines are too low to cause problems – but there can be some potentially dangerous interactions between herbal medicines and prescription drugs.

Physiotherapists

In some countries, many physiotherapists, even those in private practice, cannot treat you without the consent of a medical doctor. However, in the UK, you can self-refer to private physiotherapists if you wish.

Physiotherapists are now working in extended roles within the NHS. All physiotherapists in the UK are trained in manual therapy, including mobilizations. They are increasingly trained in manipulation. They can be very helpful to back sufferers, especially those with low back pain as well as ruptured discs and osteoarthritis.

One key factor is that physiotherapists try to learn a lot about you. 'A good physiotherapist gives you all the individualized input that you need to take care of your back for the rest of your life,' said one US survey participant, a writer who managed to control back pain for twenty years before she ran into incapacitating problems that she couldn't solve by herself. 'Even if you take full responsibility for solving your back problem yourself,' she continued, 'and I believe that everyone should have this attitude, you still have to know how to accomplish this. The road to recovery isn't always an obvious one. You can read all the books in the world and still not know what to do because books talk about the average back sufferer, and there is no such person.'

Once a physiotherapist gets to know you, not just your back pain, he or she can use a wide variety of natural corrective techniques, such as heat, cold, postural instruction, relaxation therapy and exercise therapy. Anne, a UK survey participant, said: 'I found hydrotherapy to be the most valuable. I asked the physiotherapists to give me exercises which I could continue to do in a cooler pool, at a local gym. I have continued to carry these out very successfully for three years now.'

Physiotherapists are also trained to apply modern technology to back problems, including ultrasound, electric muscle stimulation and transcutaneous electric nerve stimulation (TENS). But the value of these techniques is slight compared with what the physiotherapist can do for you by looking, listening and talking.

If you have weak or overly tight muscles, a physiotherapist's special training will usually help you correct these conditions. Is your posture bad? Do you sit properly? Are your chairs and mattress providing you with optimal support? Is your average day so stressful that you believe it to be aggravating your back pain? All these aspects of back care, and more, come under the physiotherapist's domain.

Many back sufferers in the UK survey lavished praise on physiotherapists. Sarah, a 47-year-old woman with back pain, said: 'I was taught by a patient, excellent physiotherapist how to sit, stand, walk, use stairs, kerbs, get into and out of bed, dress etc. to avoid doing more damage to my spine.'

Ben, a male UK participant, told his story: 'My trouble started when I made an awkward twisting turn whilst playing tennis. Regrettably, I did not rest long enough before recommencing tennis, gardening, etc. and suffered a severe relapse. I had most help from my health centre physiotherapist who used ultrasound and manipulation but, most importantly, taught me a number of exercises to perform regularly. I have found the following most helpful: not to persist in one activity for too long when gardening; and not to sit for long periods.'

Keep in mind that you usually need a doctor's 'permission' to be treated by a physiotherapist. Just a few words scrawled on a prescription pad will do. The doctor need not select the therapist or provide detailed instructions. And, importantly, not many doctors will turn down a politely stated request for treatment by a physiotherapist. 'I asked my GP to write a prescription for physical therapy when no relief was forthcoming from pills,' said a US X-ray technician. 'He wrote the prescription and there were excellent results within two weeks. Even the breathing exercises I learned from the physiotherapist relieve stress in general.'

In the US survey, physiotherapists were the most successful non-medically qualified practitioner for helping patients with almost any kind of back ailment.

However, there is one point to bear in mind about physiotherapists: their 'made patient feel worse' rate, of 10 per cent in the US and 11 per cent in the UK, was probably caused by pushing patients too fast in the exercise rehabilitation process, and ignoring patients' complaints about pain. It is crucial that you judge whether the pace of prescribed exercise is helping or hurting you.

	US survey	UK survey
Number of people treated	140	933
Responses	%	%
Provided dramatic long-term help	34	18
Provided moderate long-term help	31	19
Provided temporary help	8	36
Ineffective	17	16
Made patient feel worse	10	11

How to Find a Physiotherapist

If you need a physiotherapist, your doctor or hospital consultant will refer you to one. Some GP practices have their own physiotherapist. If you are in a position to pay for your own treatment, there are a large number of physiotherapists across the UK offering treatment in dedicated physiotherapy and sports injury clinics as well as many who will treat people in their own homes. To find a local private practitioner within the UK, consult the Chartered Society of Physiotherapy (see Useful Addresses, p. 463). Chartered Physiotherapists have the letters 'MCSP' after their name to show that they are members of this society. The Organization of Chartered Physiotherapists in Private Practice (OCPPP), an occupational group of the CSP for private practitioners, also has a listing service of private practitioners working in the UK. Some large employers run occupational health schemes for their employees that may include provision for physiotherapy treatment, and private medical insurance schemes for individuals through the independent healthcare sector will often include physiotherapy treatment. Check with the scheme providers for eligibility.

Chiropractors

Yes, manipulation helps. No, chiropractors are not quacks. In fact, in the US survey chiropractors were considered more effective than most medical doctors. Chiropractors are considerably less common in the UK than the USA. Nevertheless, 678 respondents to the UK survey consulted chiropractors and, of these, 71 per cent obtained some degree of relief from their back pain.

Before we look at just how well chiropractors handle back problems, let's briefly explore who they are, what they're trained to do, and what philosophy underlies this branch of healthcare. The chiropractic profession was born in America nearly a century ago. From 1868 to 1953 the American Chiropractic Association believed that the interruption of psychic energy from the brain was the cause of many ailments and diseases. The current theory holds that irritated nerve roots, or interruptions of nerve impulses, cause most problems. Manipulation, which is said to restore the body to its natural state of well-being, is the predominant form of treatment.

In the UK some people may be confused about the difference between chiropractors and osteopaths, and the professions are similar in many ways. The main differences are:

- Chiropractors work mainly on the spine; osteopaths work on the spine but also on the whole body, including peripheral joints.
- Chiropractors use more manipulative techniques; osteopaths may use manipulation in conjunction with soft tissue and mobilization (stretching of joints) techniques.

There are basically two kinds of non-medical practitioners – those who work with or for physicians, as most nurses and physiotherapists do, and those who work independently of medical doctors on the basis of different healing philosophies, the way chiropractors tend to do. Medical practitioners, however, have in the past been sceptical of chiropractors' heavy emphasis on spinal manipulation.

Of course, back pain cares nothing for theory. So here are facts and figures, and unprecedented opportunities to learn from the experiences of other back sufferers.

According to most survey participants, chiropractors can help you get temporary relief from minor or moderate low back or neck pain. But for severe, chronic low back pain, you shouldn't expect miracles. In addition, the most effective chiropractors consider advice about lifestyle, stress and exercise to be as important as manipulation in the long run.

	US survey	UK survey
Number of people treated	422	678
Responses	%	%
Provided dramatic long-term help	14	19
Provided moderate long-term help	14	14
Provided temporary help	28	38
Ineffective	33	15
Made patient feel worse	11	14

Manipulation Alone: Unsuccessful Long-Term Results

US survey results show conclusively that manipulation does not relieve back pain in the long run. To see this point more clearly, look at the way US back sufferers compare the effectiveness of manipulation alone with the success of total chiropractic care:

	Manipulation only	Total chiropractic care
Number of people treated in the US survey	333	422
Provided dramatic long-term help	5%	14%
Provided moderate long-term help	7%	14%
Provided temporary help	44%	28%
Ineffective	34%	33%
Made patient feel worse	10%	11%

Contrary to popular belief, manipulation alone is seldom the key to long-term success under chiropractic care. This means that if you see a chiropractor who relies exclusively on manipulation, you are likely to be helped for just a few days or weeks at a time, no matter how many months or years you continue treatment.

'The only thing about receiving manipulation treatments is that you have to keep seeing the chiropractor to keep from getting worse, but not necessarily better,' wrote a US housewife who had been receiving adjustments of specific areas of her spine for 12 years.

A shop-owner commented, 'Manipulation just works for a while. It's not a cure-all by any means.'

What Accounts for the Relative Success of Chiropractic Care?

'Holistic' is the word that came up repeatedly when US back sufferers who favoured chiropractic care tried to explain why it was effective. In short, these survey participants felt that they, and not just their back problems, were being treated.

Some typical comments illustrate this point.

A bricklayer with low back pain: 'My chiropractor offered nutritional advice, rather than drugs, and put me on an excellent yoga programme to strengthen my muscles. He also encouraged relaxation exercises and the use of a B vitamin for stress, as well as regular exercise such as swimming.'

A New York truck driver: 'Regular chiropractic adjustments offer steady improvement if used regularly and if combined with the kind of programme that I received – stretching and strengthening exercises and advice about nutrition.'

Gillian, a UK survey respondent, said: 'I have been with my chiropractor now for six months or more. I go every two to three weeks, depending on problems.'

Chiropractor–Patient Rapport

The chiropractor's relationship with patients also explains the relative success of the profession in helping back sufferers. Hundreds of unsolicited comments from US survey participants show, unquestionably, that patients relate more comfortably to chiropractors than to doctors. They tend to like chiropractors as individuals and can talk to them about their feelings and their lives. A good practitioner-patient relationship apparently helps the back sufferer because the most effective 'treatment' for back pain takes the form of talking and listening, of advice rather than procedures.

Advice about daily living habits, stress and exercise is considered vital by back sufferers. This advice takes time for a practitioner to dispense. And chiropractors are more willing and able than doctors to spend this time with their patients. Survey participants were emphatic about this point.

A health educator said, 'My chiropractor has always been very concerned and helpful to me regardless of what my problem is. I would pay his fee just for an opportunity to talk to him.'

A librarian: 'I felt for the first time in my life, in terms of medical treatment, that I was in competent and non-antagonistic hands.'

Chiropractors Are More Specific about What's Wrong with You

When you're in pain, it is natural to want an answer to the question, 'Exactly what's wrong with me and what can be done about it?' The more severe the pain, or the longer it lasts, the greater the need for answers. Whether it helps and is medically legitimate, chiropractors almost always offer their patients specific descriptions of what is wrong and how the problem can be corrected. By comparison, medical doctors usually give a generalized diagnosis such as low back syndrome.

If you believe in basic chiropractic concepts, the chiropractor's specific diagnosis is comforting. It builds your confidence. It removes the disquieting feeling of not knowing what's wrong. For some people, a specific diagnosis lowers stress and anxiety about back pain.

For example, a farmer who regularly put in long, physically demanding hours suffered pain in his hips and lower back. When doctor after doctor failed to come up with a specific diagnosis, he rejected all their advice (which may have been sound and helpful) and sought the help of a chiropractor. The chiropractor explained the origin of the problem as 'a malformed hip due to premature birth,' and the patient accepted this diagnosis. More to the point, the patient accepted an exercise programme (which had also been proposed by a medical doctor) that put him on the path to good health.

'The chiropractor was the only one who seemed confident about his diagnosis,' said a computer programmer, who stopped worrying about his low back pain after a chiropractor diagnosed his problem as a 'bilateral sprain of the sacrolumbar'. Before this, each of three medical doctors had diagnosed the problem in a different way – kidney infection, hypertension and low back strain – leaving the patient increasingly concerned and distressed.

Then there was the case of a young mother who was unhappy about being told by medical doctors that she simply had a 'bad back'. Although she still reported having 'a lot of discomfort' after chiropractic care, she was less worried in part because she finally had a name for her ailment: 'Subluxation T11, T12, C3 and 4, manifesting as myospasm, radiculitis associated with curvature and complicated by loss of cervical curve.'

Another survey participant, a potter, went to an orthopaedic surgeon to seek help for pain in her neck. The orthopaedic surgeon called the problem a 'pinched nerve'. The patient, dissatisfied with what she felt was a vague and rushed diagnosis, went to a chiropractor. The chiropractor's diagnosis of 'misalignment of neck and spine' was termed 'valid' by the patient, because, as she put it, 'He took the time to show me the X-rays, and I could see it for myself.'

This all sounds very positive but many chiropractors tend to use X-rays as a diagnostic tool even though they have limited use in diagnosing back pain, as they do not show the soft tissues. X-rays should only be used when appropriate (according to criteria established by the Royal College of Radiologists) because they involve exposing the patient to significant levels of radiation. (For more on the risks and benefits of X-rays, see pp. 127–9.)

Other Things to Know about Chiropractic Care

The US survey results show that 56 per cent of back sufferers who saw chiropractors received some help, while an even better 71 per cent of UK participants gained some degree of relief. Yet chiropractors can also make patients feel worse. The 11 per cent 'made patient feel worse' US figure (and 14 per cent UK figure) associated with chiropractic treatment is based on reports of a temporary but substantial increase in pain from manipulation, without any improvement in the condition after the pain subsided.

High cost and contracts

In the US survey, it was the high cost of chiropractic care that bothered survey participants most – not the cost per visit but the long-term nature of the treatment. In the USA, it is not unusual for a chiropractor to schedule regular 'maintenance' visits to ensure that problems don't recur. A few chiropractors even ask the patient to sign a contract agreeing to regular treatments for one or two years. Most survey participants who mentioned contracts objected strenuously to them. 'The chiropractor's greed put me off,' a factory worker commented, 'especially when I was told I had to sign a contract for two years of treatment.'

Unorthodox procedures and advice

About 5 per cent of chiropractic patients in the US survey reported what they believed to be unusual, even bizarre, advice or treatments. To illustrate:

- 'The chiropractor told me that I must have headaches because of my spinal curvature. I almost never have a headache. But I felt that with repeated suggestions I would, so I stopped the treatments.'
- 'I was told that my low back pain was caused, in part, by the locking of one of the pumping mechanisms affecting my cerebrospinal fluid.'
- 'My chiropractor prescribed non-prescription pills for "liver flushes". I still don't know why my liver needed flushing.'
- 'Once, when I had acute pain, I had my tailbone manipulated through my rectum by a chiropractor. The relief was amazing.'

In summary, chiropractors are neither miracle workers nor quacks. They are legitimate, professional dispensers of back care. And, in general, they treat back pain more successfully than many kinds of medical doctors.

Osteopaths

Osteopaths diagnose and treat problems with muscles, ligaments, nerves and joints. Treatment involves gentle, manual techniques – easing pain, reducing swelling and improving mobility. Osteopaths spend a large amount of their time dealing with the pain and suffering caused by back problems. In many cases they can help considerably in pain relief and lifestyle management. As well as advice on exercise, you may also be given dietary advice. On your first visit the osteopath will discuss and record your medical history in detail. A series of observations on your mobility, posture and testing of points of weakness or excessive strain will then be made. Further investigations may include an X-ray or blood test. (For advice on the risks and benefits of X-rays, see pp. 127–9.) Osteopaths complete four or five years of training in anatomy, physiology, pathology, biomechanics and clinical methods.

The practice of osteopathy is quite different in the USA (there, osteopaths are medical doctors who can prescribe drugs and perform surgery) so the US survey results for osteopathy are not included here. In the UK survey osteopathy had a good track record for a majority of patients, with 74 per cent experiencing at least temporary relief or better.

Bill, from the north of England, advised back pain sufferers to 'try osteopaths and chiropractors, if only for temporary relief', while James said: 'The person who has given me the best on-going relief is an osteopath. His diagnosis of what was going on was spot on.'

In summary, osteopaths will take on severe and chronic problems that other practitioners have given up on. And in the UK survey, they had a similar success rate to that of physiotherapists.

Number of people treated in the UK survey	613
Provided dramatic long-term help	19%
Provided moderate long-term help	17%
Provided temporary help	38%
Ineffective	18%
Made patient feel worse	8%

How to Find an Osteopath
The majority of osteopaths work in private practice although an increasing number work alongside GPs so it may be possible for your doctor to refer you to an osteopath on the NHS. It may also be possible to claim for a course of osteopathy if you have private health insurance. To find an osteopath, consult the General Osteopathic Council (see Useful Addresses, p. 463). By law, osteopaths must be registered to practice.

Acupuncturists
There are many theories as to why acupuncture works. Traditional Chinese medical texts claim acupuncture corrects energy imbalances. There is strong scientific evidence that acupuncture

stimulates the body to produce endorphins – its own painkillers. But some doctors maintain that the effect from acupuncture is purely psychological – you think it will work, so it does.

Also, as with many therapies, no one knows who will benefit from acupuncture. One patient with sciatica will get relief; another patient with a comparable problem won't. The same holds true for other kinds of back pain.

What is clear from both surveys is that acupuncture does work in some cases. (Alison, a UK respondent, said she was 'an avid supporter of acupuncture'.) And it provides relief slightly over half the time. Occasionally, it eliminates pain for a patient's lifetime.

In most acupuncture treatments, thin needles are inserted into points along meridian lines designated by ancient practitioners as channels of energy. There were no complaints about pain from the insertion of the needles, which is most often described as a pinprick sensation that lasts an instant. During the treatment, patients say, a barely perceptible current or flow of pressure from one insertion point to another can be felt, but no pain is associated with this, either. Some practitioners stimulate the needles using their hands; others attach electrodes to drive currents through the energy channels.

If you are wary of needles used for injections, rest assured that there is no comparison. Acupuncture needles are as thin as fine wires. They usually produce no bruising or bleeding. You are likely to feel comfortable, even relaxed and drowsy, during treatments, which can last anywhere from 15 to 45 minutes.

If you have not improved after five to ten sessions, you can assume that acupuncture – or at least the particular kind of treatment you are receiving – will not help you.

Most acupuncturists in the US survey were medical doctors, a phenomenon that underscores the growing acceptance of acupuncture as a bona fide medical procedure. In the UK the two main health professionals who practise acupuncture are GPs and physiotherapists. If you decide to try acupuncture, make sure you get the most out of the venture by contacting the Acupuncture Association of Chartered Physiotherapists or the British Acupuncture Council (see Useful Addresses, p. 463) for a list of recommended therapists in your area. There is no government legislation in the UK covering acupuncture at present. This means that unfortunately anyone can currently provide acupuncture treatment without any professional acupuncture training whatsoever. The British Acupuncture Council maintains standards of education, ethics, practice and discipline to ensure the health and safety of the public at all times. It is also committed to promoting research and enhancing the role that traditional acupuncture can play in the health and well-being of the nation.

Although acupuncturists are usually practitioners of last resort for chronic back sufferers, as the survey results show, being treated by an acupuncturist *is* worth a try and has far more healing value than a placebo. A total of 54 per cent of people in the US survey, and 61 per cent of those in the UK survey, found some degree of relief. This figure is even more encouraging than it appears, because some of the US patients in the 'temporary relief only' group were pain-free for up to two years. By comparison, the temporary relief gained from most other forms of treatment, including many prescription medications, usually lasts a few hours at best.

Acupuncturists in the US survey who were medical doctors were neither more nor less successful than non-physician practitioners. The important variables were the number of years' experience with acupuncture and the time invested in advising patients about exercise, stress and day-to-day living habits.

In conclusion, acupuncturists may well be helpful in providing pain relief but it is essential to seek a practitioner who is appropriately qualified. All kinds of back pain can respond favourably to acupuncture, even chronic pain that has worsened over the years. The most successful acupuncturists combine acupuncture with exercise and lifestyle advice, and acupuncture may work for many kinds of back ailments. At least five to ten treatments may be needed to determine effectiveness in individual cases.

	US survey	UK survey
Number of people treated	25	483
Responses	%	%
Provided dramatic long-term help	16	10
Provided moderate long-term help	20	9
Provided temporary help	32	43
Ineffective	28	29
Made patient feel worse	4	9

Massage Therapists

As a rule, individuals trained in massage provide neither the self-care advice nor the treatment needed for significant improvement of back problems. Yet there is no denying that a good massage is a relaxing pleasure – which can take the edge off low-grade pain caused by tight or tired muscles. One UK survey respondent said: 'I find regular back massages with arnica cream, followed by an arnica oil rub, give me the only long-term relief from what is constant pain.'

The best way to find a good massage therapist is through a recommendation. Short of this, consult your local Yellow Pages, looking for small ads that emphasize 'medical massage'. Newspaper advertisements that proclaim the attractiveness of massage personnel – or that use phrases like 'total discretion' and 'assured privacy' – are offering sexual stimulation, not backache relief.

	US survey	UK survey
Number of people treated	22	325
Responses	%	%
Provided dramatic long-term help	5	9
Provided moderate long-term help	5	16
Provided temporary help	63	56
Ineffective	27	12
Made patient feel worse	0	7

Physical Fitness Instructors

The fitness boom has resulted in the creation of thousands of spas and health clubs. The chances are that you have at least one such facility near your home, complete with an exercise expert who is willing and able to work with back sufferers.

Three key factors determined the relative success that US survey participants had with physical fitness instructors:

1. Self-assessment. If you have serious back problems, say so. Heroic attempts to join a class of superfit people got participants into trouble. You need to assess the specialized training or the instructor who will be working with you.

2. Self-protection. Ask questions; the degree of back care expertise among physical fitness instructors varies widely. (Some

physical fitness experts are exercise physiologists with expertise in treating back conditions; others have no such training.) Also, if the instructor seems uninterested in your special circumstances, move on. The risks are too great. Find someone who takes the time to learn about your back and then proposes a sensible progression of exercises. Participants called this kind of individualized programme the best insurance they could buy.

3. Self-indulgence. If going to a health club is fun and relaxing in general, and you feel as if you're 'getting away from it all', you'll benefit more than you would by doing the same exercises at home.

One UK survey participant had great success with Pilates: 'The best thing I ever did was join a Pilates studio that specialized in back injuries. Going two to three times a week made me stronger and relieved my pain in ways that medication and everything else never did. Doing anything else to try and relieve back pain was short-lived until I consistently went to the Pilates sessions. Please recommend this to your readers.'

Most importantly, remember the collective wisdom of all survey participants: only you can judge how fast and far you can go with exercise. If you have to compete with someone, compete with yourself. Do not push yourself to keep up with other members of an exercise class.

In conclusion, if you're functioning well but have a nuisance level of chronic backache, or episodes of pain a few times a year, physical fitness instructors are quite likely to give you successful results. However, the US survey respondents (58 per cent of whom gained dramatic long-term relief) were a lot more positive about fitness instructors than those from the UK (of whom 39 per cent gained temporary relief).

	US survey	UK survey
Number of people treated	17	157
Responses	%	%
Provided dramatic long-term help	58	19
Provided moderate long-term help	24	21
Provided temporary help	0	39
Ineffective	12	8
Made patient feel worse	6	13

Nurses

'I got more advice from my orthopaedic surgeon's nurse, while putting on my hat and coat after an appointment, than I did from the orthopaedic surgeon himself,' reported a young US mother. The nurse gave her helpful tips on how to cope with her infant and her back at the same time. For example, the nurse asked the patient how she lifted the baby and how she positioned herself while bathing the baby – then suggested ways to perform these procedures without back strain.

Many nurses have long experience with people who suffer from back pain. The nurse may have some answers for you, or at least the time and inclination to talk.

If you work for a large corporation with a physical fitness programme, you may be fortunate enough to find a nurse specifically trained in practical aspects of back care. Of the nine US survey participants who sought help from nurses, five saw corporate nurses who provided them with a comprehensive – and successful – rehabilitation programme.

In summary, all nine US survey participants treated by nurses were helped substantially. Meanwhile, in the UK survey, 65 per cent of respondents gained some degree of pain relief from nurses.

Number of people treated in the UK survey	136
Provided dramatic long-term help	7%
Provided moderate long-term help	14%
Provided temporary help	44%
Ineffective	29%
Made patient feel worse	6%

Reflexologists

These practitioners apply pressure to particular areas on your feet or (occasionally) your hands in order to 'rebalance energy in your body' and stimulate natural healing processes. All parts of the body are thought to be 'reflected' in the feet and hands and stimulating relevant areas is said to influence their corresponding organs and systems.

Like aromatherapy, reflexology may be particularly good for providing temporary relief of stress-related back pain.

Reflexology is unregulated at present. This means that anyone can call himself or herself a reflexologist and set up a school or college or open a register. Reflexology organizations are currently working towards self-regulation, seeking agreement on educational and training standards, a code of ethics and disciplinary procedures. The International Federation of Reflexologists (see Useful Addresses, p. 463) keeps a register of practitioners from training schools accredited with them. Ask your reflexologist if he or she belongs to a professional association.

Reflexologists did not feature in the US survey. But they provided temporary pain relief for almost half the UK patients who consulted them, though a quarter found them ineffective and 7 per cent felt worse.

Number of people treated in the UK survey	157
Provided dramatic long-term help	7%
Provided moderate long-term help	12%
Provided temporary help	49%
Ineffective	25%
Made patient feel worse	7%

Pharmacists

Pharmacists did not feature in the US survey but just over 70 per cent of UK respondents gained some degree of help from them.

Number of people treated in the UK survey	138
Provided dramatic long-term help	10%
Provided moderate long-term help	12%
Provided temporary help	49%
Ineffective	24%
Made patient feel worse	5%

Psychotherapists

Psychotherapists did not feature at all in the UK survey. In the US survey, more than 300 participants felt that stress played a role in increasing their back pain. Yet only six of these back sufferers went to a psychologist or psychiatrist for help. Of the six, four felt that their backs were slightly improved in the long run by 'talk therapy'. Many more psychotherapists (14) were involved in the survey as participants than were cited as practitioners (6). Still, if you feel that emotional problems are causing your back pain or making it worse, talking to a psychotherapist might help.

Occupational Therapists

These practitioners will show you how to protect your back and how best to go about your daily activities, with the help of special aids and techniques. To find an occupational therapist, you could start by asking your GP if you are eligible for free occupational therapy within the NHS. If not, there is a list of private, registered occupational therapists available from the College of Occupational Therapists website (see Useful Addresses, p. 463).

Occupational therapists did not feature in the US survey but were rated quite highly in the UK survey, providing some degree of relief for 66 per cent of patients.

Number of people treated in the UK survey	131
Provided dramatic long-term help	9%
Provided moderate long-term help	22%
Provided temporary help	35%
Ineffective	23%
Made patient feel worse	11%

Alexander Teachers

You have backache because you are misusing your body – standing and moving incorrectly, according to the theory of the Alexander technique. And this misuse can be brought about by physical or emotional factors, both of which can be treated by Alexander teachers. Bad posture can cause back pain. And to the extent that it affects your back problem, postural therapy may help.

The technique is named after Australian-born Frederick Matthias Alexander, a nineteenth-century actor who created it in ten years of exhaustive self-exploration. Doctors' advice could not keep Alexander from losing his voice on the stage, so he worked at correcting his total musculoskeletal technique until he cured himself.

No strong opinions, for or against, were expressed by the half-dozen participants in the US survey who tried the Alexander technique. All were chronic back sufferers in search of help for a long-standing problem. None found substantial relief in the Alexander technique.

'Alexander technique helped me to hold myself correctly and that helped some,' a reading teacher commented. 'But, in retrospect, I probably would have done as well if I had tried to change my lazy posture habits myself.'

In summary, if you have a posture problem, the Alexander technique might be worth looking into.

'Helped just a bit' reflects the reaction of most US survey participants who tried this treatment. However, one UK respondent said that Alexander technique provided 'the best all round help'.

Number of people treated in the UK survey	125
Provided dramatic long-term help	18%
Provided moderate long-term help	14%
Provided temporary help	33%
Ineffective	27%
Made patient feel worse	8%

Aromatherapists

Aromatherapy uses oils extracted from plants, known as essential oils. Each plant oil has a particular scent and is thought to have specific healing properties. The essential oils can be bought over the counter for self-treatment (e.g. by putting a few drops in your bath) or they can be diluted in a carrier oil and applied in a massage by an aromatherapist. (If you treat yourself, check the safety precautions carefully.)

Aromatherapy seems to be most effective for relieving stress, so some people may find it helpful for stress-related backache.

Aromatherapy is an unregulated profession. This means that anyone can call himself or herself an aromatherapist and set up a school or college. Aromatherapy organizations are working towards self-regulation, seeking agreement on educational and training standards, a code of ethics and disciplinary procedures. The Aromatherapy Organizations Council (see Useful Addresses, p. 463) will provide a list of member associations and training establishments. Ask your aromatherapist if he or she belongs to a professional association.

Aromatherapists did not feature in the US survey. They provided temporary relief for over half the UK patients who consulted them, though nearly a quarter found them ineffective and 7 per cent felt worse after their treatment.

Number of people treated in the UK survey	131
Provided dramatic long-term help	7%
Provided moderate long-term help	9%
Provided temporary help	54%
Ineffective	23%
Made patient feel worse	7%

Yoga Instructors

To the extent that stretching and strengthening your body is helpful – and most survey participants agree that it is – yoga instruction can be an excellent way to ease back pain. To the extent that stress contributes to back pain – and most survey participants feel that it does – yoga instruction scores again. The yoga philosophy of never forcing or straining, and of moving in a meditative manner, has obvious value. But yoga philosophy also encompasses the harmony of mind, body and spirit – a concept that is foreign to many people.

Yoga instructors achieve the best results with back sufferers who are not incapacitated by pain and who are receptive to yoga's spiritual message. People in the survey who tried to avoid philosophical concepts by studying yoga through books, articles and tapes got some help – but not nearly as much as those who worked with a yoga instructor.

Emily, a UK respondent, said: 'I picked up the courage to join a gym, tried out a yoga class and learned new coping mechanisms.

Yoga in particular has helped a lot with all the little aches and pains we suffer secondary to the main back problem. It has changed my mindset from "I can't" to "I can and I will".'

Bill, also from the UK, commented: 'I do yoga exercises regularly to strengthen my back and stomach muscles and try to listen to what my body says.'

A word of caution: many yoga exercise positions are too difficult (and risky) for back sufferers who are not fully active and functioning reasonably well. In fact, it is advisable not to practice yoga whilst you are experiencing back pain. However, once you are able to perform normal everyday activities, yoga offers day-to-day help for the rest of your life.

Try this simple form of yoga therapy suggested by several survey participants. It involves nothing more than deep abdominal breathing that has helped many back sufferers to relax and tone up abdominal muscles. Try it during your peak work hours. Five minutes is optimal; even a few breaths are useful. However, you should take care not to breathe deeply for the entire 5-minute period, as this could cause you to hyperventilate. To avoid this, you should alternate deep breaths with regular breathing.

Sit, stand or lie down in a comfortable position. Start by taking a deep breath from your abdomen (put your fingers on it at first to make sure that it, and not your chest, is expanding). Now inhale through your nose for 6 seconds . . . hold your breath for 3 seconds . . . then exhale through your mouth for 7 seconds. When you exhale let yourself go limp. After a few minutes, you should feel both invigorated and relaxed.

Although the formal research evidence for its success has yet to emerge, yoga provides very effective backache relief for non-incapacitated backache sufferers – with twenty-one out of forty-five US survey participants reporting significant long-term improvement. The US results were more positive than those from the UK. Nevertheless, 74 per cent of UK respondents gained some degree of relief.

	US survey	UK survey
Number of people treated	45	226
Responses	%	%
Provided dramatic long-term help	51	16
Provided moderate long-term help	42	21

Yoga Survey	US survey	UK survey
Provided temporary help	3	37
Ineffective	0	16
Made patient feel worse	4	10

Homeopaths

Homeopathy is based on the principle of 'like cures like.' So, for example, a homeopath will treat a fever with a substance that, if taken in normal quantities, would produce a fever. Homeopathic remedies are often diluted many times, until there is no detectable trace of the original substance. This is because homeopaths believe the greater the dilution, the more 'potent' (precise and active) the remedy.

Simple homeopathic remedies are available from health shops and pharmacies, with instructions on how to take them.

Many homeopaths in the UK are non-medically qualified. Other practitioners may be doctors, nurses, dentists or veterinarians who have taken a postgraduate course in homeopathy. With a referral from your GP, you can claim private health insurance for homeopathic treatment.

In November 2000, the British House of Lords' Select Committee on Complementary and Alternative Medicine placed homeopathy in the top five complementary therapies, and homeopaths are working towards statutory regulation.

However, homeopathy is still the subject of much debate. In 2005, the *Lancet*, a medical journal, published the results of research showing that homeopathic treatment had the same success rate as a placebo but a spokeswoman from the Society of Homeopaths said: 'Many previous studies have demonstrated that homeopathy has an effect over and above placebo.'

Homeopaths did not feature in the US survey. They provided temporary relief for about a third of the UK patients who consulted them, though over 40 per cent found them ineffective.

Number of people treated in the UK survey	84
Provided dramatic long-term help	12%
Provided moderate long-term help	7%
Provided temporary help	34%
Ineffective	42%
Made patient feel worse	5%

Faith Healers

Faith healers offer healing through the power of prayer, often accompanied by the 'laying on' of the healer's hands. If you wish to find a faith healer, you could try contacting the National Federation of Spiritual Healers (see Useful Addresses, p. 463). This organization is self-regulating, with its own code of conduct and complaints and discipline procedures. Their website includes a list of healers in different parts of the UK.

Faith healers did not feature in the US survey. For 16 per cent of UK survey respondents, they provided dramatic long-term relief but 36 per cent found them ineffective and 14 per cent felt worse after seeing them.

Number of people treated in the UK survey	83
Provided dramatic long-term help	16%
Provided moderate long-term help	7%
Provided temporary help	27%
Ineffective	36%
Made patient feel worse	14%

Chiropodists/Podiatrists

Make sure that the length of your legs is measured during any examination for back pain. A difference of 1.3 cm (½ inch) is considered significant, although some US survey participants and their podiatrists felt that even 16 mm (⅟₁₆ inch) could cause a problem. In these cases, a simple heel lift can work wonders. So can an orthotic, which is a prescribed insert for your shoe (for more on these, see p. 80). Podiatrists also relieved participants' back pain by advising them about proper shoe height and support. You may be eligible for treatment from a podiatrist within the NHS – you can check this with your GP. If not, the Society of Chiropodists and Podiatrists (see Useful Addresses, p. 463) has a list of registered private practitioners.

Over 70 per cent of UK survey respondents who consulted these practitioners received some form of pain relief. For back pain caused by short-leg syndrome, they may be able to provide instant relief.

Chiropodist/Podiatrist Survey

Number of people treated in the UK survey	72
Provided dramatic long-term help	26%
Provided moderate long-term help	18%
Provided temporary help	28%
Ineffective	25%
Made patient feel worse	3%

Nutritionists

According to these practitioners, nutritional deficiencies and food sensitivities can contribute to a number of chronic health problems. They often recommend elimination diets. Certain foods are removed and then re-introduced in groups until one of them causes a reaction. If particular foods are identified as triggers, you will be advised to avoid them. Nutritional therapists may suggest various diets, as well as vitamin and mineral supplements (sometimes in higher doses than conventional doctors approve), herbal remedies and enzymes. Patients are frequently advised to avoid wheat products, dairy products and sugar. On this subject, Sally, a UK survey respondent, commented: 'I've stopped eating fruit and sugar (apart from bananas) . . . I'd really recommend people who've got backs that are slightly arthritic to say goodbye to sugar. It's hard but worth it . . .'

Nutritional therapy is an unregulated profession, which means that anyone can call themselves a nutritional therapist, open a training school or start a register. If you wish to consult a nutritional therapist, you could try contacting the British Association of Nutritional Therapists (see Useful Addresses, p. 463). This is a self-regulating professional body that holds a nationwide register of practitioners.

The British Society for Allergy, Environmental and Nutritional Medicine (see Useful Addresses, p. 463), whose members are medically qualified doctors, only accepts patients with a doctor's referral.

Almost 60 per cent of UK survey respondents who consulted these practitioners received some form of relief, though around one-third found them ineffective.

Nutritionist survey

Number of people treated in the UK survey	48
Provided dramatic long-term help	23%
Provided moderate long-term help	19%
Provided temporary help	17%
Ineffective	33%
Made patient feel worse	8%

Herbalists

Herbalists use parts of plants to treat a wide range of health problems. Herbal remedies are also available from health shops and pharmacists in the form of tablets, oils, ointments and teas. If treating yourself with over-the-counter remedies, you should always discuss it with your doctor beforehand, follow the safety instructions and choose products from well-known manufacturers.

UK herbalists are working towards making herbal medicine a legally regulated profession. If you wish to consult a herbalist, it's best to look for a practitioner who is registered with the National Institute of Medical Herbalists (see Useful Addresses, p. 463).

Over 40 per cent of UK survey respondents who consulted these practitioners experienced temporary relief, though a quarter found them ineffective and 14 per cent felt worse after treatment.

Number of people treated in the UK survey	48
Provided dramatic long-term help	15%
Provided moderate long-term help	4%
Provided temporary help	42%
Ineffective	25%
Made patient feel worse	14%

Tai Chi Instructors

Tai Chi is a blending of martial arts and dance that can help increase your strength and flexibility if your ability to move is not overly restricted by pain at the outset. The instruction covers an intriguing way to progress from so-so to excellent shape. 'Tai Chi movement, in addition to regular back exercise, is essential,' commented a rehabilitation counsellor who improved with this combination.

This intricate and disciplined form of exercise originated centuries ago in China. Tai Chi exercises are more reflective than vigorous. They will barely raise your pulse rate, according to cardiologists who have prescribed Tai Chi for their patients. Yet, after a workout, you feel as if you have reaped the rewards of vigorous exercise. Overall, the effect is one of relaxation and pleasure, a good bet for back sufferers who need a therapeutic routine to follow and who believe that stress is a major factor in their back pain.

According to a carpenter who suffered chronic, but not incapacitating, low back pain, 'Tai Chi is the total solution to my back pain. It is a relatively painless treatment that has been the most thorough way for me to take control of my discomfort and has eliminated pain altogether for long periods of time.'

Two other US participants were equally enthusiastic about this graceful discipline that exercises virtually every part of your body – even your eyes.

All in all, for the overstressed, fairly able-bodied back sufferer, Tai Chi is a good way to enhance and complement your back exercise programme.

Number of people treated in the UK survey	44
Provided dramatic long-term help	23%
Provided moderate long-term help	11%
Provided temporary help	36%
Ineffective	23%
Made patient feel worse	7%

Kinesiologists

Few complementary therapies are as potentially useful to back sufferers as kinesiology – the study of the principles and mechanics of movement. Applied kinesiology involves the use of a wide range of non-drug, non-surgical procedures, ranging from manipulation to massage to exercise. But what stood out most in the minds of US survey participants who had kinesiology treatments was the kinesiologist's interest in and knowledge about muscles. For example, five out of six participants reported that muscles in their backs, hips or legs were measured and tested for strength and flexibility; and that specific, corrective movements and exercises were prescribed after evaluation.

The eight kinesiologists seen in the US survey were chiropractors who had received an additional degree in kinesiology – the study of the mechanics and anatomy of movement. They were able to help six of the eight participants, which is impressive, considering that all of these patients were severely limited by low back pain, sciatica or a ruptured disc. UK survey participants were not quite as enthusiastic about these practitioners, though 66 per cent gained some degree of relief from their treatment.

Kinesiologists usually employ similar techniques to those used by chiropractors, including a gentle form of manipulation. But their expertise in the area of movement seems to give them a substantial added advantage.

Note: Chiropractors who advertise the use of kinesiology usually do not have a degree in kinesiology. One disabled back sufferer, a US health educator, was in severe pain during the five years that she saw chiropractors, orthopaedic surgeons, neurosurgeons and physiotherapists. After a few months of treatment by a kinesiologist, she made a complete recovery. 'Applied kinesiology – heat, massage, acupressure, gentle adjustments and stretching exercises – finally helped me,' she said. It probably won't be possible to find a kinesiologist in your local Yellow Pages, but you may be able to contact one via the UK branch of the International College of Applied Kinesiology (see Useful Addresses, p. 463).

Applied kinesiology integrates the advantages of manipulation and individualized exercise with knowledge about how to put your muscles in good working order. With their special training in muscles and movement, these specialists can alleviate many kinds of back pain.

	US survey	UK survey
Number of people treated	8	41
Responses	%	%
Provided dramatic long-term help	50	20
Provided moderate long-term help	25	10
Provided temporary help	12	36
Ineffective	12	20
Made patient feel worse	0	14

Shiatsu Therapists
(Also Called Acupressure Massage Therapists)

The massage technique used by Shiatsu massage therapists is often referred to as acupuncture without needles, because the same meridian lines, or 'channels of energy' used in acupuncture are the focus – but thumbs are used instead of needles.

Depending on how tight your muscles are, and on how vigorous your Shiatsu therapist is, you can expect acupressure to create mild discomfort during treatment. Pressure is usually applied with the balls of the thumbs. The procedure works you over from head to foot, without necessarily concentrating on the affected area. For example, if you have low back pain, the therapist may emphasize working on points in your legs and feet in order to help your back.

Contrary to popular belief, Shiatsu is not an ancient practice but a twentieth-century Japanese innovation. And it does not necessarily involve the therapist walking on your back. Indeed, judging from US survey participants' comments, individuals with major back pain should definitely not allow anyone to walk on their backs.

In summary, Shiatsu therapists often provide the interest, skill and health approaches that help minor to moderate low back pain. Survey participants also report surprising success with do-it-yourself techniques for 'pushing away' pain.

	US survey	UK survey
Number of people treated	20	43
Responses	%	%
Provided dramatic long-term help	35	23
Provided moderate long-term help	15	2
Provided temporary help	40	40
Ineffective	0	21
Made patient feel worse	10	14

How You Can Treat Yourself

Shiatsu is far too complex a skill and an art form to be mastered from a book. However, many US survey participants found it easy to learn how to use pressure to relieve pain themselves in small areas of muscle tissue that feel 'knotted'. Here is some of their advice:

1. For minor to moderate pain from muscle spasms in areas that you can reach comfortably yourself – neck, lower back, buttocks, hips, thighs – push gently with the ball of your thumb for about 20 seconds all around the knotted area. Then apply pressure on the knot itself for 7 seconds. There will be some pain. If it's more than the slight wincing variety, use less pressure or stop. If the pain is not intense, you can use this procedure twice a day.

2. For major muscle spasm that all but prevents you from moving, have someone else 'press out' the affected area for 7 seconds in each spot. At times, this can be as effective as a muscle-relaxant injection. And, according to US survey participants, it is almost always more effective than muscle-relaxant pills when you have specific areas of tightness.

Five Shiatsu therapists in this survey referred to themselves as holistic massage practitioners, meaning that their training included more than Shiatsu or Swedish massage. These practitioners were skilled in at least one other kind of deep massage therapy – connective-tissue massage or polarity massage, for example – as well as in stress-reduction techniques. If you get a strong recommendation from a friend about a holistic massage practitioner, you may well benefit by seeing this specialist.

Although Shiatsu is unregulated, meaning that anyone can call themselves a shiatsu practitioner, the Shiatsu Society (see Useful Addresses, p. 463) maintains professional standards of practice and training and provides a list of accredited practitioners throughout the UK.

Hypnotherapists

These practitioners will put you into a hypnotic trance in order to help you overcome back pain. Once you are in a trance, the hypnotherapist will address your unconscious mind. For instance, people with arthritis may be told that they can turn the pain down like the volume on a radio.

If you decide to consult a hypnotherapist, make sure that you see an appropriately trained and experienced practitioner who belongs to a regulated association with a code of ethics and practice. Your GP may refer you to an NHS psychologist who practises hypnotherapy or you could contact the National Council for Hypnotherapy (see Useful Addresses, p. 463).

Half of UK survey respondents who consulted hypnotherapists experienced some form of relief but 40 per cent found them ineffective.

Number of people treated in the UK survey	40
Provided dramatic long-term help	22%
Provided moderate long-term help	5%
Provided temporary help	22%
Ineffective	40%
Made patient feel worse	10%

Naturopaths

Naturopathy is based on the principle that the body has a natural ability to heal itself. Like many other complementary therapists, naturopaths believe that body, mind and spirit are interrelated. Naturopaths believe that stress, too little sleep, lack of exercise and fresh air and too many 'toxins' (from processed food and environmental pollution) cause imbalances that can affect the whole person and lead to various health problems.

Numerous drug-free treatments are used by naturopaths to treat back problems and most other disorders and diseases. Techniques include manipulation, massage, diet, stress-reduction techniques and exercise. If there is a naturopath near you who comes recommended by another back sufferer, you might get some long-term support and relief. In some US states, naturopaths are recognized as family doctors, and in Germany there are several thousand state-licensed naturopaths.

In the UK, naturopathy is an unregulated profession, which means that anyone can call themselves a naturopath. If you decide to consult one of these practitioners, make sure that he or she is a member of the British Naturopathic Association (see Useful Addresses, p. 463). This is the professional body of naturopaths who are registered with the General Council and Register of Naturopaths (GCRN).

Three out of four US survey participants got long-term help for minor but chronic low back pain from these practitioners.

Number of people treated in the UK survey	35
Provided dramatic long-term help	26%
Provided moderate long-term help	9%
Provided temporary help	30%
Ineffective	26%
Made patient feel worse	9%

Dance Instructors

Dance movements are too strenuous and advanced for most people with back problems. However, if you're up to it, dance instructors (teachers of modern dance and ballet) know how to transform your body from so-so to excellent condition and do wonders for your back in the process.

The nine out of ten US survey participants who gained some degree of relief by following the advice of a dance instructor expressed the following views:

- If modern dance is to your liking, it is a wonderful way to fine-tune your body and protect it against recurrences of back pain.
- Modern dance lifts your spirits and provides a healthy outlet for stress.
- It is dangerous for anyone in pain, or even anyone who can't already do a wide range of back exercises, to try modern dance.

They also had the following in common:

1. They went for instruction after a painful episode had ended, not in the throes of back pain.
2. They enjoyed the idea of learning to dance and of practising at least three times a week.
3. After a month, they experienced substantial improvement in their posture, abdominal strength and overall flexibility, along with a substantial reduction in back pain.

'The warm-up exercises in modern dance are precisely those recommended by chiropractors I've seen,' said a publisher's administrative assistant. 'Dance is a great form of relief with just the right combination of freedom and structure needed for a healthy body and mind. I recommend it strongly as a creative way to deal with back pain.'

In conclusion, modern dance offers an invigorating form of help for back problems. But it is very definitely not for anyone still recovering from back pain. You should also look for an instructor who shows some understanding of back problems.

	US survey	UK survey
Number of people treated	10	29
Responses	%	%
Provided dramatic long-term help	50	24
Provided moderate long-term help	40	10
Provided temporary help	0	31
Ineffective	0	24
Made patient feel worse	10	10

Rolfers

Rolfing, developed in the USA, is a form of massage designed to improve posture. Treatment includes instruction on movement and breathing.

If you're not ready for the equivalent of an energetic workout, you are not a candidate for Rolfing – a deep tissue massage described by one pleased US survey participant as, 'Like someone was trying to reshape my muscles.'

Push hard enough on tense muscles and you will feel discomfort. Offer resistance to a force being applied to your body and you will ultimately feel tired, even exhausted. Combine both these sensations and you have some idea of what Rolfing feels like.

Rolfing does get results, though. The most impressive pain relief from Rolfing was reported by a massage therapist with bad low back pain. Her comment about the treatment: 'Rolfing helped quite a bit. But, after a few years, the pain returned.'

Because of the degree of pressure exerted, one US participant with sciatica reported an increase in pain lasting several days. And even some patients who were helped by Rolfing did not complete the full series of treatments. (Usually ten sessions are prescribed.) They stopped because they felt the discomfort from the procedure had become greater than the relief.

With Rolfing, you know your body is being worked on. There is discomfort as fingertips, knuckles and elbows apply pressure. This raises two questions: Why the painful sensation? Is the treatment worth it?

The discomfort comes from having to probe deeply into your muscles to free them of tightness, adhesions and malfunction, Rolfing patients say. In theory, this makes sense, because if the muscles that support your spine are not working properly, you could have back pain. In the UK survey, fourteen participants got some form of relief, and a third of the respondents got dramatic, long-term help. However, only one of the eight US survey participants who tried Rolfing got long-term results, and four got nothing positive at all. Massage therapy is an unregulated profession in the UK, which means that anyone can call themselves a massage therapist or Rolfer. For this reason, you would be well advised to look for a practitioner who is registered with the British Massage Therapy Council (see Useful Addresses, p. 463).

In summary, Rolfing may be uncomfortable but is sometimes an effective way to temporarily relieve minor or moderate – but not disabling – low back pain.

	US survey	UK survey
Number of people treated	8	18
Responses	%	%
Provided dramatic long-term help	0	33
Provided moderate long-term help	12	28
Provided temporary help	62	17
Ineffective	12	17
Made patient feel worse	12	5

Feldenkrais Therapists

Considered by some to be a psychotherapist and by others to be a kind of posture, movement and awareness instructor, the Feldenkrais therapist did not appear to provide back sufferers in the US survey with substantive help. One, a renowned foreign correspondent and author, said she had been personally instructed by Moishe Feldenkrais, the founder of this therapy, without anything like the success she later obtained from back exercises prescribed by a young orthopaedic surgeon just starting his practice.

Like yoga, Rolfing, Tai Chi and other disciplines, Feldenkrais therapy attempts to integrate physical, mental and spiritual approaches to well-being. The aim is to learn to move in a way that will help your back and improve your self-esteem.

An educator with chronic low back pain felt that 'Feldenkrais therapy was very helpful. It unlocked tight muscles and tissues.' However, none of the other four US survey participants who underwent Feldenkrais therapy found it useful or even relevant to helping resolve chronic back ailments.

Only one of five US survey participants said they had been helped in the long run. However, UK survey respondents rated it more positively, with almost 60 per cent gaining some degree of relief.

Number of people treated in the UK survey	22
Provided dramatic long-term help	27%
Provided moderate long-term help	9%
Provided temporary help	23%
Ineffective	27%
Made patient feel worse	14%

Biofeedback Instructors

Does anything give you conscious control over the physical factors that cause back pain? Is it possible to will a muscle to stop going into spasm? Can your mind prevent muscles from contracting, eradicate the sensation of pain, or keep stress from hurting your back?

The answer in many cases is yes, through biofeedback. This does not mean that biofeedback alone will cure back pain, but it can aid your overall recovery. Just as you can be taught to raise the temperature of your fingers or toes with the help of a biofeedback device, so you can be taught to ease or prevent the tension that aggravates back pain. But why not just use stress-reducing approaches like meditation or visualization? Why is a device needed to help you relax?

The technology usually consists of an electrical device that resembles a stereo tuner and connects to some part of your body via wires and electrodes. These monitor one or more vital signs, from heart rate to skin temperature, and the machine gives out a visual or auditory signal as the reading changes.

The value of the device, whether it is a £1 thermometer or a £10,000 electronic unit, is to measure specific information about your body – heart rate, for example, alpha brain waves, muscle tension, galvanic skin response or the volume of blood in your veins – and then give you auditory or visual cues as the measures change. This feedback enables you to test new ways of 'thinking relaxed' until the biofeedback gadgetry you're using tells you that you *are* relaxed. The instructor can also theoretically help you learn how to control yourself on many 'involuntary' levels, such as increasing the flow of blood to an injured body part.

Biofeedback can also be used as an adjunct to exercise therapy. Some physiotherapists in the UK use biofeedback when helping people learn core stability exercises (see p. 175). In this case, biofeedback can help people learn to recognize faulty movement patterns, in which some muscles are working too hard, while others are underperforming.

The value of biofeedback in reducing back pain has not been scientifically documented. But US survey participants were definitely able to articulate its benefits in an overall programme of back care.

'Biofeedback offered me ways of calming myself with resultant reduced muscle tension and less pain,' said a metallurgist who simultaneously used acupuncture and exercise. 'Overall, though,' he added, 'acupuncture and an exercise programme did the most for me to curb low back pain.'

A social worker with low back pain also found biofeedback a useful part of her recovery programme. 'Biofeedback was effective because it dealt with the true cause of my problem – tension. It showed me how to deal with tension properly. Overall, though, yoga was the greatest help because I've learned to see that mind and body need to be in harmony.'

And a professor who functions despite chronically painful spondylolisthesis reported, 'Anxiety and tension do affect my back and I have worked with a psychologist using biofeedback techniques to control and relieve tension in my back. This has helped. But I think depression is a big problem, too, as well as anxiety and frustration.'

Biofeedback was especially useful for survey participants with low back or neck pain caused in part by emotional stress. But this doesn't mean that any of the gadgets you see advertised are worth owning.

For one thing, all biofeedback treatments covered in this section were professionally supervised – and participants felt that the quality of the biofeedback instructors meant much more than the sophistication of the biofeedback equipment. Moreover, according to research supported by the American National Institute of Mental Health, 'Biofeedback devices purchased and operated by consumers have not proven themselves to be valid means of treatment.'

The recommendation of a health practitioner or friend is probably the best way to find competent biofeedback instruction. Overall, biofeedback instructors help occasionally – more through personal interaction than by the technology they apply. Virtually anyone with a machine or gadget can claim to be a biofeedback instructor. So ... caveat emptor. Judging by the overall reactions from survey participants, it would seem that practitioners who don't use biofeedback, but who are receptive, compassionate listeners, will assist you as much with stress-related back pain as will the average biofeedback instructor.

Biofeedback did not feature at all in the UK survey but eight out of ten US survey participants benefited somewhat from biofeedback when it was part of a total back-care programme. It seems to work best for low back and neck pain, though technology and gadgetry are less important than the skill and concern of the therapist.

Number of people treated in the US survey	10
Provided dramatic long-term help	0%
Provided moderate long-term help	50%
Provided temporary help	10%
Ineffective	40%
Made patient feel worse	0%

Section 3
Back Treatments

The passage through the medical system can actually be harmful. For many people with long-standing back pain, the therapies they have received, and the various opinions they have been given, actually contribute to the distress and disability.

Dr Charles Pither, quoted in *Sunday Times Magazine* article, 2002

I can't get the same answer twice about what I should and shouldn't do to help myself.

A survey participant

Chapter 5
Back Pain Treatments – From A to Z

*Acupuncture • Back Exercises • Braces and Supports • Chymopapain
• Cold Therapy (ice alone, combining cold and heat) • Dimethyl Sulfoxide
(DMSO) • Electrical Stimulation Therapy • Foot Orthotics • Foot
Reflexology (also called Reflex Zone Therapy) • Gravity Inversion (also called
hanging or anti-gravity) • Heat • Injections (cortisone, trigger point, muscle-
relaxant) • Manipulation • Marijuana • Massage (Shiatsu or acupressure,
Swedish) • Medication (analgesics, anti-inflammatories, muscle relaxants)
• Nerve Block Injections • Nutrition and Vitamins • Sclerotherapy
• Self-Help Stress Reduction • Surgery • Transcutaneous Electric Nerve
Stimulation (TENS) • Ultrasound Therapy • Yoga*

Only in the field of back care, where the variety of treatments is as extensive as it is bewildering, could yoga, surgery and acupuncture attract roughly equal numbers of individuals desperate for relief. And only in the field of back care, where documentation about treatment effectiveness is generally so scarce, could there be so many people promising to banish pain in so many different ways – injecting it (trigger point, cortisone and muscle-relaxant injections), numbing it (cryotherapy) and healing it with spiritual power (meditation).

Some of the most widely debated and unorthodox ways to control back pain are explored in this chapter. You'll find last-resort ways to combat chronic pain, from sclerotherapy to nerve block injections. You'll learn about techniques that are quite new to most back sufferers, including chymopapain injections for ruptured discs and gravity inversion for many different kinds of back pain. You'll hear what back sufferers are saying about the results of their illegal experimentation with substances such as marijuana and DMSO (dimethyl sulfoxide, an industrial solvent) to treat back pain.

Although you may have heard of most of the treatments in this chapter, you probably don't have enough information to decide whether any one of them will help or hurt you.

Take manipulation, for example. Is it the quackery some doctors claim, the cure-all some chiropractors proclaim, or something in between? Just what is its value?

How about heat? Should you use it? If so, when and for how long? Is wet heat really better than the old-fashioned heating pad? Analgesics are routinely prescribed for severe back pain, but do they work? How about anti-inflammatory drugs and muscle relaxants? How does aspirin compare with analgesics that are only available on prescription?

Are back supports worth trying? What can massage do for you? Are simple back exercises the answer for most back sufferers?

Here, at last, are answers to these and many other questions, provided by almost 500 US back pain sufferers and more than 2,000 UK survey participants.

Acupuncture

Acupuncture can be practised using a traditional Chinese approach, inserting fine needles into acupuncture points situated along energy channels called meridians. Alternatively, a technique called 'dry needling' can be used, where needles are inserted into trigger points. Either way, once the needles are in, they are 'stimulated' (usually by hand, occasionally by a mild electrical current) which triggers the body to make its own natural painkillers, called endorphins.

By reducing your level of pain, acupuncture can reduce your need for painkillers and therefore the likelihood of suffering unpleasant side-effects from medication. However, as acupuncture treats the pain rather than the cause of the pain, it is best viewed as a useful addition to a full back-care programme that includes exercise. It should not be seen as a 'cure in itself'.

If you are wary of needles used for injections, rest assured that there is no comparison. Acupuncture needles are as thin as fine wires. They usually produce no bruising or bleeding. You are likely to feel comfortable, even relaxed and drowsy, during treatments, which can last anywhere from 15 to 45 minutes. (For more on acupuncture, see pp. 39–41.)

A total of 54 per cent of US survey participants who tried acupuncture treatments were helped by them, and 61 per cent of UK respondents gained some degree of relief.

In conclusion, acupuncture works for most kinds of back ailments. However, at least five to ten treatments may be needed to determine effectiveness in individual cases.

	US survey	UK survey
Number of people treated	35	535
Responses	%	%
Provided dramatic long-term help	6	8
Provided moderate long-term help	17	10
Provided temporary help	31	43
Ineffective	43	31
Made patient feel worse	3	8

Back Exercises

Much has been written about the preventive and rehabilitative aspects of exercise for back sufferers. In fact, over the last two decades, more than a thousand US books and magazines have featured an X-minutes-a-day exercise programme, each one promoted as the plan for you.

Since most people with activity-limiting back pain do back exercises on a regular basis – and still have limitations – it is obvious that the whole story about back exercise hasn't been told. So let's try to sort out the misconceptions from the facts by examining some commonly held but erroneous beliefs about exercise and back pain.

If you are athletic and fit you won't have back pain. False. The physical fitness boom that took hold in the USA in the 1970s, galvanizing some 55 million Americans into regular fitness activities, did not banish back problems by any means.

Incapacitating back pain among weekend athletes is common. According to the US Health Insurance Association, an estimated 20 million sports injuries, including back injuries, occur each year. And, according to survey participants, racket sports such as tennis and squash, with their sudden lunges, starts and stops, seem to be especially risky for back sufferers.

Any reputable book, magazine article or printed sheet handed to you by a doctor can teach you the back exercises you need. This is only half true. Roughly half the US respondents who got advice this way were not helped much by it – and about 10 per cent were injured by it. If you have low back pain that is more annoying than incapacitating, and if you are in relatively good shape, the chances are that a conservative plan that progresses slowly may help you a great deal. But if you have activity-limiting episodes of back pain, or chronically disabling back pain, you probably need an exercise plan prescribed specifically for you, lest you risk serious injury, or fail to make progress.

Around 55 per cent of participants in the US survey reported exercising regularly, from four to seven days a week, with the vast majority exercising daily. And many of these people exercised after simply being handed a sheet of exercises or told to get a certain exercise book.

Around 15 per cent of US participants were told to exercise . . . did so at first . . . but stopped after they felt they had improved. 'I should exercise, but I'm lazy about it,' they said.

Of the remaining 24 per cent, 13 per cent were totally unaware of the therapeutic value of exercise; 5 per cent were reportedly told *not* to exercise; and 6 per cent stopped exercising after finding that the activity made them feel worse.

In conclusion, for the vast majority of back sufferers, appropriate exercises are essential to lessening or ending back pain. People with debilitating back pain have far more success with individually prescribed exercise programmes than with exercise routines in self-help books and articles or in health club classes. (See the low back exercise programme in Chapter 8, and see Chapters 9 to 12 for advice about exercises for ruptured disc, arthritis, neck pain, scoliosis, sciatica and spondylolisthesis.)

Number of US survey participants who exercised regularly	278
Provided dramatic long-term help	45%
Provided moderate long-term help	32%
Provided temporary help	10%
Ineffective	7%
Patient felt worse	6%

As for specific exercise advice, both US and UK survey participants' experiences show that there are two very simple 'non-back'
exercises that help just about everyone with back pain – walking
and swimming. Even the twenty-six US back sufferers who couldn't
lead normal lives because of back pain all improved in the long
run by following their practitioners' advice to walk or swim regularly. At least half an hour of brisk walking every other day is recommended, or building up to 15 minutes of non-stop swimming
three times a week. The UK survey results were remarkably
similar for both swimming and walking, with around 70 per cent
of participants getting back pain relief from these activities. One
respondent, Jane, had this advice for others: 'Keep active.
Consider exercise that keeps you mobile and flexible such as
walking, swimming, dance, use simple stretching and flexibility
exercises, plan a short simple routine to do each day.' And
another, Michelle, advised: 'Walking or swimming often relieves
back pain. Don't do high-impact sports like running. Avoid anything that demands jerky movements.'

Number of UK survey participants who had tried swimming	575
Provided dramatic long-term help	9%
Provided moderate long-term help	20%
Provided temporary help	40%
Ineffective	18%
Patient felt worse	13%
Number of UK survey participants who had tried walking	815
Provided dramatic long-term help	10%
Provided moderate long-term help	21%
Provided temporary help	43%
Ineffective	14%
Patient felt worse	12%

Personally tailored exercise advice is most likely to be forthcoming, participants say, from one of the following exercise experts:

1. Physiotherapist (practitioner trained in natural means of
   rehabilitation, who usually requires a doctor's authorization
   to treat you)

2. Sports medicine specialist (medical doctor trained to prevent and repair sports injuries, including back problems)
3. Kinesiologist (expert in the principles and mechanics of movement)
4. Yoga teacher*
5. Physical fitness instructor.*

* Not all yoga teachers and physical fitness instructors have the experience or the desire to work with back problems. On the other hand, some physical fitness instructors have advanced degrees in exercise physiology or kinesiology, and may be especially qualified to prescribe exercise.

Braces and Supports

Supports for your back are really supports for your abdominal muscles. If these muscles aren't strong enough to keep your tummy 'in', your spine will not be adequately supported and all kinds of back problems can ensue. However, overuse is self-defeating and risky, weakening the muscles needed to support the spine.

'A simple rubberized brace with Velcro fasteners provided instant relief for the first few weeks I was out of bed,' commented a chemical engineer who was recovering from a bout of severe low back spasms.

'I wear a girdle when I know I'm in for a taxing day,' said a waitress and Karen, a UK participant, made the following comment: 'If my back is really concerning me I do find that a strong panty girdle is of immense help until the inflammation subsides.'

Many different kinds of back supports and corsets are available, including some that you can purchase at a surgical supply shop without a prescription. However, most survey participants who were helped by these aids used back supports that had been prescribed for them.

The risks of supporting yourself artificially are clear. 'After wearing a brace for two months, and not exercising, my muscles were so weak that my back pain worsened greatly after the brace was removed,' commented a professional athlete who had been through disc surgery.

Emily, a UK respondent, also had a very negative experience: 'When I first sought medical help, I was prescribed a corset. It might have given some temporary relief and re-educated my posture. But long-term it caused more harm then good, weakening all the essential muscles, causing upper back pain from new bad habits (bending above the corset level) and promoting this self-image of disability and weakness. When, years later, a newer-generation consultant told me to bin it and go to physio "rehab", the pain got worse initially but then as I grew stronger I became much more positive and felt more able to cope with "normal" activities.'

In summary, if your muscles are strong enough to provide you with a built-in back support, you will only weaken this natural mechanism by using an aid. But if you're not in shape, a support may help you until you feel well enough to strengthen your muscles through exercise. Supports can provide some relief during acute episodes of back pain but they are not usually recommended by UK healthcare professionals and should only ever be used as a very temporary measure.

	US survey	UK survey
Number of people treated	70	370
Responses	%	%
Provided dramatic long-term help	0	7
Provided moderate long-term help	6	12
Provided temporary help	50	47
Ineffective	32	24
Made patient feel worse	12	10

Chymopapain

Chymopapain, an enzyme found in papaya, is sometimes used to treat sciatic pain caused by a herniated disc that would normally require surgery. It was approved for use by the US Food and Drug Administration in 1982, is quite widely used in Canada and occasionally used in the UK. The drug has been controversial ever since it was introduced, but some patients have found it very effective. However some people are highly allergic to chymopapain, so it is important to have an allergy test before starting treatment.

Injecting this papaya extract to remedy ruptured disc pain is less traumatic, invasive and costly than surgery, as long as it is administered by an appropriately qualified and experienced medical practitioner. However, as with surgery, it is important to remember that chymopapain is just one step in the recovery process. It is not in itself a cure.

Number of people treated in UK survey	29
Provided dramatic long-term help	17%
Provided moderate long-term help	11%
Provided temporary help	42%
Ineffective	20%
Made patient feel worse	10%

How It Works

Chymopapain injections sound almost too good to be true. 'One injection completely cured me without the need for surgery,' said an estate agent in the US survey.

A chymopapain injection is administered under local or general anaesthetic by a neurosurgeon, orthopaedic surgeon or anaesthetist. You lie on your side on an X-ray table. Depending on whether you are awake or asleep, different techniques are used to pinpoint the exact area where the gel portion of your disc has broken through its casing and is putting pressure on a nerve root. The injection itself takes about 5 minutes. The entire procedure, from entering to leaving the treatment room, takes about half an hour.

If the injection is successful, the chymopapain dissolves the gel from the ruptured disc, thereby lessening pressure on the nerve root. This should relieve the pain in your legs almost immediately.

Some patients who get chymopapain injections leave the same day they are treated, but most are hospitalized for one to four nights for observation or for treatment of back pain caused by the procedure itself. Disc surgery patients, on the other hand, are hospitalized for an average of eight days. And chymopapain patients have another advantage over disc surgery patients. They are usually back in full swing in six weeks, while surgery patients may need three to six months to resume the activities they pursued before the ruptured disc episode.

Some Negatives about Chymopapain

Allergic reactions

In the clinical trials that led to approval of chymopapain in the US, two out of 1,400 patients died because of allergic reactions to the enzyme. Such fatalities could probably have been avoided by proper testing to identify allergic patients and by giving them preventive medication. About 1 per cent of patients who have chymopapain injections have an allergic reaction, although most are not fatal.

Severe back pain

About one-third of chymopapain patients develop excruciating back pain from the injection. The pain lasts up to 48 hours and occasionally longer. Muscle relaxants and locally injected anaesthetics used to ease this pain don't provide much relief.

Inaccessibility to injection

Even when a myelogram or CT scan can locate a ruptured disc, a syringe cannot always reach the offending gel.

Not an all-purpose substitute for back surgery

Numerous back ailments such as degenerative disc, spinal tumours, spinal stenosis (a narrowing of the spinal column) and spondylolisthesis cannot be treated with chymopapain.

Like any other pain-relieving treatment, chymopapain 'doesn't change the conditions that brought on the problem initially. But it does offer you a less invasive and debilitating alternative to disc surgery and an opportunity to rehabilitate your back and avoid future problems.

Success rates vary from hospital to hospital. More to the point, they vary from doctor to doctor. And it is extremely important to find one of the relatively few doctors who have had a lot of successful experience using chymopapain therapy. Don't assume that any competent surgeon or anaesthetist has adequate training in chymopapain therapy.

Cold Therapy
(Cryotherapy)

Almost everyone who has back pain can warm up to the idea of soothing sore, aching muscles with heat. But who ever heard of curling up in bed with a shockingly cold ice pack?

But even if ice sounds bad, or temporarily feels bad, remember that it can do wonders for your back pain, especially when you have marked inflammation or 'burning pains'. Ice also relieves certain kinds of chronic back pain, especially for people with nerve root irritation. US survey participants who used ice advise you to apply it immediately after you have strained a muscle in your back. Don't stop after the first 24 to 48 hours, but use it on a regular basis as long as there are muscle spasms causing pain.

	US survey	UK survey
Number of people treated	14	437
Responses	%	%
Provided dramatic long-term help	0	4
Provided moderate long-term help	0	8
Provided temporary help	64	66
Ineffective	36	15
Made patient feel worse	0	7

Tom, a UK survey respondent, made the following comment: 'I have had two bouts of back problems. The first was at its worst when driving and may have been caused by muscle tension. This was helped by using cold packs on the back muscles.'

UK respondents were also asked specifically about their experiences with self-help treatment using cold packs and the results were as follows:

Number of people treated in UK survey	591
Provided dramatic long-term relief	6%
Provided moderate long-term relief	9%
Provided temporary relief	66%
Ineffective	14%
Made patient feel worse	5%

The easiest way to apply cold therapy at home is to take a packet of frozen peas (still in the wrapper), cover it in a damp tea towel and place it on the painful area for up to 20 minutes, checking the skin condition throughout. Note: It is important not to lie on the ice pack, as the pressure could give you an ice burn.

Why Use Ice?

1. Cold, like heat, is a counter-irritant, so you tend to feel the cold, not the pain. Moreover, when applied long enough, cold numbs all sensation.
2. Cold reduces swelling and bruising, and slows the nerve conduction, which in turn slows down the pain signals passing through your body.
3. Cold 'shocks' a muscle spasm into relaxing.
4. Cold lessens inflammation from muscle strain, which eases pain and can end the pain-spasm cycle.

How to Use Ice

The only real disagreement among US survey participants about using ice revolves around how to use it.

Typically, participants under a chiropractor's care used a 5-minutes-on, 5-minutes-off, 5-minutes-on technique. This total of 10 minutes' application was then repeated every 2 hours.

Patients under the care of a medical doctor or physiotherapist usually applied ice for 10 to 20 minutes at a time, two or three times a day.

What should you do? These rules of thumb evolved from discussion with US survey participants:

- If you're using ice to reduce the swelling and inflammation of a newly incurred strain, apply ice cubes in a plastic bag for up to 10 to 15 minutes at a time, every 2 hours, for the first 36 hours.
- If you're using ice to treat chronic muscle spasm, apply an ice bag for 10 to 15 minutes, two or three times a day.
- Try substituting an ice massage for an ice pack. To do this, you need a paper cup and a friend. Fill the paper cup with water and freeze it. Then tear off the top 2.5 cm (1 inch) of the cup and have someone massage the affected area, in circular motions, for about 15 minutes, always moving towards the heart.

- Note: Even though no survey participants who used ice were injured in the process, there is a risk of ice burn or even frostbite. Therefore, never apply ice directly on your skin, unless someone is continuously moving the ice from one area to another.
- If you're using ice cubes, put them in an ice bag or plastic bag and place a thin towel (a damp tea towel works well) between the bag and your skin. If your skin turns red, that's a warning. If it becomes white or numb, discontinue use.
- If you have arthritis or another medical condition, don't use ice unless it is recommended by a specialist.

Combining Cold and Heat

The previous chapter discussed the widespread use of heat in combating back pain and relieving tired, aching and sore muscles. Several back sufferers have successfully combined heat with ice to relieve severe and chronic low back pain, including both spasms and soreness. They first take a warm bath or shower, or use a heating pad, to relax and relieve soreness and pain. Then they use cold treatments on the areas that continue to spasm and hurt. The result? Much more pain relief than when just heat or cold therapy was used on its own. Also, survey participants who combined heat and cold found this form of therapy particularly relaxing.

Dimethyl Sulfoxide (DMSO)

For more than two decades, astonishing tales have circulated about low back sufferers who thumbed their noses at the law and received miraculous cures by applying an industrial solvent called DMSO (dimethyl sulfoxide) to their skin. And for more than two decades, US medical authorities have pointed out that there is no proof that DMSO works, only proof that it can be hazardous.

Itchy, blotchy, red skin and nausea are the most common problems among DMSO enthusiasts. Irreversible damage to the eyes of laboratory animals was reportedly found in early tests. And the long-term effects of using an industrial solvent on human beings are unknown. (All but one DMSO user in this survey bought the widely available industrial solvent, instead of the purer kind manufactured 'For Veterinary Use Only' – a 90 per cent solution or gel used to reduce swelling in injuries to animals.)

After decades of claims and counter-claims, DMSO remains controversial.

Meanwhile, US survey participants have these opinions to offer:

'I have used DMSO for the past six months,' reported a telephone salesperson with sciatica. 'It takes several weeks of daily applications. But there is a decided increase in flexibility and lessening of pain.'

Said a computer scientist with severe muscle spasms in his back, 'I applied DMSO full strength (99 per cent industrial solvent solution), left it on the spasming muscle group for 25 minutes, then wiped off the excess. It noticeably helped reduce the spasming. Let me add that I've been cautioned by friends to avoid putting anything on my skin that could be soaked in with the DMSO. So I wash the area first, then wear a clean, white cotton T-shirt afterwards.'

A disabled accident victim with low back pain claims that DMSO has been a blessing unmatched by prescription drugs. 'DMSO works remarkably well,' she says. 'Apply a thin coat of it as often as necessary. Some may think it has a peculiar odour (like garlicky oysters or worse), so adding clove powder to the solution takes care of that problem.'

A musician with low back pain also praises DMSO. 'Twice-a-day applications of DMSO got miraculous results.'

No user suffered anything worse than a bad itch. But it *was* a bad itch. Said a direct marketing consultant, 'My skin itched so badly that I thought I was going to jump out of it. Even when I cut the DMSO to a 50 per cent solution with distilled water, I couldn't tolerate putting it on my back.'

A miracle painkiller? A few people think so, but there are dissenters. A housewife recovering from several operations on ruptured discs said, 'DMSO did not help my pain nearly as much as Ben-Gay [Deep Heat].'

Bear in mind that it is illegal to use DMSO for musculoskeletal injuries or arthritis pain. Nevertheless, despite the risks and side-effects, DMSO did help most survey participants who tried it.

Number of people treated in US survey	8
Provided dramatic long-term help	12%
Provided moderate long-term help	25%

DMSO Survey contd.

Provided temporary help	25%
Ineffective	25%
Made patient feel worse	12%

Electrical Stimulation Therapy

Electrical stimulation therapy is most often used by physiotherapists and chiropractors. It is almost never offered as a sole means
of treatment, but usually as a supplement to massage, manipulation or trigger point injections.

Electrical stimulation equipment comes in all sizes and shapes –
from small units that a physiotherapist can bring to your home to
hefty futuristic-looking devices. All of them work by sending an
electrical current into contracted muscle areas, causing the
muscles to contract and relax.

According to US respondents, electrical stimulation therapy
had no noxious side-effects and provided minor, short-lived
relief about half the time for spasm-induced low back pain. But
the relief wasn't dramatic enough to elicit cheers from US survey
participants, except for one occupational therapist who reported
complete relief from painful muscle spasm after one treatment
of massage and electrical stimulation therapy. Electrical stimulation therapy did not feature in the UK survey.

In summary, if electrical stimulation therapy is offered as one
element in a comprehensive back-care programme that appeals
to you, there's no harm in trying it. It might even speed up the
healing process.

Number of people treated in US survey	45
Provided dramatic long-term help	0%
Provided moderate long-term help	0%
Provided temporary help	47%
Ineffective	51%
Made patient feel worse	2%

Foot Orthotics
(Also Called Shoe Inserts, Lifts and Arch Supports)

'None of the doctors to whom I brought my back problem ever
measured my legs, with the exception of those at the National
Institute of Health in Bethesda, Maryland,' reported a film

editor. 'The correction made [by varying the height of one shoe] was the only thing that really eased my pain. My orthopaedic surgeon told me that many people go through life not knowing that one of their legs is shorter than the other. Even a slight difference can cause exhaustion and back pain.'

'The most help I've received came from a half-inch lift in my right shoe,' said a mechanic who had back pain for twenty years before he was virtually cured by this simple and very inexpensive device.

'After enough doctors tell you that the problem is in your head,' a clothing salesperson explained, 'you start to believe it. Well, their thinking was upside down. Orthotics corrected my weak and painful arches. This let me walk normally. My back pain vanished and I haven't had any major problems for ten years.'

An orthotic is a prescribed shoe insert. But for our purposes, let's define it as any corrective shoe form that can help your feet and your back, whether it's a commercially available heel lift or arch support, or a prescribed insert that runs the length of your shoe.

Clearly, anything that affects the way you stand or walk can affect your back. According to a study at Iowa State University, an extraordinary 90 per cent of low back sufferers were free of pain one year after using the kind of arch supports you can find in any chemist. Can a shoe insert relieve your back pain? If you have low back pain, it's definitely worth trying to solve the problem from your feet up. If you think your legs may be only slightly different in length, it's best to see a podiatrist, surgical appliance specialist or possibly a rheumatologist or physiotherapist. For significant differences in length, you may need to be referred to an orthapaedic surgeon.

It is important to note that orthotics do have an element of risk. Two US survey participants were made worse – with markedly increased pain – because of inappropriately prescribed inserts. Furthermore, any significant change needs to be made gradually, particularly if you have a lot of back pain at the time. Abruptly changing the way you walk can aggravate a back problem. With this in mind, and based on what survey participants said, it seems sensible to wear new inserts for only 30 minutes the first day and 30 minutes more each day thereafter.

	US survey	UK survey
Number of people treated	17	205
Responses	%	%
Provided dramatic long-term help	18	16
Provided moderate long-term help	64	21
Provided temporary help	6	31
Ineffective	12	26
Made patient feel worse	0	6

Foot Reflexology
(Also Called Reflex Zone Therapy)

Reflexology (or reflex zone therapy) holds that every part of your body, including your back, is linked to a point in your feet. Massage that point and the related area of your body will feel better.

The idea does seem to have some validity. Two US survey participants with low back pain reported moderate long-term relief through foot reflexology. Three others with low back pain got temporary relief. And none of the five suffered any discomfort from foot reflexology.

The duration of temporary relief from foot reflexology compares favourably to Shiatsu – ranging from a few days to several months – providing pain-free time to work on long-term corrective measures.

In summary, foot reflexology offers some relief for low back pain, and an impressive 66 per cent of UK respondents found it beneficial.

Number of people treated in UK survey	156
Provided dramatic long-term help	5%
Provided moderate long-term help	10%
Provided temporary help	51%
Ineffective	27%
Made patient feel worse	7%

Gravity Inversion
(Also Called Hanging or Anti-Gravity)

'Anti-gravity' is a misnomer. So is 'hanging.' But never mind that. The procedures called anti-gravity and hanging do work.

A better term might be 'reverse-gravity' or 'inversion therapy'. Your body is inverted during treatment, so that the ever-present pull of the Earth's gravity tugs at all your tissues and vertebrae from the opposite direction, often with therapeutic effects. Whether you're hanging upside down or tilted just enough so that your head is lower than your feet, the inverted position is supposed to allow gravity to decompress your vertebrae and stretch your muscles.

Naturally, anything that promises new help to back sufferers is mired in the usual profusion of confusion, claims and competing products and techniques.

Comprehensively tested and researched, the daddy of the many posture-inversion systems is the Gravity Guiding System. Now widely imitated, it was developed by an orthopaedic surgeon, Dr Robert M. Martin, who, in his youth, was a skilled acrobat and expert at handstands. Under proper supervision, the most disabled back sufferers – even an individual in the throes of ruptured disc pain – can attempt to be treated with Dr Martin's technique. In part, the procedure is similar to the vertical traction used in many hospitals, with one obvious exception. Instead of being tilted towards a standing position, you are tilted towards a standing-on-your-head position in an effort to create more space between vertebrae and to diminish nerve root pressure.

'The Gravity Guiding System is more than just a safe way to hang upside down,' a lawyer who used it said. 'It has added a helpful new dimension to my daily exercise programme and has turned a chronically bothersome back into one that is virtually pain-free.'

A film editor raved about the system: 'It helped me to stretch myself out every day when I got home from work. It's not only great for your back, but for your head, too.' (According to yoga practioners and to research done at the University of Chicago, the rush of blood to the head from inversion is invigorating and perhaps therapeutic.)

Another survey participant, a jeweller, also liked the Gravity Guiding System. 'The boots help a great deal. I recommend them along with massage, proper nutrition, attention to posture and exercises that are not too strenuous.'

Many mail order and medical supply companies now sell posture-inversion systems based on Dr Martin's idea. Some can be found on the Internet. But if you have substantial back pain, or if your health is impaired, do not use this or any other reverse-gravity device or procedure without permission from a medical practitioner. Research on reverse-gravity at the Chicago College of Osteopathic Medicine reveals that any inversion procedure may pose particular risks for people with high blood pressure or glaucoma.

Survey participants sustained no ill-effects themselves, but a few reported injuries to other back sufferers they knew.

	US survey	UK survey
Number of people treated	11	41
Responses	%	%
Provided dramatic long-term help	0	12
Provided moderate long-term help	45	15
Provided temporary help	55	37
Ineffective	0	26
Made patient feel worse	0	10

More Comments about Inversion

Many US survey participants improvised well, attempting reverse-gravity via jungle gym bars, chinning bars, back swings and all sorts of other contraptions, including one devised by a mechanical engineer who says he hung from his ice skates on a suspended wire. Mail order and medical supply companies also offer various devices, some advertised on the Internet.

The enthusiasm for inversion seems almost boundless. Said a dog trainer, 'My chiropractor told me about hanging by my feet. At first I thought he was nuts. But I must say that it really works. It seems to decompress the spine. If it is hard at first, hang from the backs of your knees.'

The least amount of enthusiasm came from a teacher who makes regular use of gravity inversion. According to her, 'Inversion is of some help but yoga is best.'

In addition, two survey participants talked about injuries to acquaintances who did inversion exercises. Said one of these survey participants, 'A friend of mine went from bed rest to a half-hour workout on an anti-gravity machine and the exercises were much more than she could tolerate. You need to be gradual about it. But once you can do some regular back exercises, then you're ready for anti-gravity.'

Heat

'Get out the heating pad.' 'Soak in a hot bath.' These two pieces of advice for back sufferers turn out to be as wise as they are common. Both of these heat treatments are simple, effective and cheap, though a hot shower may in fact be preferable to a bath, particularly if you have back pain caused by a herniated disc. This is because the position adopted in the bath is a sustained bent position, which many people may find uncomfortable. Getting out of the bath may also cause discomfort.

So, apply a hot, wet towel or or have a hot shower. You'll give the same or more relief to your tired, overworked back as you would if you invested money in hot packs or whirlpools or heat therapy treatments.

A heating pad is definitely a worthwhile investment, according to both US and UK survey participants. And although practitioners of all kinds often tend to recommend wet heat rather than dry (heating pad), the US data shows only a slight difference in effectiveness.

	Wet heat	Dry heat
Number of people treated in US survey	118	51
Provided dramatic long-term help	1%	0%
Provided moderate long-term help	0%	0%
Provided temporary help	71%	67%
Ineffective	25%	32%
Made patient feel worse	3%	1%

UK survey participants were asked about several types of heat treatment and the results showed that heat therapy was the least effective (in terms of providing some degree of relief). Heat pads were the most effective, especially for temporary relief of back pain.

	Heat therapy	Hot bath or shower	Heat pack	Hot water bottle	Heat pad
Number of people treated in UK survey	149	1,272	762	906	693
Provided dramatic long-term help	13%	5%	6%	6%	6%
Provided moderate long-term help	16%	12%	13%	11%	11%
Provided temporary help	40%	70%	69%	70%	72%
Ineffective	21%	11%	10%	11%	9%
Made patient feel worse	10%	2%	2%	2%	2%

One UK respondent, Sarah, wanted to pass on this advice: 'Use a hot water bottle at the lower back when driving and a heat pad when sitting down indoors. I find that the heat really does help with the pain and discomfort. I would also suggest not having the hot water bottle too hot, as I did not realize that mine was too hot because of the pain and burnt my back.'

There are two safety tips that should always be followed when using a hot water bottle:

1. Wrap the hot water bottle in several thicknesses of towel, to prevent a burn.
2. Do not lie directly on top of a hot water bottle, as this puts pressure over the heat source and is more likely to result in a burn.

Injections

The three treatments grouped here are the most frequently used injection procedures, although they are not always similar in technique, objective or effectiveness. Cortisone injections are occasionally useful, even curative, for inflammation and pain from arthritis, sciatica and muscle strain, but side-effects can be unpleasant and dangerous. Trigger point injections can apparently work miracles, but they usually make you feel worse before you feel better. Muscle-relaxant injections offer temporary relief only – from a few hours to a day. (See elsewhere in Chapter 5 for details on chymopapain injections and nerve block injections.)

Cortisone injections

According to most US survey participants who received cortisone injections, the procedure is a last-resort attempt to deal with painful inflammation. Positive long-term results from cortisone injections were rare in the US survey. A telephone repairman with severe hip pain from osteoarthritis received three injections, found immediate relief, and was still pain-free three years later. A housewife with sciatica, who had seen everyone and tried everything to relieve the pain, said she was cured by a single cortisone injection.

Another survey participant, a retired engineer, reported great success with cortisone injections after disc surgery. Every year or so, when pain flared up in the area where his disc had been removed, a cortisone 'lumbar puncture' saved him.

In most instances, though, relief from cortisone was fleeting – a few hours or days at most. Also, there are risks associated with cortisone and other steroids, especially when taken over time. For example, a professor who received an injection every week for a month was hospitalized with extreme mental confusion attributed to cortisone. And a housewife who received cortisone injections retained so much fluid that she gained over 27 kg (4 stone) and developed kidney problems.

	US survey	UK survey
Number of people treated	15	535
Responses	%	%
Provided dramatic long-term help	7	9
Provided moderate long-term help	7	14
Provided temporary help	40	45
Ineffective	33	23
Made patient feel worse	13	9

Trigger point injections

'When one small area of muscle near where my buttock joins my hip was touched by the doctor, it hurt like hell and pain radiated from that spot down my leg to my knee.' This statement from a computer programmer probably defines a 'trigger point' as well as or better than most technical explanations. Indeed, there is little agreement among doctors about what a trigger point is, or the mechanism behind it.

However, survey participants who had trigger point injections all said they could feel small areas of soft tissue that seemed to be knotted, were extremely painful to the touch, and radiated pain to other areas of the back, buttocks or legs. These points were injected with a solution of painkiller, often xylocaine or procaine, mixed with saline or cortisone. Participants warn that the insertion of the needle hurts about twice as much as an ordinary injection – uncomfortable but not unbearable. And for the first day or two after an injection, you can expect to feel worse before you feel better, with the trigger point area feeling bruised and swollen. But when there is relief a few days after the injection, it usually represents a major step towards recovery.

Trigger point injections require considerable expertise on the part of the practitioner, although any medical doctor can give them. And although trigger point injections have been used for decades to alleviate back pain, their effectiveness is still controversial and relatively few practitioners offer them.

	US survey	UK survey
Number of people treated	10	66
Responses	%	%
Provided dramatic long-term help	10	14
Provided moderate long-term help	0	9
Provided temporary help	40	48
Ineffective	20	20
Made patient feel worse	30	9

Muscle-relaxant injections

If specific muscles in your back are contracting or in spasm, some doctors may suggest injecting an anesthetic into the affected area. They believe this injection makes more sense than the 'shotgun' approach of prescribed muscle-relaxant pills. There is usually temporary relief from a numbing agent such as novocaine, xylocaine or procaine. And there is the added hope that during the several hours you're not in pain, the pain-spasm-pain cycle will be interrupted and possibly broken.

Survey participants stress the importance of avoiding normal activity while part of your back is numb. Until full sensation returns, you should do little.

	US survey	UK survey
Number of people treated	6	101
Responses	%	%
Provided dramatic long-term help	0	11
Provided moderate long-term help	0	21
Provided temporary help	66	48
Ineffective	16	19
Made patient feel worse	16	1

Manipulation

Manipulation, used as one element in a well-rounded programme of total back care, can reduce back pain and help sufferers to function normally. US survey participants found it better for temporary relief but 39 per cent of UK respondents gained long-term help.

The two kinds of medical specialists who use manipulation most frequently are chiropractors and osteopaths. But other specialists, including some physiotherapists and GPs, also manipulate the spine as part of their recovery programmes for back sufferers.

Although manipulation is a discipline that requires extensive training, it is also, like so many other medical procedures, an art form. Perhaps this explains why the average chiropractic patient in the US survey went to at least two chiropractors or osteopaths before finding a manipulator who got results.

Nevertheless, participants' experiences show how to cut down on the amount of running around it takes to find a practitioner skilled in manipulation. The best and surest way is to get a recommendation from another back sufferer.

An alternative approach is to arrange an appointment for consultation purposes, rather than for treatment. This allows you to gauge the practitioner's receptiveness to spending time learning about you and your problem, as opposed to getting you on the table immediately. You'll also get a chance to ask the practitioner about his philosophy of manipulation. The gentler forms produced the most satisfactory results for US survey participants. One specific technique mentioned frequently and favourably was 'directional non-force manipulation', but try not to get caught up in the manipulation name game.

There are dozens of names used for manipulation techniques. Some are technical and others imply merchandizing ploys. The differences separating one from another are usually indiscernible to lay people (and to some manipulators, for that matter). Promise-laden brochures proclaiming the unique healing powers of this or that form of manipulation are fairly common. In short, ignore claims that border on the miraculous, be sceptical about supposedly documented success rates of 90 per cent or higher, and look for a professional who is interested in you and in an overall programme of back care. You can contact organizations such as the Complementary Medical Association, the General Osteopathic Council or the Chartered Society of Physiotherapists (see Useful Addresses, p. 463) in order to find reputable, registered practitioners.

In summary, manipulation reduces pain temporarily in a majority of treatments but is not by itself a long-term solution. It's best for low back pain and neck pain, especially within the first few weeks of a pain episode. And you should beware of practitioners using manipulation to treat acute pain caused by a herniated disc.

	US survey	UK survey
Number of people treated	333	838
Responses	%	%
Provided dramatic long-term help	5	19
Provided moderate long-term help	7	20
Provided temporary help	44	40
Ineffective	34	11
Made patient feel worse	10	10

Marijuana

All the US survey participants who turned to marijuana for pain relief treated it as a prescription drug and said they did not use it regularly for recreational purposes. They approached it cautiously and used it for specific reasons.

'Illegal though it may be,' said a book-keeper with sciatica, 'marijuana helped relax me, especially during periods of extreme pain.'

A paraplegic with chronic, severe pain throughout her back found marijuana an invaluable sleep aid on occasion: 'When the pain is unbearable and I can't sleep, one marijuana cigarette makes comfort and relaxation quite easy.'

An artist who underwent disc surgery and then suffered from scar tissue pressing on his nerves said, 'When I'm in pain, nothing helps except smoking a little dope. Sometimes it's the only thing that helps me stand the pain.'

'Instead of taking a strong prescription drug, smoke a small amount of marijuana or make a tea out of it,' advised a salesperson with a ruptured disc.

'If the pain is bad, marijuana works the same as muscle relaxants without the side-effects,' noted a market researcher with severe low back pain.

An office manager with low back pain disagreed with all this advice: 'I experienced mild discomfort when I smoked marijuana. It seemed to make me more sensitive to pain.'

A computer programmer also felt that marijuana could increase back pain: 'I suggest that people with back trouble stay away from marijuana. It makes you feel the pain more.'

A waitress with low back pain found marijuana harmful: 'I suspect that the effectiveness of marijuana as a drug used for tension can create negative effects. I hold an opinion that marijuana has damaging effects to the spine. That is my idea from experience.'

In the US survey, no one had a middle-of-the-road opinion about marijuana. It either helped where prescribed drugs didn't, or it made the individual feel worse. However, in the UK survey an impressive 84 per cent gained some degree of relief from this drug.

In the UK, marijuana was reclassified from a Class B to a Class C drug in 2004. The UK government is considering legalizing it for medicinal use. However, at present, it is still illegal for doctors to prescribe it for their patients.

	US survey	UK survey
Number of people treated	8	135
Responses	%	%
Provided dramatic long-term help	0	15
Provided moderate long-term help	0	15
Provided temporary help	65	54
Ineffective	0	11
Made patient feel worse	35	5

Massage

A close relative of acupuncture, Shiatsu is applied along meridians, or pathways through which energy is said to flow through the body. Shiatsu may feel a little like 'bad medicine that must be good for you.' The pressure of the massage, usually exerted with the ball of the thumb, sometimes elicits a few ouches and grimaces from back sufferers with tight muscles. This minor pain hardly ever persists after the treatment, but excessive pressure on the lower back can be injurious and did cause an increase in pain for two of the twenty-nine US survey participants.

With its low level of long-term success, Shiatsu wouldn't normally get much acclaim in a report of this kind. But its value has to be taken seriously for three reasons.

First, its 'temporary help' rate of 69 per cent in the US survey was surpassed only by aspirin and wet heat for short-term relief.

Second, wet heat was usually the first step taken by back sufferers to alleviate pain. Shiatsu, on the other hand, was usually the treatment of last resort for survey participants with the most intractable problems. And it typically got results where heat did not.

Third, the temporary help provided by Shiatsu usually lasted long enough for participants to get involved in long-term rehabilitation programmes.

According to US survey respondents, Shiatsu, or acupressure massage, was the most successful, drug-free treatment available for temporarily relieving low back and neck pain.

	Swedish	Shiatsu
Number of people treated in US survey	95	29
Provided dramatic long-term help	2%	3%
Provided moderate long-term help	3%	7%
Provided temporary help	61%	69%
Ineffective	31%	14%
Made patient feel worse	3%	7%

Swedish massage, by comparison, with its mostly smooth-gliding movements, was soothing and relaxing, if not healing and pain-relieving. It was also virtually pain- and risk-free. The one exception – which applies only to severely disabled back sufferers – is that lying on your stomach for up to one hour, even with a small pillow tucked under you, can aggravate lumbar pain. Shiatsu also carries this element of risk. But the risk can be minimized or avoided as follows:

1. When you're on your back, put a folded towel or small pillow under your neck and head, and one or two pillows under your knees.
2. If you think you can lie on your stomach without aggravating your problem, tuck a pillow under your abdomen. If the pillow is thin, and you feel a pull on your lower back, fold the pillow in two. In any event, make sure the pillow is under your abdomen and not under your chest.
3. If you feel uncomfortable lying on your stomach, try lying in an oblique position: lie on your side, tuck a folded pillow against your abdomen, and lean into it. Keep leaning towards the stomach-down position as far as you can without turning onto your stomach. Experiment with different positions for your legs, making sure that you keep at least one of them bent.

Note: Many massage therapists, and virtually all chiropractors, feel they cannot work on you unless you lie on your stomach. So check before you go. As with every other aspect of back care, remember to believe in your judgement about yourself.

In the UK survey, participants were asked about their experience of massage in general. Like the US respondents, they found it particularly helpful for temporary relief of back pain.

Number of people treated in UK survey	737
Provided dramatic long-term help	8%
Provided moderate long-term help	15%
Provided temporary help	63%
Ineffective	9%
Patient felt worse	5%

One UK respondent swears by a combination of massage and homeopathy: 'I find regular back massages with arnica cream, followed by an arnica oil rub, give me the only long-term relief from what is constant pain.'

Medication

Pills are the most popular form of treatment for back pain. Yet, according to US survey participants, no prescription drug was significantly more useful than a placebo. (A placebo is a pill or treatment with no active ingredients or known medical value, but that nevertheless helps some of the patients who receive it.) And, of course, the harmful effects of prescription drugs can far outweigh those of placebos.

This doesn't mean that you should refuse to follow your doctor's advice about taking medication for back pain. It is to say, however, that you should carefully consider which medicines you decide to take on a regular basis, and whether or not their benefits outweigh the side-effects they sometimes cause.

Medication used to be over-prescribed for ailments such as back pain. For years, patients who went to a doctor wanted to come away with something concrete – and that something was a prescription. But this attitude seems to have changed. A survey conducted by researchers associated with Johns Hopkins Hospital found that 'patients who did not receive prescriptions reported more satisfaction with their visits to physicians than patients who did receive prescriptions. Patients may not be as prescription-oriented as many physicians believe.'

Judging from the experiences of UK survey participants, the most important point is to match the strength of the analgesic to the level of pain, thus enabling you to avoid using stronger painkillers, which are likely to cause more side-effects. However, you should also use medication early on, before high pain levels set in. (This will help you avoid taking large quantities of painkillers later on, when the increased pain has already started and it is too late for the medication to reduce it significantly.)

Ben, a UK respondent, said: 'Learn intelligent use of painkillers/anti-inflammatories. Take with food, take before pain is intense, use moderately, not dependently.'

Another recommended: 'Occasional short courses of Diclofenac tablets for periods of greater discomfort.'

Anne, another UK participant, found that medication enabled her to continue leading a relatively normal life, and had this advice for fellow back pain sufferers: 'If they help, take them! If you haven't been prescribed anything, ask your GP for Solpadol or something similar (prescription strength co-codamol, 30/500), much more effective than over-the-counter medication). (I went 3 months before another back pain sufferer told me about this, and my GP was happy to prescribe it, but hadn't thought to suggest it herself!!) Decent painkillers can make the difference between a good and bad night's sleep, and if you haven't slept well you're tense and ache more next day, which means you're even less likely to sleep the following night – and a vicious circle is set up. They can help you maintain your social life (e.g. an evening out at the theatre) by reducing your pain sufficiently to prevent it being a distraction. They can also help you return to work.'

And Catherine, another UK respondent, tells a familiar tale that also illustrates an important point about the way pain systems in the body work: 'I'm sure that other people will have had my situation: I had seen two different physios and was a mystery to my GP because I was experiencing very severe pain and yet no one could find anything wrong with me other than bog-standard mechanical back pain. I spent a lot of time researching and reading up on the Internet, and couldn't find an explanation for myself. None of the anti-inflammatories or analgesics I was taking could reduce my pain from unbearable on the bad days.

Tip 1: I was signed off work and just getting worse and worse until I asked for a second opinion from the Physio Department at my hospital. I was referred to an Extended Scope Practitioner who, rather than treating me or manipulating me, educated me about my condition and how to overcome it myself (and how the problem could be tackled in my approach as much as what I was doing physically). She was the first person to give me a real answer about what was going on – that my problem related to the tissues attached to one of my lumbar facet joints and that the inflammation had made the nerves very sensitized, hence the reason I was experiencing such acute pain. She was a life-saver . . .

Tip 2: The intense local pain I felt was accompanied by a great deal of heat both locally and throughout my body. I also felt sick and headachey. On good days, it felt as though I had a deep cut inside my tissue, running along a 6- to 8-inch area. A full dose of Celebrex and Co-codamol just dulled it slightly.

I now know that nerves can become very sensitized by disruption to normal service, such as long-term inflammation. This is not the same as nerve pain, but causes a very similar kind of pain and can be treated the same way. Once my GP knew this, he could prescribe amitryptiline, which turned my life around at the time.'

There was a big difference in the results of the US and UK surveys on medication, with most US respondents reacting negatively to prescribed drugs and most UK participants finding prescription painkillers, anti-inflammatories and muscle relaxants very helpful. This difference could be partly due to the time-lag between the two surveys. Doctors may have become more skilled at prescribing medication appropriately in the intervening period.

Guidance given by health professionals on the use of medication can also significantly affect the outcome for the patient. For instance, those people who follow advice about taking non-steroidal anti-inflammatory medication with food are much less likely to suffer gastric problems as a side-effect.

Prescription analgesics	US survey	UK survey
Number of people treated	138	943
Responses	%	%
Provided dramatic long-term help	0	11
Provided moderate long-term help	0	17
Provided temporary help	30	58
Ineffective	61	11
Made patient feel worse	9	3

Prescription anti-inflammatories	US survey	UK survey
Number of people treated	70	837
Responses	%	%
Provided dramatic long-term help	0	12
Provided moderate long-term help	2	18
Provided temporary help	24	51
Ineffective	60	13
Made patient feel worse	14	6

Prescription muscle relaxants	US survey	UK survey
Number of people treated	95	413
Responses	%	%

Provided dramatic long-term help	0	13
Provided moderate long-term help	0	15
Provided temporary help	36	54
Ineffective	55	12
Made patient feel worse	9	6

Most medicines have some side-effects but people experience them to differing extents. If you find the side-effects of your medication particularly unpleasant, it may be well worth reducing your dose or even stopping entirely. However, you should always consult your doctor or pain specialist first.

Most side-effects reported in the US survey were of the 'unpleasant but temporary' variety, although some survey participants suffered more serious effects.

Here is a list of which medicines made US survey participants feel worse – and why:

Analgesics

Side-effects included nausea and other gastro-intestinal disturbances, impairment of mental clarity. Different combinations of paracetamol or Panadol with codeine, and aspirin with codeine, were prescribed most frequently. For most US survey participants, there were no significant differences between prescription and over-the-counter drugs in reducing pain, and the majority of survey participants who took pain pills considered them ineffective. Highly potent painkillers are available and are necessary in some instances, but back sufferers raised two warning flags about them: (1) be aware of the possible side-effects of what has been prescribed for you; and (2) remember that a pill powerful enough to mute pain will also deprive you of helpful warning signals. In other words, if you take a strong analgesic, you should modify your physical activities and movements.

Muscle relaxants

Side-effects included dizziness and light-headedness, drowsiness, impairment of mental clarity. Robaxin and Parafon Forte were the brand names mentioned most frequently, but the majority of US survey participants could not remember the name of the muscle relaxant prescribed for them.

Prescription anti-inflammatories

Side-effects included gastro-intestinal disorders, including aggravation of ulcers and gastritis, as well as a few cases of rectal bleeding. Motrin, Indomethacin and Naproxen were the pills taken most frequently.

Aspirin (anti-inflammatory and analgesic)

Side-effects included gastro-intestinal disturbances. Many participants didn't include aspirin in their list of medicines simply because aspirin is used so commonly and is often not considered a 'real' medicine. In fact, most participants who mentioned aspirin said it had been recommended by a doctor. But the vast majority of medical authorities agree that aspirin is a powerful drug, and that regular, long-term use requires the approval and supervision of a qualified practitioner.

Valium (Diazepam)

Side-effects included drowsiness, light-headedness, impaired mental clarity. When Valium is prescribed for back sufferers in the USA, it is usually meant to act as a muscle relaxant with stress-reducing qualities. It is supposed to act on the part of the brain thought to influence emotional stability. Individuals who take Valium during the day should not be surprised if they cannot function as usual. Few doctors told the US respondents that it could be dangerous to drive while using Valium.

According to current medical opinion in the UK, diazepam (Valium) should definitely not be used to manage acute back pain and this suggests that it should not be used for chronic pain either. Dependence can be a major problem with this medicine.

Non-Prescription Medication and Supplements

UK survey participants were also asked about their experiences with non-prescription medicines, supplements and remedies. Of these, the most effective (in terms of providing some degree of relief) were analgesics and anti-inflammatories, and the least effective were Devil's claw and glucosamine.

Non-prescription analgesics

Number of people treated in UK survey   664
Provided dramatic long-term help   6%

Provided moderate long-term help	13%
Provided temporary help	63%
Ineffective	16%
Made patient feel worse	2%

Non-prescription anti-inflammatories

Number of people treated in UK survey	526
Provided dramatic long-term help	7%
Provided moderate long-term help	13%
Provided temporary help	62%
Ineffective	15%
Made patient feel worse	3%

Devil's claw

Devil's claw root is an anti-inflammatory herb, which has become a popular remedy for arthritis. It is thought to reduce inflammation in the joints and is available from chemists and healthfood shops in the form of capsules or tablets. It stimulates the production of stomach acid, though not as much as non-specific anti-inflammatories, so you should avoid it if you have ulcers or other gastric problems. Pregnant and breastfeeding women and children under sixteen are also advised not to take this remedy until more studies have been done.

Number of people treated in UK survey	67
Provided dramatic long-term help	15%
Provided moderate long-term help	14%
Provided temporary help	27%
Ineffective	37%
Made patient feel worse	7%

Glucosamine

Glucosamine is a chemical that occurs naturally in the body and is used to produce cartilage, tendons and ligaments (the connective tissue for our joints). It has become a popular remedy for back pain, especially pain caused by osteoarthritis, in the form of supplements made from shellfish shells (which should not be taken by anyone who is allergic to shellfish). The usual dose to treat osteoarthritis is 500 mg three times a day, or 1500 mg a day. However, you need to check carefully how much glucosamine there is in any supplement you take, as it varies considerably, and follow the instructions.

Number of people treated in UK survey	345
Provided dramatic long-term help	10%
Provided moderate long-term help	25%
Provided temporary help	28%
Ineffective	34%
Made patient feel worse	3%

Herbal remedies

Number of people treated in UK survey	113
Provided dramatic long-term help	12%
Provided moderate long-term help	24%
Provided temporary help	33%
Ineffective	26%
Made patient feel worse	5%

Homeopathic remedies

Number of people treated in UK survey	76
Provided dramatic long-term help	12%
Provided moderate long-term help	28%
Provided temporary help	29%
Ineffective	25%
Made patient feel worse	6%

Nerve Block Injections

Three participants in the US survey had nerve block injections, often consisting of alcohol or a steroid designed to numb the nerve centre that is generating the pain. In addition, several survey participants talked about the effect of nerve block treatments on back sufferers they knew.

The skill of the practitioner can make a big difference. 'The treatment of the most lasting benefit was the nerve block provided by the neurosurgeon,' said a social worker in the US survey.

'I had three injections next to the spine. I can't say it cured me, but it helped tremendously.'

Nerve block injections are usually given by neurosurgeons or anaesthetists who work on this treatment regularly. In the UK, these injections are often available through pain clinics. Other medical doctors can administer nerve blocks, but since experience is critical to success, you really need to ask a doctor about his track record with this procedure.

In summary, nerve block injections have considerable potential for relief – but also for harm. Many UK participants reacted positively to this treatment, with 81 people gaining some degree of relief. However, 25 participants found it made no difference and 16 participants felt worse.

Number of people treated in UK survey	122
Provided dramatic long-term help	15%
Provided moderate long-term help	15%
Provided temporary help	37%
Ineffective	20%
Made patient feel worse	13%

Nutrition and Vitamins

Most survey participants were uncertain about the extent to which nutrition and vitamins helped prevent or relieve back trouble. The most popular suggestions were: take calcium and vitamin C supplements, particularly after an injury or surgery; avoid processed foods, sugar, alcohol and chemical additives; and eat more complex carbohydrates, less protein and fat.

	US survey	UK survey
Number of people treated	11*	210
Responses	%	%
Provided dramatic long-term help	0	10
Provided moderate long-term help	27	24
Provided temporary help	9	28
Ineffective	64	34
Made patient feel worse	0	4

* Dozens of US survey participants experimented with nutrition and vitamins. The individuals represented here made a concentrated, long-term effort to relieve back pain by changing their nutritional habits.

Here are specific recommendations from US survey participants about the role of nutrition and vitamins in alleviating back pain.

For osteoarthritis

There is no proof that any foods or vitamins can prevent, relieve or cause osteoarthritis. It is true, though, that taking vitamins A, B, C and E and calcium seems to make some osteoarthritis sufferers feel better.

Five participants in the US survey found that adding calcium to their diet 'cured' osteoarthritis-like symptoms. Possibly, what seemed like arthritis to these individuals was really a calcium deficiency, which is fairly common in older people. Still, if you have osteoarthritis, it might make sense to try a multivitamin and calcium supplement. Beware of taking megadoses, though. It is known that megadoses of many vitamins and minerals can have serious toxic effects.

Also, in rare instances, nightshade plants like tomatoes, potatoes and peppers can cause an allergic reaction that makes muscles feel sore and inflamed. Again, consult an allergist or a practitioner trained in nutrition if you think this possibility is worth exploring.

Other supplements that US survey participants found helpful included magnesium, alfalfa and kelp tablets.

In the UK, the most popular supplements used to treat osteoarthritis are glucosamine sulphate, cod liver oil, chondroitin, Omega 3 fish oil and evening primrose oil. The research that has been carried out on these five supplements indicates that they may all offer osteoarthritis sufferers some benefits in terms of increased mobility and reduced pain.

For low back pain

There is no such thing as an 'Eat Your Way to a Better Back' diet. But there are consistent indications that a bad diet can make back pain worse:

1. Eating poorly – consuming a lot of sugar and junk foods and not receiving proper nutrition – can make you feel tired and out of sorts. And this can only make your back and the rest of you feel worse.

2. Not drinking enough liquids and not eating enough fibre can make you constipated. Constipation was mentioned by a dozen US survey participants as a condition that aggravated or caused back pain.
3. Being overweight can be hard on your back, especially if you end up with a protruding gut. A lean body hardly precludes back pain, but a few overweight back sufferers did feel better after shedding surplus kilos.
4. Alcohol and caffeine can lead to and aggravate ulcers, gastritis, colitis and other gastro-intestinal problems – all of which can cause back pain. Medical treatment for these problems helped five US survey participants to eliminate back pain.

Chiropractors offered the most advice about nutrition, according to US survey participants, and it was not uncommon for them to 'prescribe' vitamins and minerals.

Sclerotherapy

Sclerotherapy involves injecting a chemical irritant and local anaesthetic into ligaments, usually around a joint thought to be unstable. Your body reacts to this irritant by forming scar tissue, which is supposed to help stabilize your back. The procedure was used fairly commonly several decades ago by medical doctors to repair hernias (scar tissue covered the tear) and to eradicate varicose veins.

A farmer who risked losing his business because of back pain, and who had done virtually everything under the sun to keep working after disc surgery, praised sclerotherapy. 'The injection to build up scar tissue around the area of pain helped the most. It relieved the pain, and I was able to work, drive a tractor, trucks and machinery.'

A housewife who got the same level of long-term help remarked, 'The injections were somewhat painful, probably made worse because I was terrified of them. But afterwards, it was the first time in five years that I could do a normal amount of housework.'

On the other hand, two low back patients felt that sclerotherapy treatments injured them permanently. 'After the injections

I couldn't bend as well or perform my daily routines without greater pain,' a nurse reported. 'Three years later, I'm still worse off for having had those idiotic treatments.' And another farmer commented: 'After a series of sclerotherapy injections, a CT scan showed that the treatment caused a lot of scar tissue to form in my lumbar area. This is why I have more severe pain.'

The reported long-term damage to two survey participants should give readers pause for thought about sclerotherapy. If the scar tissue that results presses on a nerve root, you're in trouble. Moreover, although scar tissue resembles the fibrous tissue in muscles, it lacks the 'stretchability' of muscle and can impede normal movement.

In conclusion, these high-risk injections should only be given after thorough investigation by a suitably qualified healthcare practitioner. Otherwise they could cause significant and permanent damage. In the UK they are sometimes applied by rheumatologists.

Number of people treated in UK survey	18
Provided dramatic long-term help	33%
Provided moderate long-term help	0%
Provided temporary help	22%
Ineffective	17%
Made patient feel worse	28%

Self-Help Stress Reduction

US survey participants reported there is no single best way to reduce stress. But according to sellers of books, tapes and gadgets advocating a particular stress-reduction technique, *theirs* is the best way.

It really doesn't matter which stress-reduction technique you use. Survey participants cited here practised meditation, visualization or prayer, and each of these approaches worked to some extent. Moreover, there is virtually no risk of stress-reduction therapy making you feel worse, unless, of course, you substitute it for needed professional help.

Technique is not the key: belief is. If you believe that a method of stress reduction will help you to relax – and control back pain – it probably will. It isn't a question of tricking yourself. It is, at the very least, a respite from the daily grind – a way to treat yourself well every day and interrupt the activities that allow stress to build up to unmanageable levels.

Several survey participants had success with the following visualization/imagery technique:

- Find a time each day when you will not be interrupted. This may be easier said than done, but everything hinges on your having solitude. Even a few minutes is valuable, but half an hour is ideal.
- Clear your mind of the day's activities and problems. Lie down in any position that feels comfortable. Take a few deep breaths. As you exhale, imagine that you're in a relaxing environment – perhaps on a beach or near a lake. See yourself there. Allow the image to become real to you.
- Now, picture a soft breeze warming your body, one part at a time, relaxing you. Save your aching back for last. Then concentrate on making every part of your back become more and more relaxed.
- Imagine your back feeling well. Imagine it being well and pain-free.

In summary, any technique that provides a break from stressful activities can help your back. 'Visualization' was the most popular self-help, stress-reduction technique used by US survey participants.

	US survey	UK survey
Number of people treated	17*	128*
Responses	%	%
Provided dramatic long-term help	18	12
Provided moderate long-term help	64	16
Provided temporary help	6	51
Ineffective	12	14
Made patient feel worse	0	7

* Limited to self-taught, stress-reduction techniques used in part to relieve back pain. Survey results for other disciplines that reduce stress and back pain, such as yoga, biofeedback and counselling, are presented separately.

Surgery

Perhaps the most important fact to know about disc surgery is that you probably don't need it. For every survey participant who had disc surgery, three others were told they probably had disc problems requiring surgery but found successful alternatives.

This widespread use of 'ruptured disc' as a diagnosis isn't surprising for two reasons. First, participants with severe, chronic back pain were typically referred by a GP to an orthopaedic surgeon or a neurosurgeon, either of whom was more likely than any other practitioner to suspect a ruptured disc or suggest surgery. Second, most survey participants who were told they needed surgery received a tentative diagnosis that was not borne out by diagnostic procedures.

This was the experience of Julia, a UK survey respondent: 'I suffered acute back pain after about thirty years of "on and off" low back pain and sciatica. I had an MRI scan which showed two discs blocking nerve paths. I had sciatica in both legs and was on a morphine-based strong painkiller. My husband had to carry me to the loo and I couldn't walk for a week. I had to attend the appointment with the surgeon on crutches and was put on the list for a "discectomy". In the eight months that I waited my doctor referred me to the NHS physio and he gave me Pilates-type exercises to do. It took a long time but I am now completely pain-free, having strengthened my "inner-core" muscles.'

There is a growing consensus among medical authorities that no more than 5 per cent of back sufferers require surgery. But Dr Norman Shealy, president of the American Holistic Medical Association, is even more optimistic. He believes that fewer than 1 per cent of back sufferers have disc problems requiring surgery.

If surgery has been advised for you, survey participants' experience can help you choose a surgeon and avoid post-operative complications. The absence of skilled physiotherapy is one major reason for a poor outcome from surgery; scarring is another reason. Survey participants who didn't fare well after surgery tended to be abandoned – in spirit if not in fact – by doctors. You may also be interested to read about helpful alternatives to surgery that some of them tried.

	US survey	UK survey
Number of people treated	65	204
Responses	%	%
Provided dramatic long-term help	25	24
Provided moderate long-term help	25	21
Provided temporary help	28	23
Ineffective	8	21
Made patient feel worse	14	11

Choosing a Surgeon

For most people, disc surgery is elective surgery, even though severe pain may make them feel as though they have no choice. And that means you can probably choose your own doctor.

If the orthopaedics department is in a teaching hospital, ask if the surgery would be performed by the orthopaedic surgeon in charge of your case or by a resident. Residents have to practise on someone, but not necessarily on you.

It is extremely important to learn about the rehabilitation process. Again, try to be positive and specific with your questions. Ask about the range of time usually needed for partial and complete recovery, and what kind of physiotherapy is offered. Remember that a good physiotherapy programme is crucial; it can make a competent surgeon seem like a genius.

Disabling Post-operative Problems . . . and How to Avoid Them

Of the 33 US survey participants who failed to improve in the long run, or who became worse after disc surgery, only six felt they knew the reason for their problems. CT scans revealed that these six individuals had formed scar tissue from the surgery, and this tissue was apparently generating pain by pressing on nerve roots. In some cases, nerve root pressure causes worse pain than a ruptured disc. It seems that no one who has a disc removed surgically can avoid the formation of scar tissue. But why scar tissue is a problem for some people and not for others remains a mystery.

Most survey participants who recovered fully from disc surgery shared two key elements in their rehabilitation process: (1) ice massages during the first weeks after surgery; and (2) a supervised, daily physiotherapy and exercise programme that included an emphasis on building abdominal strength. (See Chapters 10 and 11 for tips on how to do appropriate exercises.)

How to Avoid Surgery for a Ruptured or Degenerated Disc

Talking about how to avoid surgery may seem out of place in a section about surgery, but most people considering surgery are secretly or openly wondering whether they can avoid it. Approximately half of 65 survey participants with positive myelography or CT scan results did just that. After hearing they had a ruptured disc, they opted against surgery. Most were functioning well an average of five years after the initial diagnosis. And they attributed their success in avoiding surgery to one of the following approaches or procedures, listed according to their frequency of use. (You'll find a thorough look at how best to recover from a ruptured disc, and achieve fitness, in Chapter 9.)

- Strong pain medication (Oxycodone, for example) was an important factor. Prescription pain pills don't work well for all back conditions (see pp. 94–8 for details), but in the case of debilitating, acute sciatica caused by a ruptured disc, potent pain medication is essential. Milder analgesics usually don't help true sciatica, when the pain is accompanied by 'pins and needles' or numbness and/or weakness in the leg. The result is that some patients are unnecessarily driven to surgery by intolerable pain.
- Having a supportive practitioner who wants to avoid surgery as much as you do is extremely helpful. Otherwise, you will have to deal with the physical pain and the pressure to 'get over it quickly'.
- Survey participants also stress the need for carefully planned and supervised physiotherapy, covering everything from the length of time you should walk each day to the therapeutic use of ice and graduated exercise. Professional help during this stage of your recovery is almost essential. The right help for a few weeks can enable you to take charge of your recovery more effectively.

Transcutaneous Electric Nerve Stimulation (TENS)

This device is about the size of a mobile phone. You can hook it over your belt or conceal it under loose clothing. It runs on batteries, costs upwards of £26 and sometimes as much as £70, and sends electrical impulses across the skin via electrodes.

The sensation you feel is not the least bit painful. 'Buzzing' or 'tingling' are the descriptions used most often by survey participants.

'It seems like many people are divided on the effectiveness of transcutaneous electric nerve stimulation,' reported an artist who tried it because the formation of scar tissue after surgery was causing her severe pain. 'Many feel it is all psychological,' she continued. 'But I was in pain for five months taking pills like one eats potato chips and I could get no relief whatsoever. With TENS, I was able to handle the pain and finally get rid of most medications.'

An executive with low back pain had the opposite experience. His discomfort increased: 'It felt like a vibrator on the place where it hurt.' (Note: TENS devices hardly ever cause pain; placing the electrodes differently, or reducing the intensity, might have prevented the problem in this case.)

Meanwhile, Gillian, a UK survey participant, reacted very positively: 'I find that using my own TENS machine, especially after retiring at night, for half an hour, whilst reading a book, makes for a more restful night. I also use the TENS machine first thing in the morning, if necessary. A lot of people do not seem to be aware of how it helps pain relief.'

So how does a TENS machine work? It is thought to send signals to the brain that block other nerve signals carrying pain messages. It is also believed to stimulate the production of endorphins (natural pain-relieving hormones produced by the body). One hour on, followed by one hour off, is a commonly used regime during the day, leaving the electrodes off at night.

TENS is not addictive and seems to have few side-effects. It's often recommended in the UK for pregnant women as a way of controlling labour pains, especially in early labour. It has also been recommended for treating pain after surgery but, according to the UK College of Anaesthetists, TENS isn't effective on its own as pain relief for acute moderate to severe post-operative pain.

There is also some debate as to whether TENS is effective for chronic pain, and some experts feel that more research needs to be done in this area.

If you would like to try using a TENS machine, ask your doctor first whether you can hire a machine locally before you decide to buy one. You could try your local health centre, high street chemist or hospital pain clinic.

In conclusion, US survey participants gained less relief from this device than has been reported in most other studies but 68 per cent of UK respondents found it helpful. TENS also helped some post-surgery patients cut down on prescription painkillers.

	US survey	UK survey
Number of people treated	14	573
Responses	%	%
Provided dramatic long-term help	7	7
Provided moderate long-term help	0	15
Provided temporary help	29	46
Ineffective	57	24
Made patient feel worse	7	8

Ultrasound Therapy

Ultrasound therapy uses very highly pitched sound waves that cannot be heard by the human ear. These waves are thought to have a micro-massaging effect, as the sound waves pass through the tissues. (This brings more blood to the area, which is helpful during healing.)

Philip, a UK survey participant, said: 'I visit an osteopath every 4 or 5 weeks [who is] qualified to apply acupuncture and ultrasound . . . I had an accident about 5 years ago, when I apparently damaged about four-fifths of my lower back. Following the initial pain and subsequent treatment (mainly ultrasound), I had no more problems until about 2 years ago.'

In the US survey, 62 per cent found ultrasound completely ineffective. UK survey respondents reacted more positively. However, according to international guidelines, there is little evidence to support the use of ultrasound in treating mechanical/non-specific low back pain.

	US survey	UK survey
Number of people treated	71	71
Responses	%	%
Provided dramatic long-term help	0	13
Provided moderate long-term help	2	8
Provided temporary help	35	46
Ineffective	62	23
Made patient feel worse	1	10

Yoga

Many disciplines other than yoga combine help for the spine, the mind and the spirit. But none comes close to matching the widespread appeal and positive results of yoga.

If you haven't tried yoga because it seems mystical or somehow peculiar to you – an activity associated with ex-hippies or Indian holy men – consider the following comments.

A joiner was surprised and delighted to find that yoga suited him. 'Yoga has helped my back more than anything,' he said. 'I stumbled on it by accident as a back pain remedy. I was curious and took a class.'

'Yoga is a wonderful way to keep your back limber and your whole body in good shape,' commented a domestic cleaner. 'It is such a wonderful experience – my spine and muscles feel so much improved and my head feels clearer. It is the best thing to do for your back as well as your spirit.'

A manual worker said, 'Yoga seems to have strengthened my back. It certainly brings a lot of temporary relief from tension. But if not practised regularly and carefully, I believe it is possible to harm the spine with "over-enthusiastic" yoga.'

In summary, an extraordinarily high percentage of survey participants who practise yoga get good results in the long run. However, individualized, modified yoga instruction is the key to success, since many regular yoga positions can lead to injury. Modified yoga therapy helped back sufferers with osteoarthritis, neck pain and scoliosis. (See Chapters 12–14.)

Yoga therapy survey	US survey	UK survey
Number of people treated	45	226
Responses	%	%
Provided dramatic long-term help	51	16
Provided moderate long-term help	42	21
Provided temporary help	3	37
Ineffective	0	16
Made patient feel worse	4	10

How to Get the Most Benefit from Yoga

A few survey participants learned yoga entirely on their own. But those who were helped the most got started with professional and personalized instruction.

If there is a yoga class near you, it is best to drop by and discuss your needs with an instructor. The importance of the yoga instructor's willingness to modify the therapy cannot be emphasized enough. At least two generally accepted forms of yoga therapy for back sufferers could actually cause further injury if you try them while you are in pain or before you have the necessary flexibility. One is the Cobra, in which you lie on your stomach and arch your back by raising your head and chest. The other is the Plough, where you lie on your back and raise your straightened legs up and over your body and head, until your toes touch down behind your head.

However, if you are able to do regular back exercises, and seem to have progressed as far as you can with them, yoga is an excellent way to further both your physical and emotional well-being.

If professional yoga instruction is not available to you, here are some exercises you can try on your own:

1. *Relaxation position.* This deceptively simple procedure tells you as much about the meditative yoga philosophy as does any yoga exercise. Lie on your back with a pillow under your knees. Keep your arms at your sides and your legs slightly apart. Let your body go limp, with neck, arms and legs allowed to shift naturally into the most comfortable position possible. Now think about muscle relaxation. Start with your feet, ankles and legs. Concentrate on making the individual muscles and joints relax. Work your way up your body to your

neck and head. Take a few minutes to do this. When you are finished, your concentration and energy will be directed towards the exercises to come.

2. *Stretching your spine from a sitting position*. Sit on the floor with your legs fully extended and your ankles touching each other. Raise your arms in front of you. Now slowly lower your upper body as far as you can while also lowering your hands to your knees. When you feel resistance, hold this position for a count of ten. Start with three repetitions and increase by one repetition every other day until you reach ten.

3. *Flexibility twist*. Stand with your feet close together. Raise your arms to shoulder level, keeping the elbows straight, and touch your hands together. Slowly turn your upper body to the left. When you meet resistance, hold for ten seconds. Return to the starting position. Drop your arms and relax for a few seconds. Perform the same movement to your right. Start with three repetitions and increase by one repetition every other day until you reach ten.

4. *Modified Locust*. Lie face down with a pillow tucked under your abdomen. Keeping your knees straight, raise one leg about a foot off the floor. Hold for a count of six, then lower the leg slowly to the floor. Do the same procedure with the other leg. Start with three repetitions and increase by one repetition every other day until you reach ten.

5. *Mountain*. Stand up straight with your arms by your sides. Breathe in and out gently and deeply five times.

6. *Extended Mountain*. Stand up straight with your arms by your sides. Then interlace your fingers together and extend your hands up towards the ceiling as you slowly lift your heels off the floor and come up on to your toes. Give yourself time to become balanced, then breathe in and out gently and deeply five times.

Note: None of the above exercises, except the relaxation position, should be done by anyone whose activities or motions are greatly restricted by pain.

Section 4
Categories of Back Pain

Most back pain affects the lower region of the spine. Only 10 per cent of bad backs are caused by a specific disease or problem.

Jill Palmer, medical correspondent, *Daily Mirror*

The severity of backache ranges from minor niggles to excruciating pain but the problem on a whole is remarkably widespread.

Malcolm I.V. Jayson, Professor of Rheumatology, University of Manchester

Very often, episodes of back pain will settle without any need for active treatment by the doctor, but people who have had a serious episode of back pain in their life are likely to suffer from back pain from time to time in the future. A minority of those will have relatively continuous pain.

Helen Parker and Chris J. Main, *Living With Back Pain*

Chapter 6
Your Diagnosis

Lack of diagnostic consistency among practitioners
• Ruling out serious medical conditions • How specialists' biases shape
their diagnoses • How to interpret a tentative diagnosis • Obvious spinal
anomalies may not explain your problem • How to describe your pain to a
practitioner • Diagnostic procedures (examination, X-rays, CT scans,
myelograms, MRI)

In the UK guidelines, the most frequent diagnosis for back pain is 'non-specific low back pain' (it used to be termed 'simple backache' but, as we know, it is far from 'simple!'). The maxim that you can't treat a patient without first knowing exactly what's wrong with him or her doesn't hold up in the field of back care. Most people never find out exactly what's wrong with their backs, and they get well nevertheless.

For example, a 60-year-old construction worker who saw a noted orthopaedic surgeon received a diagnosis of severe osteoarthritis of the lumbar spine – very specific. But after a few weeks of bed rest and exercise therapy, there was no improvement. A lesser-known orthopaedic surgeon then diagnosed the problem as a general weakness of the lower back – not very specific. But the result of his approach to treatment was successful.

If you look back at the introductory explanation 'About Your Back' (p. xvii), you will see that each nerve supplies both muscles and joints in the back. This can make it very difficult to pinpoint the exact cause of pain in different parts of the back, which partly explains why it's often so hard to get a specific diagnosis.

You Need a Diagnosis That Rules Out Serious Medical Conditions
When you're dealing with persistent back pain, it is essential to evaluate underlying medical causes of this pain. The chances are 95 in 100 that nothing of great consequence will be discovered.

But if you have severe or chronic back pain, don't take chances. Any disease or disorder, literally from your head to your toes, can cause back pain. And some two dozen participants in the US survey, about 5 per cent of the total, needlessly suffered back pain for years because no practitioner made a thorough effort to identify the tangible – and treatable – cause. One was a writer whose neck pain caused him great anguish for five years. In all that time, no doctor tried systematically to rule out a tangible cause of his pain. The practitioners he saw talked continually about stress as a major causal factor, until the writer himself wondered whether the pain was 'all in his head', or at least mostly caused by stress. Finally, relatively common diagnostic measures revealed a large but non-malignant tumour. When the tumour was removed, the pain eventually went with it.

A businessman who owned his own company spent years seeing virtually every famous back specialist in the US. As in the writer's case, he was repeatedly told that the problem wasn't physical but that he needed psychological help. Crippled with pain, depressed and obsessed with thoughts about suicide, the patient tried one last specialist. A treatable neuromuscular disorder was discovered. In six months a prescribed drug brought him a 90 per cent recovery. In a year the patient was fully recovered.

Colitis, an inflammation of the colon, turned out to be the cause of back pain for a secretary. She went to a general practitioner for a complete medical examination after years of chiropractic care failed to control her chronic back pain. Appropriate medication quickly solved her problem.

Perhaps the most frustrating story of this kind comes from a publishing executive who was warned by an osteopath that he would have to live in a wheelchair for the rest of his life. A 'crooked spine,' the osteopath said, 'was combining with spondylolisthesis [see Chapter 12] to produce incapacitating and irreversible leg pain and numbness.' But after ten years of agony, the last two of them disabling, the executive saw a chiropractor who diagnosed the problem as short-leg syndrome. The real culprit, again, was the lack of a thorough examination. The chiropractor prescribed a built-up shoe, and the patient was fully recovered in two months.

Finally, another cause of lower back pain, for older men, can be undiagnosed prostate cancer. Alan, a UK participant, wanted others to know this: 'My back pain started about 15 months ago and started to get more and more serious. After three months the GP decided to take a blood test and my PSA [Prostate Specific Antigen] level was almost 60! I was rapidly referred to the local hospital and prostate cancer, which had spread to the spine and other bone areas, was confirmed. I was immediately placed on hormone therapy and the back pain soon disappeared. . . I am bringing this to your attention as I was never aware that lower back pain could be a symptom of prostate cancer and feel that this fact deserves a mention in your book, particularly for the over-sixties who, I believe, should have a PSA test if the pain cannot be related to anything specific. In fact, a PSA test at least once a year for the over-sixties would be desirable. In my case it could have picked up the prostate cancer before it had spread to the bones. I am now 70 and feel very positive with my treatment. Regular massage helps to control "ageing" aches and pains in the back and elsewhere.'

Be Thoroughly Evaluated Once. Then Ignore Diagnostic Jargon and Focus on Getting Well

Some survey participants, after receiving appropriate diagnostic tests (discussed below) and after being bombarded with vague diagnoses that basically said, 'You have pain, but nothing is seriously wrong,' continued making the rounds of practitioners in search of the 'right' diagnosis – one that sounded specific, tangible and curable. Looking back, almost all of them found this to be a tremendous waste of time and money.

You should know that US survey participants who received no diagnosis did just as well in the long run as patients who received one or more diagnoses. This is because a fancy diagnosis for low back pain usually does not have specific treatment implications. For example, an author with low back pain accumulated the following labels: low back syndrome, idiopathic lumbar-sacral radiculopathy, low back derangement, lumbar strain, myositis and myoligamentous lumbar-sacral strain. All of these mean essentially the same thing: low back pain. Moreover, the patient got the best results from the practitioner who called the problem 'low back syndrome'. And the doctor didn't even mention this diagnosis until recovery was well under way and a health-insurance form forced him to give the problem an official name.

How to Know Your Probable Diagnosis Before You Are Examined

As predictably as hairdressers focus on split ends and cobblers look for run-down heels, certain kinds of back practitioners tend to diagnose with tunnel vision. The US survey results demonstrated graphically that the name of your problem may depend on the name of your practitioner's speciality, as follows.

Chiropractic diagnosis

The chances are nine out of ten you'll be told your spine is misaligned. 'Misalignment' is the specific term chiropractors use most often to describe back pain. 'Subluxation' is another, more impressive way of saying misalignment, but it means the same thing. 'Twisted pelvis' is another common way for chiropractors to describe a specific area of an improperly aligned spine. So is 'spinal curvature', indicating either a slight scoliosis (lateral curvature) or increased lordosis (an overly pronounced inward curve in the lower back). Chiropractors also talk in terms of 'pinched nerves' and congenital bone defects such as 'malformed hips'.

There is nothing inappropriate about these diagnoses. On the contrary, it reassures many back sufferers to know that the chiropractor feels something is wrong. Given a choice between having a 'bad back' or a 'subluxation of L4, L5' with a 'twisted pelvis' to boot, many people prefer the latter diagnosis. After all, they are in pain, and they want to know why.

Surgeons

When you see a surgeon, he or she is primarily interested in the question: could these symptoms be helped by an operation? If the answer is no, they will usually discharge you or refer you to another specialist. The two most common diagnoses from orthopaedic surgeons and neurosurgeons are 'low back syndrome' and 'there is nothing really wrong'. Most back sufferers who get a 'nothing really wrong' diagnosis are frustrated by it. But if you know beforehand that this diagnosis from surgeons is very common and that most surgeons are interested only in treating people surgically, you might be relieved instead of frustrated. Look at it positively. At least you have now ruled out certain known conditions and can either treat yourself or get some initial help from a practitioner who is interested in back problems that don't require surgery. And the vast majority of back problems don't require surgery.

General practitioners

The US survey found that most general practitioners and junior doctors tend to come up with a catch-all diagnosis – low back pain or muscle spasms – which usually implies treatment with prescription drugs. Low back pain, for example, is normally treated with painkillers by GPs; while muscle spasms are treated with muscle-relaxant pills.

Sports medicine specialists, physiotherapists and kinesiologists

These practitioners' diagnoses often focus on the muscular status of different parts of the body, e.g., weak abdominal muscles, tight hamstrings and weak lower back muscles. And these diagnoses have specific implications for individualized exercise therapy. However, physiotherapists will also look at joints, soft tissues, nerves, discs, and other anatomical and functional aspects when making a diagnosis.

Acupuncturists and Shiatsu therapists

In the US survey, these two specialists tended to offer no diagnosis at all. One would think this would have frustrated patients, but it didn't because the practitioners seemed so willing to try to help. And their positive attitude gave patients the feeling that they had some diagnosis – and a corresponding course of treatment – in mind. In the UK, acupuncture can sometimes be provided by GPs and physiotherapists. These practitioners would always examine and diagnose the patient first.

Holistic, alternative practitioners

For convenience, this phrase is used to describe practitioners such as holistic massage therapists, naturopaths and Rolfers, and unconventional diagnoses turn out to be the norm for this group. For example, a holistic massage therapist may attribute chronic low back pain to an excess of urea in the blood and a lack of ying energy. Meanwhile, a naturopath may claim that low back pain is due to lethargy caused by a poorly functioning liver and a lack of zinc and magnesium.

And the offbeat diagnostic beat goes on. Posture therapists will point to posture deficiencies. Feldenkrais therapists will find fault with your awareness of how you move. Rolfers will declare that your state of mind and muscles are not in the best shape. Biofeedback therapists will tell you that your life is too stressful, and so on.

The point here is to demonstrate how certain practitioners follow predictable patterns in assessing your condition and framing a diagnosis. Of course, predictability does not make a diagnosis inappropriate or appropriate. Mostly, it means that you can easily end up with more diagnoses than you would care to count, and that in most cases you need not be concerned about what your problem is called. Instead, you should focus on learning (in the following chapters) which treatments are most likely to help you overcome different types of back pain.

Tentative Diagnoses: Take Them with a Pinch of Salt

Some diagnoses are best guesses. They are subject to further diagnostic procedures, or they will be proven or disproven by the passage of time.

Take the case of a journalist who gritted her teeth and put up with many years of back pain until the problem finally overcame her. On the basis of X-rays and a clinical examination, an orthopaedic surgeon told her she had a ruptured disc requiring surgery. (In fact X-rays are usually ineffective in diagnosing a ruptured disc because the discs themselves cannot be seen on conventional X-rays.)

'The diagnosis terrified me,' she recalled. 'In retrospect, I feel that it amounted to a misdiagnosis, since I got well without surgery.'

Whether the diagnosis was incorrect will never be known. What is known, though, is that it was a tentative diagnosis. The pain in the journalist's legs could have been caused by any one of numerous conditions.

Another participant in the US survey, a businessman, had the wits scared out of him by five diagnoses, none of which was based on concrete evidence: ruptured disc, spinal tumour, compressed nerve in low back, deteriorated disc, and Wilson's Disease (a serious and rare neurological disorder).

There is nothing intrinsically wrong with tentative diagnoses. They can simply indicate that your first visit, which usually consists of history-taking, direct examination and X-rays, signals the need for further diagnostic procedures.

So don't panic needlessly about think-aloud diagnoses. They tend to be less accurate than weather forecasts. They can also give you a headache that will make your back pain seem mild in comparison. And they turn diagnosis into a multiple-choice format – 'It could be a disc, a facet joint, some arthritis or a pinched nerve' – often without regard for the patient's feelings.

In fact, the way you are told about a tentative diagnosis can be frightening, even debilitating. It is one thing to say, 'You may have a ruptured disc, Ms Jones.' But it is quite another matter to say, as a handful of doctors in the US survey did before solid evidence was in hand, 'Have an operation now or you'll be pleading for help in a few years.'

Many practitioners don't bother telling patients whether diagnoses are tentative or documented. As a result, the patient may leave the office badly shaken, rather than informed, with a first-hand and unwelcome opportunity to learn about the role of stress in back pain.

What They See May Not Be What You've Got

A renowned physician at a New York medical centre treated Arthur Klein, the author of this book. After examining Arthur thoroughly, he asked whether his back had been X-rayed recently. It hadn't. The doctor thought for a few seconds and, reasonably certain that the problem was muscular in nature, said, 'Let's skip the X-rays. Even if we find a slight abnormality, we still won't know if it is the cause of your back pain.'

This doctor's decision turned out to be sound. And his thinking makes an important point about diagnosis – namely, what your practitioner sees may have nothing to do with your problem. Take the case of the fast-food franchise manager who had low back pain for the first time at the age of 45. An X-ray showed that two of his lumbar vertebrae were fused and apparently had been so since birth. The practitioner attributed the pain to this congenital fusion. But the vertebrae had been fused for 45 years without causing back pain. Furthermore, the patient's pain vanished in a few weeks while the fused vertebrae, of course, did not. So there's no way of telling whether the malformation had anything to do with the episodes of back pain.

There are probably millions of people with visible conditions – mild scoliosis, lordosis, some osteoarthritis and congenital malformations – who don't have back pain. There are also millions of people with these problems who do have back pain. And millions of people suffer terribly despite the absence of any obvious abnormality on which to blame the pain. So remember that your spinal curve or malformed vertebra may have nothing to with any given bout of back pain.

Here are some more examples:

A book-keeper with low back pain saw three specialists, two of whom attributed the pain to a curvature in her upper back (scoliosis). The third practitioner agreed that there was a curvature but commented, 'It is ludicrous to think that this mild a curvature could be the major cause of your problem.' The patient's treatment and recovery had nothing to do with trying to correct, counter or even consider her spinal curvature.

A farmer was told by one back specialist that his sciatica had been caused by a congenital hip malformation. Another specialist noted the malformation but didn't think it was congenital or worth worrying about. The farmer recovered by devising his own treatment plan.

A 73-year-old retired hospital administrator was told that an extra lumbar vertebra was causing an unstable back with resultant low back pain. The patient asked her doctor why a structural oddity should suddenly be giving her trouble. There was no answer. There is no answer.

The moral: once you have a diagnosis that rules out serious structural abnormalities, you can probably afford to ignore the little curves and various oddities that practitioners like to point to as maybe, could-be, might-well-be reasons for back pain.

Diagnostic Procedures

The First Step: Describing Your Pain

The overwhelming majority of US survey participants felt that the quality of their dialogue with practitioners was more important in diagnosing a problem than any clinical or technical procedure. Why? Pain can't be seen, and its intensity cannot be measured. It has to be described, and you're the only one who can do it.

With this point in mind, here are suggestions from participants for making your examination more productive:

- If you've already seen several practitioners, or if your problem has lasted a long time, mention this in advance to the practitioner's receptionist, and request an appointment time that is either longer than usual or held during non-rush hours.
- Write a short chronology of your condition. This one-page report – at the most – isn't meant to take the place of your verbal explanation, but it will help you organize your thinking. And good practitioners appreciate a concisely written history.
- If a written report seems presumptuous to you, or if it's just not your style, consider making some notes for your own use.
- When you're in pain and in need of help, it's difficult to feel that you should examine the practitioner as carefully as you hope he will examine you, but try. The success or failure of treatment often hinges on your rapport with the practitioner. Trust your instincts. If you don't have a good feeling about the practitioner, no matter how esteemed his reputation, don't proceed with treatment or even with an examination. (Naturally, if you're in acute pain, you will want to get whatever immediate relief you can.)

In *Oh, My Aching Back*, a bestselling book by Dr Leon Root, the author states: 'The inability of most patients to clearly explain what bothers them is a long-standing source of grievance to modern doctors.'

Ironically, participants in the US survey had just the opposite complaint. In effect, 'Modern doctors don't listen well, don't believe that you can contribute anything intelligent, and seem put off if you can.' This situation may now be improving, as more doctors are being trained to listen to their patients. However, many practitioners are under pressure to deal with each patient within a limited time, and this may sometimes lead them to appear rather brusque and impatient. Don't be put off by this. Just give them the relevant information about your back pain, and quietly and firmly ask the questions you need to ask.

The Diagnostic Examination

Observation is the first part of examination. That is, the competent practitioner will look at your posture, gait and other movements from the moment you walk into view, as well as while taking your history and examining you. Then you will probably be asked to walk a bit, bend over gently from the waist, and bend to each side. Pain and lack of mobility, if any, will be noted. So will alterations in the movement patterns, tremors, lurching or inability to perform normal movements.

While you're lying face down on the examination table, the practitioner will perform a hands-on examination. They will palpate (lightly tap) your back to determine the extent of spasming. He or she will also probe your back, hips and buttocks to check for tightness, 'knotted' muscles, trigger points (small, extremely sensitive areas that are painful to the touch), and areas of referred pain. If lying on your stomach causes you pain, ask if you can lie on your side, or tuck a small pillow under your abdomen.

While you're on your back, the practitioner will raise each of your legs. Sharp pain felt during this procedure, as opposed to the slight pulling sensation of a tight hamstring, may indicate a ruptured disc. (It also tests the dynamics of your nervous system, known as neurodynamics or neuromechanosensitivity.)

You will also be asked to bring both knees towards your chest simultaneously. If you have a plain old backache, you'll feel pulling and tightness in your lower back. If you have a ruptured disc, you may find this to be a relatively pain-free position. Your reflexes and neurological reactions will be checked with a small rubber hammer. Lack of appropriate knee-jerk response may indicate involvement of the nerve root. The same holds true if you show an abnormal reflex when tested in your Achilles tendon area.

The chances are about nine out of ten that the findings in your examination will be negative. From your viewpoint, however, the medical word 'negative' means 'positive' – no serious disease, neurological impairment or structural abnormality.

X-rays: Their Value and Shortcomings

If you see an orthopaedic surgeon or chiropractor, you'll probably be advised to have one or more pictures taken of your back. Actually, 'advised' isn't the right word. 'Told' is more accurate. You usually don't have a choice unless you forego the examination altogether or see a back doctor who uses X-rays sparingly, or see a practitioner who isn't allowed to take X-rays, such as a Shiatsu therapist or a non-medically qualified acupuncturist.

X-rays usually don't reveal much about back pain. What can you expect X-rays to tell you about your back pain? Chances are . . . nothing at all. But some important conditions can be seen this way. Osteoarthritis, for example, shows up on X-rays. X-rays are also crucial for ruling out possible fractures.

Then there are the congenital 'spondy' conditions, as confusing as they are hard to pronounce. Spondylolysis involves incompletely formed vertebrae. If you have spondylolysis, it can evolve into spondylolisthesis, a forward shift of one of the vertebrae, causing low back pain.

Spina bifida, an opening in the spine that can be serious enough at birth to cause paralysis below the lesion, is fairly common in a very mild form that seldom accounts for back pain. X-rays will show that a portion of the spinal column failed to develop – a condition called spina bifida occulta – in perhaps 20 per cent of the population. But it is just an X-ray finding, and no one knows how this painless anomaly is related to the full-blown spina bifida, if at all.

The risks versus the benefits of X-rays

Keep these points in mind when deciding whether to have your back X-rayed:

- Fewer than 5 per cent of survey participants who were X-rayed by medical doctors learned the cause of their back pain from these X-rays.
- X-rays neither spot nor rule out many serious conditions because they do not clearly show soft tissues, such as muscles,

tendons, ligaments, discs, nerves and cartilage. For example, ruptured discs are undetectable on X-rays, and some spinal tumours are very hard to see.

- A safe level of radiation has been established – only to change time and time again as new evidence reveals new dangers. For example, when X-rays were first used, it was common to treat a strep throat with them. Years later, the treatment was found to have caused cancer. In the UK, the Royal College of Radiologists has issued guidelines about which types of X-rays are the most helpful for particular problems. Doctors use these guidelines, along with the results of clinical examination and the patient history, to decide whether or not an X-ray or scan is likely to help find a specific cause for the pain. Doctors are anxious not to expose people to high levels of radiation unnecessarily. (For example, a CT scan exposes the patient to the equivalent of the radiation in 500 chest X-rays.) For this reason, they need to be sure that the exposure will be justified by the potential benefit. X-rays of the spine are mainly used when the patient has had an accident, to check that there is no fracture or dislocation. They can also be helpful when symptoms, including pain, suggest that there could be an infection or inflammation. In addition, X-rays can show congenital bone abnormalities and changes in bone size and shape related to ageing, arthritis and osteoarthritis. They are not advised for academic purposes – they should only be used if they will change the treatment offered.

- Two of the most common causes of back pain – muscle strain and disc problems – are not visible on X-rays. A third cause of back pain – worn facet joints (the small joints that enable your movable vertebrae to function) – seldom show up clearly enough on conventional X-rays to determine the extent of wear.

In conclusion, unless a practitioner is looking for a specific abnormality or disease – as opposed to taking an X-ray 'just as a precaution' or 'just to have a look' – you probably won't gain anything in the process.

Don't get caught up in the doctor/chiropractor debate about X-rays. If you see a medical doctor and then go to a chiropractor, the chiropractor will reject the doctor's X-rays and insist on taking his own. The reverse is also true. Get X-rays from a chiropractor, take them (if you dare) to an orthopaedic surgeon, and 'I'd like to take some X-rays' is what you're likely to hear. To put it mildly, doctors and chiropractors disagree about how to take X-rays and how to interpret them.

According to US survey participants, most chiropractors take X-rays while you're standing up; they feel it's pointless to 'shoot' you when you're lying down, since most people don't feel pain when they're reclining. Doctors, on the other hand, complain that chiropractors take single pictures of small areas of the spine – too small to provide the necessary information.

In reading X-rays, a doctor will tell you there is no structural malformation, while a chiropractor will see malformation in misaligned vertebrae. Neither believes the other's judgement or accepts the other's interpretation.

Finally, if you do have X-rays taken, insist that a lead shield be placed over your reproductive organs. This should be done routinely, but it isn't always.

CT Scanner: More 'All-Seeing'

The CT (computerized tomography) scan, also known as a CAT (computer assisted tomography) scan, has been widely hailed as a landmark technological breakthrough in diagnosis. When used for back diagnosis, this scan can detect just about everything a practitioner might be looking for – ruptured disc, degenerative bone diseases, tumours, narrowing of the spine and a host of other problems.

CT is vastly more sophisticated and all-seeing than X-ray technology. The patient lies inside the CT scanner, and radiation is beamed from several directions at once to produce a composite image. The computer part of the equipment analyses the numerous views, combining them into a series of highly detailed pictures. Unlike X-ray images, a CT scan shows soft tissue as well as bone. But like standard X-ray procedures, CT scans involve appreciable levels of radiation exposure.

But not even a CT scan can show every possible view of the back, thereby leaving the way open for oversight and misdiagnosis. And even in cases where a CT scan helps diagnose a ruptured disc, patients about to enter surgery must undergo further test procedures to pinpoint the location of the protruding gel.

Because a CT scanner is costly to own and maintain, the machines tend to be clustered at major medical centres, and appointment time is limited. US survey participants reported waiting up to eight weeks for a CT scan. They also said that unless their problem was deemed 'serious' enough, their request to have a CT scan was turned down.

Myelography: What Doctors Don't Tell You

Myelography is not commonly used in the UK. However, the word 'myelogram' sends chills up and down the spines of many US back sufferers whose doctors recommend the procedure. A myelogram involves placing the patient on a tilting table and injecting a solution opaque to X-rays into the spinal column. Tilting the table disperses the injected dye throughout the spinal column. X-rays are then taken. The dye enables abnormal shapes – such as a ruptured disc or a narrowing of the spine – to show up.

About fifty participants in the US survey had one or more myelograms. Highlights of their experiences follow.

Two survey participants reported permanent harm caused by a severe inflammation of the spinal cord from an allergic reaction to the oil-based myelography solution, Pantopaque. This chronic condition, called arachnoiditis, results when drops of Pantopaque remain in the spine. Arachnoiditis is often more disabling than whatever was causing pain in the first place.

Pantopaque has long been banned in Sweden and other countries. It has been replaced in most American hospitals by water-based solutions. A water-based myelography solution can be put into the spine with a smaller needle, so there's less discomfort at the outset. It does not cause chronic inflammation, and it does not have to be removed after use. But remember, any procedure that entails inserting or withdrawing fluid from the spine can bring on severe headaches.

Ten survey participants got violent headaches after myelograms. Some back doctors mentioned the possibility of myelography-caused headaches to patients, but the duration and intensity of the pain was often glossed over. Three participants reported post-myelography headaches lasting from three to six months. About 20 per cent of patients receiving myelograms got severe headaches lasting from 24 to 48 hours.

Doctors seldom mention the possibility of injury or increased back pain from myelography. If it is mentioned, the implication is that patients who claim they were hurt by myelography are hypochondriacs or malingerers. But survey participants believe that the risks are very real, and numerous articles in medical journals seem to substantiate their claims.

'I ended up extending my hospital stay for five days due to a spinal leak from the myelogram,' said a nurse who had previously seen the same problem occur with her own patients.

'On one of three myelograms,' recalled a housing administrator, 'the nerves to my left leg were touched – oh boy! There was pain for months.'

Said a service station owner, 'The myelogram was pure hell at the time and for months afterwards.'

An editor remarked, 'They would have to catch me for another myelogram. I suffered years of pain and discomfort from it.'

You will seldom read about the extent to which myelography fails to pinpoint ruptured discs and other malformations. The percentage of diagnoses that myelograms miss is anyone's guess. According to one survey participant, a tree surgeon, 'The medical people said I had all the symptoms of a ruptured disc, but a myelogram couldn't prove it. I was told that myelograms are 80 to 85 per cent effective and that I had fallen into the 15 to 20 per cent crack.' And according to the Manual of Acute Orthopaedic Therapeutics, interpreting myelograms is 'fraught with the possibility of technical errors.'

MRI Scans: The First-Choice Test

With a combination of magnetic force and radio signals, MRI (magnetic resonance imaging) sees soft tissues – discs, muscles and ligaments – better than any existing technology. A computer collects and interprets radio signals from the body, displaying on its screen a composite image of structure and function in the examined part.

There is no pain associated with the procedure and no risk of radiation. For these reasons, MRI scans are by far the best option for investigating spinal cord and chronic spinal pain problems. Unfortunately in the UK patients often have to wait a considerable length of time for an MRI scan.

Now You Be the Diagnostician. Then Let's Move on to Getting Rid of Your Pain

At this point I hope you are clearer about the whole confusing saga of diagnosing back problems. But even if you're just clearly confused, don't worry. Pain may be invisible. But you know where you hurt. Even if you don't have a concrete diagnosis . . . even if you don't believe the one that you have . . . even if you don't know which of several diagnoses is the 'right' one . . . you do know your own symptoms and, therefore, you can 'categorize' your own pain, as long as serious medical conditions have been ruled out as the cause of this pain.

The sole aim of the rest of this book, then, is to guide you to what other back sufferers report works for specific categories of back pain. These categories – low back, ruptured and degenerative disc, sciatica, osteoarthritis, neck, scoliosis, spondylolisthesis – cover the kinds of back problems that were mentioned most frequently by survey participants. Four categories – ruptured disc, osteoarthritis, scoliosis, and spondylolisthesis – were chosen for their obvious specificity. The remaining three categories – low back, neck and sciatica – reflect how back sufferers themselves describe pain when back practitioners cannot agree on its cause.

If your back pain falls into more than one category, you'll find more than one chapter of value. If you suffer from low back pain and sciatica, for example, both those chapters should help you.

This much is certain. Whether you need professional help right now as part of your long-term, back-care programme – or whether you need immediately applicable self-treatment techniques – you will have the benefit of other back sufferers' experience in eliminating or easing virtually every kind of back pain.

Chapter 7
How to Be Your Own Low Back Doctor for Acute, Severe Pain

Eight myths about low back pain – debunked • The best mattress • How to get in and out of bed • The right position for lying in bed • How to ease pain • Techniques for stress reduction • Diet • Preparation for exercise • Posture • Avoiding re-injury

Low back pain is not considered a disease. It is called by dozens of names, from old-fashioned lumbago to the fashionable facet joint syndrome, from misalignment to lumbar-sacral radiculopathy, from muscle strain to just plain low back pain.

No one knows for sure why people suffer from low back pain. Only colds and sore throats top it as reasons for seeking medical attention. According to a national survey carried out in 2000, almost half the adult population of the UK had experienced low back pain lasting at least 24 hours at some time during the year. In 2003/04, nearly 5 million working days were lost in the UK through bad backs. Yet there is no national research foundation worrying or wondering about it. It is, in short, the UK's biggest and most baffling pain. *And it can be controlled or greatly reduced.*

You've no doubt heard that before. And you probably wouldn't be reading this book if the promise of this or that 'X Minutes a Day Surefire Formula for Eliminating Back Pain Forever' programme had come true. But the advice offered here is of a different sort, based on the actual experience of US and UK survey participants with low back pain. They know all too well that no pill or potion, movement or motion is usually the single key to ending your troubles; that some little-known, self-help healing approaches work wonders; that an array of widely publicized treatments are ineffective and dangerous; that you can't necessarily end your back pain by yourself overnight. Many of you will make remarkable strides in just days or weeks, but not everyone can. If you are a chronic back sufferer, it may take months to recover, but it can be done. Some of you may also need professional treatment and advice at first. And knowing when and how to get professional help is an essential but often overlooked aspect of self-care.

This chapter will teach you how to become your own low back doctor. About 80 per cent of US survey participants with low back pain have either eliminated pain completely or have reduced it enough so that it no longer seriously limits their lives. And we believe that what they know can help even the most disabled low back sufferers. Certainly, they can help you discover what steps you should take right now to keep your own back in good shape for years to come.

Eight Myths about Low Back Pain – Debunked

So much misinformation plagues people with low back pain that it seems sensible to begin this chapter with facts, all based on the US survey results, that dispel some well-established but unfounded myths.

1. Myth: You must know exactly what is wrong with your lower back in order to have a good chance of resolving the problem.
   Fact: If you're in generally good health, an exact diagnosis is usually as meaningless as it is difficult to attain. What is meaningful is the nature of the treatment, not the terminology of the diagnosis.
2. Myth: Back specialists agree about what causes low back pain.
   Fact: There is little agreement. People with bad posture, weak abdominal muscles and unmanageable stress get low back pain. But so do people with correct posture, strong abdominal muscles and well-handled stress. All that's known is that some treatments and approaches work extremely well, while others are grossly over-rated.
3. Myth: Most patients are too lazy to do back exercises even if they are prescribed by their practitioners.
   Fact: Nearly three-quarters of low back sufferers in the US survey report doing back exercises regularly (at least four times

a week), and most of these individuals exercise daily, even though their practitioners did not prescribe an exercise regime.

4. Myth: Any good-quality book, article or instruction sheet from a doctor can teach you what you need to know about exercise therapy.

   Fact: People with chronic, activity-limiting back pain recover more fully after receiving instructions and individualized attention from exercise experts. (The best of these experts are mentioned in this chapter and fully described in Chapters 3 and 4.)

5. Myth: If you need professional care, choose either an orthopaedic surgeon or a chiropractor.

   Fact: Neither orthopaedic surgeons nor chiropractors were rated tops for low back pain by the back sufferers in the US survey.

6. Myth: Most people solve their low back problems with the help of medical doctors.

   Fact: Most people start their treatment with medical doctors but complete it with a non-physician practitioner – many of whom have more training than doctors in musculoskeletal disorders and exercise therapy.

7. Myth: The most widely used treatments for low back pain are always the most effective treatments.

   Fact: Some extremely popular treatments, including prescription drugs, have little value for many back sufferers – and may have the potential for harm.

8. Myth: Eighty per cent of back sufferers recover within two months without any treatment.

   Fact: This figure – which appears in many books and articles on back pain – is misleading. The key is the word 'recover'. The truth is that 80 per cent of back sufferers do get back on their feet within a matter of weeks. But the quality of their recovery is too often incomplete and temporary. Most of them continue to have episodes of recurrent back pain in the months and years that follow. What's more, 'within two months' is a long time if you are the one who has to endure those weeks or months of pain, or if you lose your job during that time. In the UK, in the course of a year, around 3.5 million people experience back pain for the first time and for 3.1 million of those people their pain lasts throughout the whole year. By this time, many have stopped seeking health-care and are in control of their symptoms themselves.

How to Relieve Acute, Severe Low Back Pain

Important: The remainder of this chapter is devoted to those of you who recently have been incapacitated with low back pain. However, it is also valuable if your activities have been severely limited for a long time. If your pain is chronic, but you can function in most ways, you may want to skip to the next chapter.

Sometimes it happens out of the blue:

'While shaving one day, I bent over the sink and experienced a stabbing pain between my hips,' said a lawyer. 'It took me 10 minutes to get from the bathroom to the bedroom, which was only about 20 feet away.'

A garden centre worker had a similar tale: 'I was lifting a small plant. My back wasn't properly lined up, as I was bending over at the hips. I suffered a muscle strain so severe that I could not sit or stand and had to actually crawl into the doctor's office.'

Sometimes it happens after days or weeks of warning signs:

'I had been packing and lifting cartons for two weeks in preparation for moving,' a pizza restaurant owner reported. 'My back felt like hell, but then it had always been a bother. I was a little worried about it, but I figured, "I can stand the pain. It's just the price you have to pay." Besides, I was doing my back exercises. Then one morning I woke up and couldn't believe the pain. There was no way I could move. I could barely breathe, the pain was so intense. It took me almost an hour to get out of bed.'

'Back pain was nothing new to me,' a sales representative said, 'but if you had told me I could have been out of work for six weeks with it, and not even have something like a ruptured disc, I would have laughed. After putting in a lot of overtime, though, and gritting my teeth about the pain all that time, I got up from my chair, reached for my attaché case to leave for home, and wound up being taken to the hospital in an ambulance.'

How to Get Rid of the Pain

Here are some of the most frequently asked questions, followed by answers from back sufferers who recovered quickly and learned how to prevent relapses of low back pain.

Q: Should I Seek Professional Help?

A: When your back is really hurting so badly that you can't move, you're bound to want to ask your doctor or a back specialist for help. But when your muscles go into spasm and contract to a point that you can barely move, the effort required to get to a practitioner's office usually offsets the value of any treatment. The car journey, the wait to see the doctor, the need to stand or sit for a long time – can all make matters worse. In short, your severely contracted muscles are telling you to stay put. (The pain is usually eased in the short term by lying down flat and then getting up and walking around. Try to avoid prolonged periods of sitting.)

If you are in more pain than you can stand, or if there is any chance that you have a serious medical condition, then you need professional help. But you should try to have your practitioner make a house call.

This is easier said than done, but your GP may be prepared to come to your home, especially if he or she has treated you before. And some cities and towns have an emergency service, listed in the telephone directory, specifically designed for people in your situation.

If you want to increase the odds of a bedside visit, survey participants suggest that you *don't* say, 'I'm in too much pain to move,' even though that may be the case. Drastic descriptions may land you in a hospital accident and emergency department, which can be a disastrous place for a back sufferer. Instead, say something like, 'I seem to have a bad case of muscle strain. But when I try to get up the pain gets worse.'

Q: What Kind of Mattress is Best?

A: Most survey participants use a firm mattress with a 2 cm (¾ inch) plywood bed board between it and the box spring. But many of those who expressed the most enthusiasm about their sleeping arrangements suggest omitting the box spring and putting an extra-firm mattress on a platform bed.

If you have the option, don't use a brand-name mattress. Instead, have a foam-rubber company make you a 15 cm (6 inch) thick, extra-firm mattress. It's less expensive than purportedly corrective mattresses and at least as firm and comfortable.

Futon mattresses on platforms are the next choice of US survey participants. But if your hips, buttocks or thighs are painful, you will probably find the futon too thin and hard, and the cause of unwelcome pressure.

If your bed is too hard (as may be the case with some 'orthopaedic beds'), try placing a duvet between the under-sheet and the mattress. This gives a softer surface, especially for a more petite sleeper. Remember that what feels firm to someone of 50 kg (8 stone) is very different to what feels firm to someone of 115 kg (18 stone).

Of the 15 US survey participants who turned hopefully to water beds, 8 switched back to firm mattresses and bed boards, complaining that the bed couldn't be made hard enough to suit them. They also said that the water produced a 'rolling action' that made it difficult for them to control their movements and positions. (However, this has become less of a problem with more recent advances in water-bed technology.) The other 7 were happy with their water beds so long as the mattresses were kept 'filled to the top' and 'firm'. They said the water enabled the spine to align more comfortably, and that the floating sensation eased the pressure on the spine and muscles. You can also regulate the temperature of water beds, which can be an advantage.

Some back sufferers give up mattresses altogether and take to the floor when their back pain flares up. But lying on the floor is not recommended for incapacitating pain and muscle spasm, primarily because getting up from and down to the floor may add to your pain. Also, if your low back pain is accompanied by pain and spasming in the hips and upper legs, even a carpeted floor can put too much pressure on inflamed and sensitive areas, causing more pain and spasm. If, however, you find yourself stuck between a hard floor and a sagging mattress, take the floor until you can make other arrangements.

Q: What Is the Best Way to Get in and out of Bed?

A: The stoop-and-roll technique works best, even when you can barely move:

Stand with your back to your bed, close enough so that the backs of your legs touch it. Look straight ahead, pull in your abdominal muscles, keep your back straight, and sit. (Don't twist around to see where you will land.) Then, in one easy, fluid motion, using your arms and hands to help support and guide you, roll onto your side and swing both legs onto the bed.

Never flop backwards onto the mattress from a sitting position. Also, never leave your legs dangling off the bed, as that position is guaranteed to make your back arch painfully.

To get up, reverse the process: ease your way over to the edge of the bed, remaining on your side with your knees bent. If you're lying on your right side, place your left palm on the mattress next to your right shoulder. Then, in one easy motion, push down on your left palm, swing yourself into an upright position, bring your legs off the bed, and put your feet flat on the floor. Now keep your back straight and stand up, pushing off with your hands if that makes it easier for you.

One way to help yourself when getting in and out of bed is to reduce the distance you have to stoop or rise by raising your mattress to a height of 75 cm (2 feet 6 inches) from the usual 60 cm (2 feet). An admittedly expensive way to do this is to buy an old-fashioned poster bed, as most are 15 to 25 cm (6-to-10 inches) higher than modern beds. Other ways to give yourself a lift: replace the detachable legs of a low, modern bed with taller legs, or have a taller platform bed designed for you. Then, when you feel well enough to do household tasks again, the extra height will facilitate making the bed each day and changing sheets.

Q: How Long Should I Stay in Bed?
A: In the past, doctors used to advise patients to rest until the pain eased. However, it is now known that this advice was not helpful. You are more likely to develop chronic (persistent) back pain if you stay in bed for more than a few hours. Here is a rule of thumb for you to follow: just as soon as you can move around in bed without severe pain, former back sufferers suggest, try walking for a few minutes. You'll feel achy, but if there's no substantial increase in pain, you're on your way. Carry out your normal activities as far as possible. You may not be able to do this at first if the pain is severe. However, you should try to get back into normal activities as soon as you can. As a rule, it's best not to do anything that causes a lot of pain. Gradual increments

are the key. The next time you're up, don't walk until you drop. If you do too much right away, you risk a serious setback. However, you will have to accept some degree of discomfort when you are trying to keep active. Try setting a new goal each day. For example, you could try walking around the house on one day, a walk to the shops the next, and so on.

Here is a brief case history showing how one back sufferer dealt with the difficult question 'How long should I stay in bed?'

A piano tuner awoke one morning barely able to move. The episode was like many he had experienced in the past. It took him 15 minutes to get out of bed. A hot shower loosened up his back enough to keep him going. From experience, he knew that lying in bed, or remaining motionless for long, would just make him worse. And he was right. He made it through the day and his pain was gone in a week.

Q: Is There a 'Right' Position to Assume while Lying in Bed?

A: Yes, because you can take the strain off your back by lying correctly. Lie on your side and keep your knees bent. Put a small pillow under your head. The pillow should be just plump enough to keep your head and neck level with the rest of your spine. Put another firm pillow between your legs so that it holds apart your knees and your feet.

You should not lie absolutely still. When your muscles are contracted and spasming, even a little movement can help you maintain some flexibility. For example, you can slowly and gently straighten out your legs and return them to a flexed position. Move your arms and torso a bit. Shrug your shoulders. Virtually any kind of shifting around, no matter how slight, can make you feel a little better.

It's also a good idea to change position as you need to. The most basic way to change your position – and ease tightness and pressure – is to shift from one side to the other. To do this, keep your knees bent, roll slowly onto your back, and then roll onto your other side. Also, try lying on your back with a small pillow under your neck (but not under your shoulders) and two or three big pillows under your knees. The majority of acutely incapacitated low back sufferers are more comfortable in the side position, and if they have one-sided leg pain it is usually preferable to lie on their side with that leg uppermost.

Don't try to sit up in bed to read or prop yourself up on an elbow to eat or drink. And don't lie on your stomach. If you must do so for an examination, tuck a folded pillow under your abdomen.

Q: What Can I Do to Speed Up My Recovery from Acute Back Pain?

A:
Use ice
You can reduce the severity of muscle spasms by repeatedly icing the affected areas during the first 48 hours. Your best bet is to fill a plastic freezer bag with ice cubes, wrap it in a damp tea towel, and apply it to your lower back for 10 to 15 minutes every 2 to 4 hours. If your hips, buttocks and upper legs hurt, use ice on these areas, too. If it's awkward to hold the ice bag in place, you can affix it with masking or surgical tape or a tubigrip bandage. However, you should never lie on an ice pack, as it could cause an ice burn. (See pp. 76–8 for more details about using cold therapy safely.)

Try acupressure
You can reduce spasming by giving yourself Shiatsu (acupressure) treatments. You can also combine Shiatsu with ice, as follows:

Apply cold anywhere that hurts, from your lower back to your knees, for 5 minutes. Next, apply pressure to these same places with the ball of your thumb (if you can reach), using small circular motions for about 10 seconds on each spot. Then re-apply ice for 5 minutes more.

Apply heat
About 48 hours after the onset of pain, try using heat to relax your muscles and facilitate healing through increased blood flow. If you have spasming after heat treatments, apply ice to the painful spots. (Some people find that ice continues to soothe them

more effectively than heat long after pain begins. If your body responds better to cold than to heat, stick with the ice pack.)

Hot baths, hot showers, hot water bottles and heat pads were all considered very effective by survey participants, for short-term relief of pain. Rosemary, a UK respondent, made the following comment: 'I find showering rather than bathing is better. I get more backache getting out of a bath and from cleaning it after use. I also find the continued hot water in a shower more beneficial than a warm bath cooling as you sit in it.'

Have a good massage

This is another drug-free muscle relaxant that will help your muscles unwind. A professional massage is best. But even a partner with little experience can raise your spirits and possibly rub away some tightness. Have your partner use a light oil and a fairly light touch. Too much pressure on your lower back could make matters worse at this point. Your partner should concentrate on three areas – your legs, back and neck – massaging towards the heart, using either a long, continuous, gliding motion with the palms or a circular motion with the fingertips and palms.

Q: How Can I Reduce the Stress of Being in Pain?

A: There is no question that back pain causes stress. And this stress, in turn, can magnify your pain. To minimize and control the effect of the stress-pain cycle, try some of the following stress-reduction approaches suggested by US survey participants:

Do deep breathing exercises for a few minutes each hour. Inhale through your nose for 6 seconds; hold your breath for 1 second; exhale through your mouth for 7 seconds. Keep your eyes closed, and expect to feel more relaxed each time you exhale.

Visualize a state of relaxation and well-being. Once or twice a day, when you know you're not going to be interrupted (many survey participants suggest that you unplug your phone or take it off the hook), try to give yourself a vacation from pain. Concentrate on the thought that the pain is diminishing and leaving your body. Start with your forehead and facial muscles. Tighten them. Then let them relax completely. Using this same procedure, work your way down, relaxing your neck, shoulders, arms, chest, abdomen, pelvic area, legs and feet. Now work on your back. Picture it relaxing, starting from the shoulder blades and working down. As an aid, some survey participants visualized a ray of sunlight touching each area that they wanted to relax. Others imagined a silky fabric or soft breeze helping each area to unwind and become pain-free.

Meditate, letting your mind go blank until you're unaware of pain or any thought or feeling. Laugh. Find something to make you laugh or smile. Read a funny book, watch a comedy on TV, rent a DVD or two, and watch films that take your mind off your troubles and put you in an upbeat mood. Listen to music that relaxes you.

Pray. Believe that your pain is easing and that you are on the road to recovery.

Q: Must I Adjust My Diet while I'm Recuperating?

A: According to US survey participants, the biggest risk you face from poor eating habits while inactive is constipation. Just being less active can, and often does, cause constipation, which in turn makes some people's back pain considerably worse.

To help avoid constipation, you need to drink plenty of water. And make sure you get enough fibre and roughage by eating a variety of wholegrain foods, raw fruit and raw vegetables.

Of course, what you eat and how much you eat affect your weight, and many back specialists believe that excess weight can sometimes contribute to back pain. According to survey participants, however, weight is often not a critical factor in back pain. Of the eighteen people in the US survey who dieted as part of their total programme of back care, none felt that weight loss was nearly as important in reducing back pain as other factors mentioned in this chapter. Obviously, to be grossly overweight is to beg for a variety of medical problems. But weight loss alone is probably not a major factor in alleviating back pain.

Q: When Can I Start to Exercise and What Exercises Should I Do?

A: As soon as your contracted muscles have eased enough for you to move around in bed and be up and about for even a few minutes, you can try some of the pre-exercise 'positions' that survey participants found especially useful. They are small but meaningful steps that you can take even before your pain has lessened enough to allow you to exercise. In a week or two, when you have mastered these positions, you will be ready to attempt the exercises in the next chapter.

Position 1: Basic exercise position

From the foetal position, with both knees bent, simply roll onto your back. Position your feet flat on the mattress, with your heels about 15–45 cm (6–18 inches) from your buttocks.

If you have been in severe pain, and the muscles and ligaments in your lower back have contracted, holding this position for a few minutes will set the stage for correcting the exaggerated 'S' curve in your lower back, called swayback or lordosis, that contributes to back pain.

Keep your arms at your sides when you're in this position. But, for just a moment, to appreciate your ultimate goal, slip one hand, palm down, between the small of your back and your mattress. Then do it again after you've been in this position for a few minutes. The curve in your lower back should now be a trifle flatter just from the pull of gravity.

If you can lie in this position comfortably for 5 minutes, try Position 2 later in the day or the next morning.

Position 2: Basic position with pelvic lift

Assume Position 1, but this time use a towel under your buttocks to raise your pelvis slightly, thereby flattening your lumbar curve a bit more.

Fold a bath towel once and slide 2.5 cm (1 inch) of the folded towel under the edge of your buttocks, at the point where they join your thighs. Do this for 2 minutes, once in the morning and once in the evening. If the position doesn't cause you discomfort, add 1 minute more each time, until you reach 10 minutes in the morning and 10 minutes at night.

At this point you can drop Position 1. You may discover, though, that even after you are recovered and exercising regularly, Position 2 will still be useful, helping to relax your back when it's tired.

Position 3: Basic position with knees clasped

When you can maintain Position 2 for 10 minutes twice a day, you might find, as many survey participants did, that it is useful to increase the amount of stretching you get from this position. Immediately after completing Position 2, keeping the towel under you, bring one knee up towards your chest and hold it in place with your hand. Now bring the other knee up. Clasp your hands just below both kneecaps. Gently, very gently, pull your knees towards your chest just a few centimetres. Hold for a count of six. Return to the Basic Position. Repeat these steps six times. The slight amount of stretching involved here might be considered 'exercising' but the real point is simply to relax in a comfortably flexed position, not to try to draw your knees towards your chest as much as you can.

Position 4: Basic position with legs supported

This position is a slightly more difficult alternative to both Positions 2 and 3, primarily because you have to get up from and down to the floor. But because your legs will be supported, you might find it more relaxing and pain-reducing. If so, substitute it for Positions 2 and 3, and do it twice every day – more often if it makes you feel better.

Begin by lying in the Basic Position on a carpeted floor (or on a gym mat or two folded blankets) with your feet in front of a sofa or a chair. Support your neck with a folded towel, or support your head and neck with a small pillow. Put both legs, one at a time, on the chair seat or sofa. Your feet and calves – but not your thighs – should rest on the elevated surface. If you're using a chair with a hard seat, you will feel more comfortable with a towel or blanket on the seat.

Q: How Do I Gradually Get More Active?

A: Try the following suggestions:

- *Walk your way out of pain.* As you recuperate, walk as much as you can. Sitting puts much more strain on your back than standing. It slows rather than hastens your recovery. Walk on level ground. When you venture outside the first few times, avoid steep gradients and uneven terrain. Walking up or down hills causes a noticeably greater strain on low back muscles. And uneven ground – like rocky or gravelly areas or beaches – tends to jar your back and make it difficult to relax and stride comfortably. These are best tackled when your back pain has eased.

- *Stand with your weight unevenly distributed.* Most people with low back pain are much more comfortable if they shift their weight from one foot to the other when they have to stand for any length of time, for good reason: when you shift most of your weight to one leg, and bend that leg slightly at the knee, you lessen your lumbar curve. But don't favour one leg for more than a few minutes at a time. Shift back and forth as your comfort level dictates. If possible, use a footstool, a book, your child's stuffed animal or anything else that's lying around to prop up your foot. This further reduces your lumbar curve. Again, don't favour one leg; switch back and forth.

- *Also, wear a pair of well-made shoes.* Don't pad around in old slippers, clogs or run-down trainers. Your footwear should have at least a 2.5 cm (1 inch) heel and contain a cushioned heel and arch support. (Virtually all good shoes have these features; running shoes are also acceptable.)

Q: Once I'm on the Road to Recovery, How Can I Maintain Good Posture?

A: Keep three things tucked in – your abdomen, bottom and chin – and the rest of your body will tend to line up properly.

The more your bottom juts out, the greater your lumbar curve and back pain. Tucking in your chin is important, because it helps you to maintain a proper cervical (neck) curve. Position your chin too high, or let it droop too low, and you'll add to the strain on your neck and the rest of your spine. The importance of good posture cannot be emphasized enough. US survey participants mentioned it more than any other factor as a way to speed up recovery from acute episodes of low back pain. It gets instant results, costs nothing to learn, and will do more for you than most professional treatments.

One UK respondent said: 'sucking in the stomach and walking tall, without raising shoulders, I find helps.'

Face what you want to see. While lying, standing or sitting, turn your entire body, not just your head, towards anyone or anything you're looking at. Otherwise, the top part of your spine (your neck) will be going one way, and the lower part another way, which may increase spasming.

Q: How Can I Avoid Re-injuring My Back?

A: *Adopt easy-on-the-back dressing habits.* Low back sufferers re-injure their backs more from reaching the wrong way to put their shoes on than from lifting heavy objects. With this in mind, survey participants recovering from acute, severe low back pain recommended the following:

- Keep your next day's clothing – including your shoes – within reach of your bed. This way, you can start your day with relaxation and pre-exercise positions, not a hunt for what to wear. You can also give your back a break when you get dressed – as the next paragraph explains.
- If you are still very tight and prone to spasming, put on waist-to-feet clothing – underwear, socks, skirts, trousers – while lying on your back in bed. You can even put your shoes on this way, using an old towel to keep your sheets clean.
- If you feel comfortable enough to sit while putting on your socks and shoes, bring your feet to you, while keeping your back as straight as possible. Minimize bending from the waist to put on footwear. If need be, support the weight of your legs by propping your feet on a chair.
- *Keep your hands close to yourself.* Don't reach out to pick up objects or perform an activity, no matter how light the object or easy the activity. For example, don't extend your arm fully to pick up a child's toy, water a plant, or answer the phone. Sidle right up to objects; the closer your arms are to your sides, and not to what you're reaching for, the better for your back. If you can't avoid reaching – to turn on a tap, for example – turn to one side. It's easier to bend sideways than forwards.
- Also, until your back has recovered, don't reach above your head for objects. If no one can help you, use a stepladder. Reaching for high objects arches your back – and that can cause trouble.

Chapter 8
How to Be Your Own Low Back Doctor for Chronic Pain

Two case histories • Attitude: taking charge of the problem and changing your life accordingly • How to lift and carry (from groceries to children) • Sitting (how to select a good chair for relaxation or desk work, how to make a car seat more comfortable) • Exercise (how to structure an individualized exercise regime; complete instructions for a safe, eleven-step exercise programme based on survey participants' experiences)

Important: This chapter is specially designed to help you get rid of chronic low back pain – the discomfort and limitations that have bothered you for months or years.

If your low back pain is caused by a ruptured disc (Chapter 9), osteoarthritis (Chapter 11), spondylolisthesis (Chapter 12) or scoliosis (Chapter 12), I suggest that you read one of these chapters first, then follow the guidelines in this chapter.

If you are currently incapacitated with acute back pain, see Chapter 7 first.

If you have chronic low back pain – and most participants in both the UK and US surveys did – the chances are that you . . .

- Suffer some degree of discomfort every day
- Don't know what to do or where to turn to improve your condition substantially
- Find that certain days and weeks are more painful than others – and not always for obvious reasons
- Exercise on a regular basis (or at least know that you should) but aren't sure that the exercises you do are helping your back as much as possible

- Hardly expect a cure to drop into your lap, but are weary of getting simplistic and uninformed responses to your questions.

Two Paths through Pain

Two cases offer some valuable insights.

Case 1

Kevin, a 34-year-old, long-distance independent lorry driver, had devoted his career and his life's savings to running his own business. But now it seemed that he might lose everything he had worked so hard for, because of a chronically and increasingly painful lower back.

Every year Kevin suffered two or three episodes of low back pain. Each episode either reduced his driving time or kept him off the road entirely. As the years passed, Kevin's pain grew worse. The muscle-relaxant pills prescribed by his GP made him more drowsy than comfortable. A back support that worked at first hardly helped at all now. Exercises that used to make him feel better caused severe spasming. And acupuncture wasn't making any difference.

Kevin asked his doctor to recommend a specialist. His GP, predictably enough, referred him to an orthopaedic surgeon. The orthopaedic surgeon examined Kevin thoroughly, found no 'pathological anomalies' and told him that the only real answer was to get out of the haulage business.

Kevin went through the roof. 'How would you feel if I told you that the only way to get rid of your back pain was to give up being an orthopaedic surgeon?' he yelled.

The orthopaedic surgeon was sympathetic but repeated his contention that sitting in a lorry for long periods of time was extremely hard on Kevin's lower back. His recommendation stood.

Remarkably, by the time Kevin told me his story, his back had become pain-free.

'Did you change your job?' I asked.

'No, although I thought long and hard about it,' he replied. 'I was unbelievably depressed and frustrated at first. A couple of weeks passed and I was driving, with my lower and middle back taped up to hold out for the rest of the run, when a Peggy Lee song came on the air about "Is that all there is?" The thought struck me. I couldn't believe that all modern medicine could offer was changing my job.'

'How did you turn around a condition that had been deteriorating for eleven years?' I inquired.

'After the orthopaedic surgeon,' Kevin answered, 'I went to a chiropractor. I tried manipulation and other treatments for six months. Each treatment made me feel better and I thought I was coming along. But then the amount of relief started lasting for just a couple of hours, rather than a few days or a week. I felt I wasn't really improving overall, and I was losing time and money by seeing the chiropractor three times a week, so I stopped.'

'What did you do then?'

'Nothing. I mean, I didn't see anyone else. Who was I supposed to see? Instead, I talked to people with back problems and looked at some back books. By this time, my friends and relatives were clipping out and sending me any articles they saw about back problems. It took a long time to get better, but I got there. It was touch and go for two years, a lot of trying to figure out what I should and shouldn't do – everything from how I sat when I drove to doing back exercises that would help rather than just keep the status quo, to little things you can do for yourself without making yourself feel like an invalid or basket case.

'People should be realistic,' he added. 'Anything that causes you as much trouble as my back caused me, and for such a long period of time, is going to take a lot of changing. The question is what to change and how. And, for me, there was also the question of whether I would work it out first or drive my family and myself crazy in the process.'

Case 2

Maggie, a 51-year-old management consultant, had been bothered by low back pain since she hurt herself leaning over a sofa to force open a jammed window. That was twenty years ago.

At the time I talked to Maggie she rated her pain at 7 on a scale of 0 to 10 (0 being pain-free and 10 being totally incapacitated). The long meetings and luncheons with clients required in her business were particularly hard to take. She had been doing back exercises every day for 15 years – a wide variety of exercises learned from many different practitioners and books – and she felt these definitely helped stop her pain getting even worse.

Maggie had been examined or treated by eleven practitioners over twenty years. When she first experienced pain her GP had prescribed rest and medication. Soon afterwards the parade started.

'After I saw my family doctor, I went to a neurologist, who prescribed more rest and more drugs. I took pain pills and muscle relaxants, the biggest change from these being that I couldn't think straight. The neurologist thought I might have a ruptured disc and sent me to a neurosurgeon. No luck there, so I decided to go it on my own. But after ten years of managing pretty well, including swimming every day at a health club and doing a lot of exercise, things started going downhill.

'I went the chiropractic route at this point and made some progress. Not enough though. A few years ago, my pain was consistently bad enough to affect my business. I couldn't make long plane trips and it was torture to sit through all-day meetings.

'A few months ago, I went to see a well-known back specialist. He sarcastically diagnosed my problem as "treadmillitis" – running from doctor to doctor – handed me a sheet of exercises to do and told me to stick with him or any other competent doctor of my choice and get the problem resolved once and for all.

'I've also tried acupuncture, naturopathy, psychotherapy and massage. I've had it. I don't know what to do now,' Maggie concluded.

'Did the exercises from the latest doctor help?' I asked.

'I think they're actually making things worse,' Maggie replied. 'But I'm so frustrated I'm doing them anyway.' Further conversation with Maggie revealed that she accepted everyone's judgement but her own about how to get well. She was always trying the 'latest' exercise programme. A water mattress suggested by a friend was bothering her back. She didn't take a back cushion to meetings or use a special carry-on seat for her frequent plane trips because such items embarrassed her, she said. Her footwear was appropriate for meetings but inappropriate for her back. Indeed, Maggie concluded that there were a dozen things she could do to help herself. And when I last spoke to her, she was doing those things and was in better shape than she could remember for ten years.

Kevin and Maggie are 2 of the 240 chronic low back sufferers in the US survey. Their stories demonstrate patterns of success and failure, but both offer proven, concrete approaches that you can apply right now to cut short the recovery process and banish chronic low back pain from your life. Since chronic low back pain is dramatically affected by what you do every day, I will begin with those daily activities, functions and attitudes that have the most to do with back problems.

Some of these points may seem mundane or even silly. But they play a crucial role in resolving low back pain. In fact, collectively, they may be more important than any other factor in determining whether your low back pain will continue, worsen or improve. As you study these points, you might find it useful to tick the ones you particularly need to act on. Then, after completing this chapter, you might come back to the ticked-off points and plan your corrective strategy.

Having the Right Attitude

Reviewing the comments of survey participants who had found a way out of years or even decades of chronic low back pain, one thing above all stood out – their attitude.

It wasn't simply a belief that they would get well, although that was important. It wasn't anything mystical. They had simply made up their minds to put themselves in charge of ending their back pain. They listened to the experts without awe and with the knowledge that they themselves ultimately knew more about their bodies than anyone else possibly could. Those who sought professional care did so for a limited time and acted as partners in the treatment, not as helpless victims looking to be cured. And all made the resolution of back pain a high priority in their lives.

These former back sufferers rejected as nonsense any claim of instant pain-banishing magic. They also rejected the idea that low back pain was common and inevitable. (Some noted that back pain is uncommon in many societies, including Japan and other Far Eastern countries.) They refused to believe that low back pain was the price they had to pay for walking upright, pointing out that walking upright a lot is a great way to avoid back pain.

They shunned the myth that low back pain is part of growing older. (The majority of back sufferers are under the age of 45.)

In essence, these former back sufferers took charge. They listened, learned, then decided for themselves what they needed to do to get well. They became their own low back doctors.

The Most Popular Tips for Preventing Low Back Pain

In the section of the US survey that asked, 'What are your most helpful tips for other back sufferers?' advice about lifting topped the list. The most often-stated advice was, in a phrase, to bend your knees and not your back. More emphatically, as one survey participant put it, 'Never bend from the waist, not even to pick up a pin.'

Some of the following advice about lifting is standard; you may have heard it before. Other suggestions are more unusual but equally useful. You will also receive advice about how to handle the three most common 'back breaking' lifting activities mentioned in this survey – lifting a baby, lifting shopping, and lifting heavy objects around the house and garden.

How to Pick Up and Carry Miscellaneous Objects

- Position your feet about shoulder-width apart with one foot a shoe length in front of the other. This position makes it easier to keep your back straight, to get up and down, and to maintain your balance.
- Keep whatever you're picking up close to your body. A 4.5 kg (10 lb) object extended just a few centimetres away from your body can strain your back.
- Make sure that you don't strain your neck by sticking your chin out. Keep it tucked in.
- Always bend your knees rather than your back.
- If you need to lift a heavy object, get help. It is much better to wait for help than to struggle alone and risk further damage to your back.

Carrying Shopping

It may be neat and efficient to have all your shopping packed into a single cardboard box, but a heavy box is a disaster for lifting and carrying. Instead, it's best to carry heavier items in a rucksack on your back and have bulkier, lighter items packed into two bags of roughly equal weight, with handles. It is much easier to carry shopping with your arms at your sides than to clutch bags to your chest. Lifting your arms while holding heavy packages puts more strain on the back, participants say.

You would have thought that driving to the supermarket would solve your shopping problem. However, taking a car on shopping outings can actually cause back sufferers more problems. When you have to walk home with your shopping, you tend not to take most of the store with you. Not so when you're driving. This leads us to one of the Top Ten Back Wreckers in our survey: getting shopping into and out of a car boot. If the boot of your car was at the level of your rear window, you wouldn't have a problem. Unhappily, though, no one has designed a car with the floor of the boot at this height.

So, even if you're driving, avoid heavy boxes. Avoid bags that are weightlifters' specials or else, when removing objects from the boot, you'll be bending perilously at the waist and leaning forward to grab the bottom of the bag or box. And that could lead to trouble. Also, lift bags out of the boot, one at a time, by the handles, or skip the boot altogether if you can and put your shopping on the back or front seat close to the door.

If you are suffering an acute episode of back pain, have your shopping delivered. Don't worry about treating yourself with kid gloves. If it's strenuous exercise you want, work out under supervision at a gym. From what survey participants tell us, it seems safer to bench-press 45 kg (100 lb) than to grunt and lift a 9 kg (20 lb) box of shopping off the floor of your car boot.

Four female UK survey participants had the following tips:

'Use the disabled trolley, and put up with the filthy looks. Accept any help with lifting that's going, or with big shops. Let someone else do it if you can. (Lifting and twisting at the same time is an absolute no-no!) It really doesn't matter if you run out of cabbage; have sprouts instead. For small shops I take the bike so I don't have to carry things. If you qualify, apply for a blue badge.'

'Shopping is a problem. I can only do this by car. Choose a car that is easy to load/unload. I have a little Daewoo Matiz hatchback, no sill to lift bags over, comfortable height for me. Fortunately most supermarkets now have more of the smaller, higher-level trolleys. Do not use the deep ones, it really is asking for trouble. And if you need help loading or unloading, you've got to ask. Sometimes I leave the non-perishables in the car till someone can help me carry them in.'

'Never pick up anything big or heavy yourself or reach high up to get anything off a shelf. I did this once and will never do it again. I always ask for help and just say I have a very bad back, could they get something down for me, and then if it looks big or heavy I ask if they will carry it to the car for me. Most places are happy to help if you are just polite.'

'If my back is really bad I'll do an Internet shop from Tesco or Asda, which is a brilliant service.'

Lifting and Carrying Babies and Children
To have them is to love them. And to love them is to want to pick them up, hold them over your head, and delight them by giving them piggybacks and rides on your shoulders.

Not to be able to do these kinds of things is the most heart-breaking situation a back sufferer can encounter. With this in mind, here is some advice from survey participants about mini-mizing your back problems and maximizing your pleasure with your children.

- Avoid the cradle or Moses basket on a stand. It is cute, charm-ing and possibly an even greater plague for back sufferers than car boots. The Moses basket is precisely the wrong height – too high to let you kneel on the floor and comfortably reach your baby, and too low for you to reach your baby without bending yourself out of shape.

   One solution is to use a big wicker laundry basket instead; line it with soft blankets and place it on the floor or at the level of a changing table – about midriff high. Fastening it securely to a platform or a sturdy, low table may do the trick. When the child is big enough for a cot, don't lean over the bars to lift the baby in or out. Instead, drop the collapsible side, get down on your knees, and go from there.

- Playpens are another macabre invention designed without parents' backs in mind. If you can't avoid playpens, at least get one with a side that folds down in seconds, allowing you to kneel, rather than lean over, to pick up your child.

- Changing tables take up space and aren't cheap, but most survey participants with children consider them essential. If you don't have one, you can kneel and change the baby on the floor or on a low bed.

- Sit in a rocking chair to feed or lull your baby to sleep. Rocking chairs have been popular with back sufferers for a long time. The backs of these chairs are usually straight. The rocking movement, according to some back sufferers, may ease stiffness and discomfort for you, while helping to calm the baby.

- The least stressful way to carry an infant a long distance is on your back in a carrier. It may seem impersonal not to wear the carrier in front where you can see your child, but babies don't seem to mind, and your back will thank you.

- Avoid the hip carry. A mother of twins in the US survey routinely used to pick up and carry her two-year-old twins, one on each hip, until a doctor who was a friend of the family pointed at her and exclaimed, '*That* is your back problem.' The hip carry was used by many mothers and fathers in this survey. And most realized at some point that the technique was causing them pain.

- If your child and your back are acting up at the same time, and your child wants to be held, try to comfort him or her while you're kneeling or while both of you are lying down.

- Piggyback rides are easier on you if your child can climb up on a chair and then grab hold of you while you're standing.

- A top-of-your-shoulders ride isn't the worst thing for your back. It's lifting your child onto your shoulders that's the real problem. Have your child get on a chair and climb on your shoulders while you are kneeling with your back to the chair.

Felicity, a UK survey respondent, had some very useful advice on this subject: 'Young children do learn about your capabilities and will adapt: does it really matter if they have odd socks on and you can't reach to sort them out? Some things simply have to go by the by and in a way this gives you energy to concentrate on doing the best you can.'

Sitting

'Take a seat and make yourself comfortable,' the receptionist at a prestigious rehabilitation clinic told the strong-backed husband of a low back sufferer. He did – in a plush, leather chair whose rounded back defied all attempts to get comfortable. An hour later, when the doctor was ready to see the patient – who because of her low back pain had chosen to stand rather than sit – the husband was sorry that he hadn't made an appointment for himself.

As every reader of this book already knows, sitting is hard on the back. Most low back sufferers would probably agree that the problem is not that we evolved into creatures who stood upright but that we decided to 'take a load off our feet' and sit down at work, in the car and just about everywhere else.

A Good Chair Gave Some Survey Participants More Help than a Good Back Specialist

US survey participants were almost unanimous about what constituted a good chair.

Overall qualities

Look for a straight-backed chair with a back tall enough to support your lower and upper back, arms to support the weight of your arms, and a seat that is firm enough to keep you from sinking in, wide enough to shift around in, and deep enough to support your thighs almost to your knees.

The back of the chair

Most chairs that you find in homes, offices and restaurants have as little backing as a bikini. Either there is enough room between the slats for a small child to crawl through or there is nothing but air at the point where the small of your back is yearning to make contact.

And, as if all this weren't bad enough, most chair backs aren't straight either. They are almost as curved as the inside of a barrel, or they tilt back just enough so that you're neither reclining nor able to sit up straight.

Nevertheless, think straight and insist on adequate support when you shop for your own chair. Make sure the back of the chair extends down to, or almost to, the seat. Also see to it that the back of the chair is at least high enough to make contact with your head, so that it can adequately support your upper back and neck.

The seat

A chair seat should be firm enough for you to sit on without more than about 1.3 cm (½ inch) of give. For well-padded individuals, a hard seat without any cushioning is fine. The depth of the seat – measured from back to front – should be about 45–60 cm (18–24 inches), depending on your size. You want enough seat depth to support about three-quarters of your thighs. Less will create a pull on your lower back; more, extending to your knees or beyond, will also play havoc with your back.

When considering the depth of a chair, assume that you might be using a back support, which will take up some of this measurement. In fact, if the only problem with a chair is that it has too much depth, that's easy to solve. Add a firm pillow, a back support or both.

Chair arms

Your chair should have them. Chair arms take the weight of your arms off your back. They're not critical, but they are helpful. If you have to make do without them, rest your arms in your lap.

The back support

Most secretarial and executive desk chairs have lumbar-support contours, but even the best of them aren't as effective for low back sufferers as the unadorned straight-backed chair with the back support of your choice – a rolled-up towel, cushion, pillow or commercially available backrest. Anything that provides the hollow of your back with something to rest on tends to relieve (or prevent) nagging low back pain.

UK survey respondents had the following advice for fellow back sufferers:

'I have had prolapsed disc problems for over thirty years. I never sit on a low soft chair otherwise I can feel my sciatica start straight away. I invested in a Parker Knoll orthopaedic chair with a lumbar support many years ago and it has been of great benefit. I have a "Backfriend" folding seat which I find invaluable. If I go visiting I always ask for a dining chair to sit on or I sit on the floor.'

'When confronted with dining chairs without lumbar support – in hotels etc – use a "Backfriend", remain at the table for as short a time as possible. All my own upright chairs slope BACK and offer LUMBAR SUPPORT. These all relieve tremendously the likelihood of pain in my mid-back building up – but make me a social eccentric!'

There is one difficulty with straight-backed chairs – namely, it isn't always possible to use them. For example, a straight-backed chair would be impractical to use at a desk, especially if you have to move back and forth between your desk and your typewriter or computer, turn to talk to people, or rummage through files.

For working at a desk, you might want a rolling office chair with a built-in lumbar support. Scores of different brands and models, ranging in price from modest to extremely expensive, are available at office furniture and department stores, and over the Internet.

How to Choose a Good Desk Chair

1. Never buy a desk chair sight unseen or seat untried. Sit on it for 30 to 45 minutes before buying it. One survey participant was reluctant to do this for fear of making a nuisance of himself. Another survey participant was mistaken for a sales-person sitting down on the job. But it's your back and your money. And an actual trial is the only way to make an intelligent selection.

2. Check the position of the lumbar support area. This is the part that bulges a bit toward you and should fit right into the small of your back. Lumbar supports tend to be positioned too low on most chairs, making contact with your sacrum (the protruding bony area of your spine directly below your lumbar curve) instead of with your lumbar curve. If the back support is adjustable up and down, that's a plus, but it's not a guarantee that the chair will feel right to you.

3. Try out the tilting action of the back of the chair. Does it support your weight when you're sitting up straight? Or does it tilt back too easily under your weight and prevent you from sitting straight? You want to be able to vary your position

from time to time by tilting back into a reclining position. But to reiterate, if the chair cannot support your weight and keep you at a 90-degree angle, the undesired tilting will cause you back pain.

To maximize your comfort, think of other constructive ways to vary your position when you're sitting at a desk, and try to get up and move about at least every 20 minutes.

When you're not at your desk, and want to get away from a straight-backed chair, you might consider a reclining chair. They were popular among survey participants who wanted the comfort of an easy chair without its usual feet-down, sink-in-and-suffer quality. Reclining chairs are almost never as good as the best straight-backed chair, but they are usually better than other easy chairs for two reasons. They tend to have firm seats, and the reclining action puts your knees above your hips.

Legal Requirements for Office Seating

In the UK, employers are legally obliged to ensure that their employees are working in a safe and healthy environment. This obligation also applies to temporary staff and home-based employees.

By law, office chairs (those used at workstations) must:

- Be stable (i.e. have five legs, arranged in a star shape)
- Allow the user easy freedom of movement and a comfortable position
- Be adjustable in height
- Have a seat back that is adjustable in both height and tilt; the seat back should move independently of the seat to allow for a more comfortable seating position.

There are a number of things you can do to make your own workstation healthier and safer for your back. For instance, you should always arrange your working area to suit you, whether you are working at home, in the office or sharing a desk. Remember to alter the height of your chair so that your shoulder and elbows are completely relaxed. Make sure that your thighs are roughly at right angles to your body or sloping slightly down. Use a footrest if your feet don't reach the floor. The top of your screen should be at horizontal eye level. If not, adjust it using a monitor arm or screen raiser. If you use your computer often, your computer screen and keyboard should be directly in front of you so you don't have to twist to use them. Position the screen at arm's length. And if you use a laptop, plug it into a separate screen when in the office.

Further tips for a healthy back include:

- Changing your position every 20 minutes
- If you are sitting down, standing up and stretching, and walking away from your desk briefly (e.g. to do some photo-copying or filing)
- Standing when taking alternate phone calls
- Leaning backwards and forwards to avoid staying in the same position for too long, and using the full range of movement of your chair.

UK survey participants made the following comments:
'ENSURE YOUR WORKSTATION IS RIGHT FOR YOU! Ensure that your chair and screen height are correct and, if necessary, that you have a foot support. If necessary, use a back cushion for your chair.'

'If you are working at a computer make sure you have a DSE [display screen equipment] assessment and that you have the correct chair – with lumbar support if applicable. If you need an orthopaedic chair, using JobCentrePlus can save you money, as they will pay for part of the cost. It is worth everything to invest in the correct chair if you suffer from back pain.'

How to Keep Your Car Seat from Driving You to a Back Doctor

An acquaintance of mine, a strapping, clean-living fellow in his thirties, recently threatened to put his furniture-removal business up for sale. If you do a lot of driving, you can probably guess what caused him to think about selling a successful enterprise. It wasn't the lifting, even though he routinely picked up many heavy items during the course of a day. It was sitting behind the wheel that did the damage. According to survey participants, car (and lorry) seats are only outdone in terms of back discomfort by restaurant seats, soft couches and sofa beds.

What can you do about this? If you're wealthy, perhaps buying a Volvo or Mercedes will help. US survey participants mentioned the unusual comfort of these cars, though Joanne, a UK participant, preferred the Renault Scenic: 'Ensure you choose a car with a good sitting posture when you next buy a car – I like the Renault Scenic as the sitting position is similar to a chair with my legs bending at the knees rather than stuck out too far in front and applying too much leverage on my spine when I brake. Remember to check out the access to the boot too. Can you load up your shopping easily?'

But wealthy or not, there is a great deal you can do to improve your comfort in a car.

1. *Buy or make your own car seat.* Probably the best way, and certainly the cheapest, is to buy two pieces of plywood from a lumberyard – one that is seat-sized, the other tall and wide enough to support your back. If you're handy, cover both pieces of wood with 1.3 cm (½ inch) of firm foam rubber and a cover, then connect the two pieces of wood with hinges. If you're not handy, simply place a chair back support or rolled-up towel between your back and the backrest board, and a seat cushion or a thrice-folded beach towel on the seat board.

2. *Get as close to the wheel as you can without discomfort.* Never mind the image of the racing-car driver who holds the wheel at arms' length, or the feeling many of us have that the only people who sit close to the wheel are nervous wrecks who drive at 50 km (30 miles) per hour on motorways. The point is that sitting close to the wheel will elevate your knees and enable you to place your free foot flat on the floor.

3. *Sit at a right angle.* Tilt the back of your seat so that it is nearly perpendicular (90 degrees).

4. *Use the armrest on the driver's side if you can.* You might also want to create an armrest to support your other elbow. Nothing fancy is needed – a towel-covered box, a couple of cushions or pillows – just about anything that comes up to armrest height will do.

5. *If your back starts to feel tired, do something about it immediately.* Move around in your seat, readjust your back support, stretch, try reclining the back of your seat a bit – and take a break every half hour. Just a few minutes of walking and shaking loose the kinks will help immensely.

James, another UK respondent, had these helpful tips to offer: 'When driving, ensure that your car seat is comfortable and supportive and that you are in a correct driving position. If not, try lumbar supports, wedges or whole seat cushions (orthopaedic). Drive only so long as you are comfortable. Break up long car journeys . . . Get out of the car, stretch, do exercises (if possible) such as gentle bending, shoulder shrugs and head rolling.'

Exercise

'I did my back exercises faithfully for ten years,' reported a professor in the US survey. 'And they helped. A doctor gave them to me, and if I stopped doing them for a few days, my low back pain got noticeably worse. Still, over the course of the ten years, my overall condition slipped a bit. Working out with weights started to cause me pain. I could still do everything. But some days were bad and my back really hurt. I had to watch myself more, be more cautions about things like raking, shovelling, and sitting too long. The idea of having to be even a little less active bothered me, so I went to a back doctor with a big reputation. It seemed to me that he knew less than I did about backs and exercise. Finally I found a doctor who was an exercise expert and he individualized an exercise programme that has made a tremendous difference.'

Like this professor, many back sufferers in the US survey relapsed but then made progress again after years of 'doing the right exercises' failed to prevent deterioration. Obviously the exercises weren't right for them.

There were also many survey participants who recovered successfully from low back pain in large part by piecing together their own exercise programmes. The comments of a draughtsman typify this approach: 'I've created my own back exercise programme,' he said. 'I learned a few exercises from a physical therapist [physiotherapist] and a couple from a chiropractor. But most exercises I picked up from doing a lot of reading and talking to other people with back problems.'

Both these approaches to exercise therapy – learning on your own and receiving a professionally individualized programme – are reflected in this section. Each exercise is accompanied by variations, to help you customize your own programme. Collectively, these exercises have done the most good for the most US survey participants. Equally important, they caused no known setbacks or injuries. These exercises aren't a cure-all – no exercise programme is – but they can give you the strength and flexibility you need to function much more effectively.

To reiterate, these exercises, along with other suggestions described in this chapter, will probably provide you with all the help you need. But 25 to 50 per cent of this book's readers will probably not achieve maximum gains without professionally prescribed, individualized exercise therapy. If you do go down the professional route, a single examination/consultation and a few demonstration sessions may be all that you'll need. This next point should be obvious, but it's worth stating anyway: you can be certain that seeking professional exercise therapy is decidedly not a case of your failing to take responsibility for your own problem. It is, instead, a proven way that some chronically limited individuals can, and should, help themselves. As Dr Hans Kraus states in his landmark book *Backache, Stress and Tension*, an exercise programme 'is a craft, even an art'. He adds, 'An exercise prescription should be regarded as potent medicine, which it is if properly given.'

I agree. And here, for the majority of low back sufferers, is the right medicine to promote optimum back fitness.

The Most Important Back Exercise is a Mental One

It has been said a hundred times by participants in this survey, and could be repeated a thousand times more, that your approach to back exercise – your attitude and preparation for exercise – is at least as important as the mechanical components of the exercise therapy itself.

US survey participants offer these ways of thinking about exercise:

- Exercise therapy, no matter how cautious it may seem to you, is almost always more beneficial than anything you can put into or onto your body.
- Try to ignore two mass-media concepts about exercise: (1) that it must be vigorous and competitive, and (2) that results have to be instantaneous. Back exercise runs counter to both these beliefs. As one survey participant put it, 'Slower is better, gradual is faster, and vigorous is self-defeating.' Properly done, back exercise will bring you small but noticeable improvement in a few weeks. And in three to six months, you can feel like a new person.
- It's OK to think that back exercises aren't exciting or that they are like bad-tasting medicine that is good for you. 'I consider back exercise to be about as scintillating as going to the bathroom . . . but just as essential,' said one low back sufferer. Of course, other survey participants disagree. They look forward to their 15 to 30 minutes a day of exercise. For them it's quality time – time when they are alone, quiet, in touch with themselves, meditative, doing something good for themselves. The latter perspective certainly makes things easier. In any case, it is important that you exercise intelligently.

Some Other Suggestions to Help You Get the Most out of Your Exercise Programme

1. *Try to perform back exercises daily.* About 70 per cent of low back sufferers in the US survey felt that they had to exercise every day either to achieve maximum fitness or because they felt, 'If I don't make it a habit, I may not exercise at all.'
2. *Adjust the pace to your needs.* If you haven't been exercising regularly, or you're recovering from an acute episode of low back pain, you can speed up your progress with a twice-a-day exercise programme – once in the morning and once in the evening. Not everyone can find the time to do this, but survey participants recommend it highly. Then, at the point you're exercising to maintain rather than reach a high level of fitness, reduce your programme to once a day.
3. *Exercise when and where you like.* Pay no attention to what people say about the great importance of exercising at the same time every day, in the same room, and on the same surface. This

kind of sameness is unnecessary and even counter-productive for many back sufferers, who believe it smacks of the same compulsive, driven behaviour that aggravated their backs in the first place. What's more, a rigidly fixed routine can quickly become boring and stifling enough to be dropped. A beautician who exercises strictly as a preventive measure commented, 'I do back exercises three days a week in a gym (once alone and twice as part of a group), two nights a week on my bed, and two nights a week on the living room carpet with my husband. According to what I've been told by back specialists, my routine, or lack of routine, is almost sinful. I say, nonsense.'

4. *Establish a logical exercise sequence.* Even though they may scoff at having the same time or place for exercise, most survey participants believe that an exercise regime should always be done in the same sequence. A sense of logic and order – warm-ups, increasingly difficult stretching and strengthening, then cooling off – seems a necessary part of the therapy.

5. *Create a good exercise environment.* Your exercise room should be warm and free of draughts. If it isn't, turn up the radiator or put on an electric heater about half an hour before exercising. Keep overhead lights off. Put the telephone out of reach and turn it off if possible. Tell the kids not to disturb you. (There's no harm in trying.) Try to free your mind from the problems of the day. Wait at least two hours after eating a heavy meal to exercise, an hour after a light meal or snack. It's not a good idea to watch TV while exercising. Apart from being distracting, watching TV while exercising can put a strain on your neck. Consider playing your favourite music instead.

6. *Try warming up before doing back exercises.* Some survey participants felt that a warm shower or the use of a heating pad just before exercise enabled them to stretch more easily, get more from the therapy, and increase their rate of progress. Furthermore, most survey participants agreed that starting their exercises immediately after waking up didn't give them enough time to warm up. If you must exercise first thing in the morning, move around in bed, then walk for a few minutes before you begin.

7. *Get the most out of your exercises safely.* Stretch to the point of resistance, then try to move just a fraction beyond it. But

don't 'go through' pain. Overstretching is worse than not exercising at all. It can cause great harm, including torn muscle fibres, spasming and pain. Stay in touch with yourself and within yourself. Plan to expand slowly but continuously your limits of strength and flexibility. You can make tremendous progress this way.

Exercise 1: Breath of the Yogi
For relaxation and abdominal toning

According to survey participants, this first exercise simultaneously relaxes and energizes your body, thus preparing you for the rest of the exercises to come. Lie in the Basic Position (on your back with your knees up, feet flat, arms at your side). Inhale through your nose. Allow the breath first to expand and fill your abdomen, then your chest. If you're not used to deep abdominal breathing, put a hand on your abdomen when you inhale; if your abdomen rises, you're breathing properly. Exhale through your mouth . . . slowly. Inhaling should take at least 8 seconds, exhaling 12 seconds. When you exhale, let yourself go limp. Repeat three times.

Exercise 2: Pelvic Tilt
To improve posture by reducing your lumbar curve and strengthening your abdominal and buttock muscles

Stay in the Basic Position. Slide one hand, palm down, between the surface you are lying on and the small of your back (lumbar curve). The space or hollow that you feel is what you're going to flatten away when you achieve the Pelvic Tilt. Then push down and try to squash your hand. This movement automatically tilts up your pelvis. If you're having trouble getting the feel of this exercise, pretend that you're trying to pull in your abdominal muscles so that they touch your spine. Relax.

- *Frequency:* Week 1 – three repetitions of three seconds each; by the end of Week 2, three repetitions of six seconds each; by the end of Week 3, six repetitions of six seconds each.
- *Advanced Version 1:* Lying in the Basic Position, push down, contracting your abdominal muscles, and squeeze together your buttocks. This buttock-clenching motion raises your

pelvis and flattens your back. A handful of survey participants with unusually weak abdominal muscles found this variation easier to do than the basic Pelvic Tilt.

- *Comment:* If human beings had perfectly straight spines, instead of an 'S' shape, their movements would be severely limited. So the problem is not that you have a curve in your spine, but that your lumbar curve is probably exaggerated – a condition called lordosis, or swayback. At the other extreme, some people, including back sufferers who have been bedridden for years, may have an overly elongated (flattened) 'S' curve. If you're one of these people, you won't be able to slide your hand between a firm mattress and the small of your back when you're in the Basic Position. And you will find that the Pelvic Tilt is either uncomfortable or pointless to do. For most low back sufferers, however, the Pelvic Tilt is an essential way to flex and strengthen the back.
- *Advanced Version 2:* Stand about 30 cm (12 inches) away from a wall and gently lean your back into it. Then try to flatten your lumbar curve by contracting your abdomen and buttocks. Some survey participants found this awkward or uncomfortable to do. Others raved about its value, not so much as an exercise but as a way to take the strain off their backs after they had been sitting for a long time. We suggest that you use this manoeuvre any time during the day that your back needs a brief respite.

Exercise 3: One Knee-to-Chest
To stretch the lower back

Note: Do not attempt this exercise if you have had a hip replacement.

Starting in the Basic Position, slowly bring one knee towards your chest as far as you can, without using your hands and without straining. Since you will be stretching slowly and fluidly, it will take you a few seconds to reach your limit. When you reach it, hold for one second. Then return your knee to – and through – the starting position, sliding your heel until your leg is fully extended and flat on the floor. Wobble the leg a few times, moving your ankle a bit to the left and right. (This 'shaking loose' procedure helps keep you relaxed and flexible during the exercise.) Slide the leg back up to the starting position. Repeat this entire procedure with your other leg.

- *Frequency:* Week 1 – three repetitions of 5 seconds each; by the end of Week 2, six repetitions of 5 seconds each; by the end of Week 3, ten repetitions of 5 seconds each.
- *Comment:* This is the most basic of low back stretching exercises. It seems simple, and it is. But don't underestimate its value. Most survey participants felt that if the knee-to-chest exercise were the only exercise they did, it would keep their backs in reasonable shape.

Exercise 4: Knee Spread
To stretch hip, groin and buttock muscles

Remaining in the Basic Position, and without exerting any effort, allow both knees to spread apart and lean downwards towards the floor. The weight of your legs will spread your knees apart. When you feel resistance, hold for 3 seconds and return to the starting position.

- *Frequency:* Week 1 – three repetitions of 3 seconds each; by the end of Week 2, four repetitions of 5 seconds each; by the end of Week 3, six repetitions of 5 seconds each.
- *Comment:* If you have tighter-than-average muscles, or if you're unusually tight now because of a recent episode of back pain, don't let your knees spread apart as far as they will go. Stop when you feel the slightest pulling sensation. Then stretch a little more each day until you achieve a wider but still comfortable position.

Many back books suggest a hip-stretching exercise that involves dropping both knees over to one side until they rest on the floor. This exercise will stretch your hips. But, as it also twists your torso and arches your back, many survey participants feel it does not belong in a gentle back exercise programme.

Exercise 5: Knee-to-Shoulder
To stretch your hips, buttocks and lower back

Note: Do not attempt this exercise if you have had a hip replacement.

Lie on your side in the foetal position. Bend both legs at the knees slightly. Relax your arms, elbows bent, with your hands resting near your face. Slowly slide your top leg towards your shoulder. When you feel resistance, drop your knee on the floor, relax your leg completely for 1 second, then slide it back to the starting position. Do the number of repetitions suggested below. Then turn onto your other side and repeat the exercise.

- *Frequency:* Week 1 – three repetitions; by the end of Week 2, six repetitions; by the end of Week 3, ten repetitions.
- *Comment:* Aside from the obvious stretching value of this exercise, it gets you off your back and prevents stiffness from exercising in one position for too long.

Exercise 6: Modified Bent-Knee Sit-ups
To strengthen your abdominal muscles

Return to the Basic Position. Tuck in your chin and pull in your abdominal muscles while inhaling. As you start to exhale, simultaneously raise your head and reach your hands up towards your knees. You'll know you've raised your head far enough when you can see your navel. Hold this position for 1 second, then return to the Basic Position. Relax for a moment. Repeat.

- *Frequency:* Week 1 – three repetitions; by the end of Week 2, six repetitions; by the end of Week 3, ten repetitions.
- *Advanced Version 1:* Instead of keeping your arms at your sides, and then extending them towards your knees as you raise your head, fold your arms across your abdomen. This increases the level of difficulty slightly. Also, with your arms in this position, you'll actually be able to feel your abdominal muscles contract and strengthen. We suggest you try this variation a month after being able to do the easier version.
- *Advanced Version 2:* Clasp your hands behind your head. Raise both your head and shoulders until they are just slightly off the floor. Hold this position for 3 seconds rather than just 1 second.
  Note: Take care not to force your head forward, as this will flex the neck too much. You can guard against this by keeping your elbows open wide, rather than bringing them in close by your ears.

- *Comment:* Every US survey participant interviewed, and every back practitioner who treated these survey participants, agreed that strong abdominal muscles were essential for low back fitness. However, there was also widespread disagreement about what was required to make your abdomen strong enough to help hold your spine in place and allow you to maintain good posture. A slight majority of survey participants believed that the modified half sit-up recommended here would provide you with the strength you need without causing you harm.
- A handful of survey participants and back practitioners felt that deep breathing alone could sufficiently firm up your abdominal muscles. A slightly larger group believed that doing isometric contractions (pulling in your abdominal muscles for a few seconds; then pushing out) would do the job. And about 25 per cent of back sufferers and back specialists believed in more strenuous abdominal-building exercises, such as full bent-knee sit-ups, sit-ups on slant boards, and sit-ups done from an inverted position.

Note: Don't even attempt straight-leg sit-ups. They put excessive strain on your lower back and take away from your efforts to strengthen your abdominal muscles.

By following this suggested plan, and exercising twice a day, you'll be doing 20 modified half sit-ups a day. At that point, if you're pain-free, you may choose to switch to bent-knee sit-ups, with your feet held down by a partner or hooked under a desk or sofa. However, based on the comments of survey participants, these are not recommended for most back sufferers. Modified half sit-ups will safely give you all the abdominal strength you need to perform a full range of daily activities, from extensive sitting to manual work and athletics.

Exercise 7: Single Knee-to-Chin: Extra Stretch
To stretch your lower back

Note: Do not attempt this exercise if you have had a hip replacement.

This exercise is the same as Exercise 3 – with one important difference: after you raise one knee towards your chest as far as you can, clasp your hands just below that knee and apply gradual upward pressure. By using your hands and arms this way, you'll find you can move your knee several centimetres more towards your chest and stretch your lower back more fully.

- *Frequency:* Week 1 – three repetitions of 3 seconds each; by the end of Week 2, six repetitions of 6 seconds each; by the end of Week 3, ten repetitions of 6 seconds each.
- *Advanced Version 1:* Keep one leg fully extended and flat on the floor during the exercise. This enables you to stretch the lower part of your spine even more. However, it also increases the risk of injury to your lower back. So if you're in the process of rehabilitating your back, this variation is not recommended. But if you want to get from fit to fitter, add this version to your routine after a month of doing all the exercises in this chapter.
- *Advanced Version 2:* As you bring your knee to your chest; simultaneously raise your head and try to touch your chin to that knee. This variation increases the amount of flexing you do. It also strengthens your abdominal muscles. The only major drawback, according to survey participants, is a psychological one. In all other exercises I've mentioned, there is no set 'athletic goal', such as having to touch your chin to your knee. And the absence of this kind of goal is a plus, because it allows you to find and slowly expand your own limits. If you're in reasonably good shape, try the variation I have just described, but don't get competitive and over-stretch in an effort to 'do it successfully'. You have but one goal: progress. I suggest that you try adding this variation to your routine two months after being able to do all the exercises in this chapter.
- *Comment:* If you watched a group of people do the exercises and variations described in this section, you would note tremendous differences in the degree to which people can stretch. Some people can touch their knees to their chests on the first try; some take six months to do it; others are never able to do it. It doesn't matter which group you fall into. Simply move to your point of resistance and try, gradually, to expand it.

Exercise 8: Knee-to-Shoulder
(Repeat Exercise 5)

Exercise 9: Both Knees-to-Chest
To stretch your lower back

Note: Do not attempt this exercise if you have had a hip replacement.

Starting from the Basic Position, put your knees together, clasp your hands around them, and pull them towards your chest. If it's awkward to clasp your hands around your knees while you're lying in the Basic Position, raise your knees a few centimetres first and then clasp them. When you feel some resistance, pause. Then try to gently stretch your way past that level for 6 seconds. If you can't stretch any farther without pain, then just hold the position for 6 seconds.

- *Frequency:* Week 1 – three repetitions of 6 seconds each; by the end of Week 2, six repetitions of 6 seconds each; by the end of Week 3, ten repetitions of 6 seconds each.
- *Advanced Version:* Same as above except that you keep your knees shoulder-width apart rather than together and clasp a hand around each knee. With your knees apart during this exercise, you'll be able to stretch farther than you can when keeping them together. Based on the experience of survey participants, we recommend that you substitute this variation for the knees-together version after you can comfortably do all the exercises in this chapter.
- *Comment:* If you've never done back exercises before, it may seem that bringing both knees to your chest does no more or less for you than the single-knee-to-chest exercise. Not so. When you actually perform these stretching exercises, you'll feel differences. And you'll discover that the differences will add new dimensions to your flexibility and suppleness.

Exercise 10: Modified Half Sit-ups
(Repeat Exercise 6)

Exercise 11: Hamstring Stretch
To stretch the backs of your thighs

If your hamstring muscles are tight, and they most likely are if you have low back pain, it is important to find a way to stretch them without straining your lower back in the process. That is why, although the following exercise is probably the safest way to stretch your hamstring muscles, I suggest that you *don't* do this exercise until you have first done all the preceding exercises for one month.

Start in the Basic Position. Raise one knee towards your chest. Fully extend and straighten your leg toward the ceiling at a 45-degree angle. Then, keeping your knee straight, try to move your leg up towards a 90-degree angle.

Frequency: Week 1 – three repetitions of 3 seconds each; by the end of Week 2, six repetitions of 6 seconds each; by the end of Week 3, ten repetitions of 10 seconds each.

Comment: The safety feature here is initially to extend your leg at a 45-degree angle – even though you can go higher. At this angle there is virtually no risk of overstretching your hamstrings. It's better to wait until your flexibility increases before attempting to extend your leg all the way up to a 90-degree angle.

There are three other commonly used hamstring-stretching exercises, none of which is recommended by most survey participants. But I will briefly describe these variations, because you're likely to run into them and should know why they might not be advisable.

1. A straight-leg lift done from the Basic Position, locking your knee and raising your straightened leg from the floor toward 90 degrees
2. Sitting in a chair, bending from the waist, and lowering your head towards your knees
3. Sitting on the floor with your legs straight out in front of you and leaning forwards

Survey participants felt strongly, however, that these movements, compared with the recommended exercise, placed unnecessary stress on the lower back and hips.

Two Useful Core Stability Exercises

The following exercises are easy to do and are widely recommended by physiotherapists in the UK. Researchers have found that the abdominal muscles play an important role in supporting the spine. Strengthening these muscles therefore helps prevent and treat lower back pain. The transversus abdominis muscle has received particular research attention. And it is now accepted that this muscle is vital to developing core stability and that learning to use it correctly to support the spine and maintain good posture is very beneficial. For all these reasons, abdominal-strengthening exercises and transversus abdominis co-ordination exercises are increasingly being used in lower back pain prevention and treatment programmes. The multifidus muscle runs vertically on each side of your spine and also helps to support your lower back.

Transversus Abdominis

Start on all fours, on the floor. Ensure that your shoulders are over your hands and your hips are over your knees. Your back should be flat. Now pull in your stomach, drawing in your belly button up towards your spine. You should only move your tummy muscles, not your back. Hold this position for 10 seconds, then slowly let go. Repeat ten times. Once you've learned how to do this exercise, you can do it sitting, standing or even in bed.

Multifidus

Stand up and put one foot forward as if you are walking. Place your weight on the back foot and tighten your stomach muscles (as in the transverses abdominis exercise). If you wish, place your thumbs on your low back, on either side of your spine. Slowly rock forward onto your front foot, allowing your back heel to lift slightly. You should feel the weight shifting from your back leg to your front leg. Hold this position for 10 seconds, then slowly let go. Repeat ten times. Once you've learned how to do this exercise, you can also do it sitting.

This chapter has given you a lot of general advice about living with chronic low back pain. If you follow the tips provided here by survey participants, you will probably find that your level of pain decreases and that daily life becomes easier. The next three chapters are designed to provide more specific guidance for particular conditions. They cover three relatively common problems: ruptured discs, neck pain and osteoarthritis-based back pain.

Chapter 9
How to Recover from a Ruptured Disc

Advisability of surgery – laminectomy, discectomy • Outcomes of surgery
• Outcomes of non-surgical treatments • Dangers of some manipulation
treatments for acute disc pain • Chronic disc pain: specific exercise advice
• Individualized exercise therapy • Walking and swimming as alternatives to
back exercises • Gravity inversion • Spinal fusion

'The pain I felt during this time was something I hope not to experience again in my lifetime,' said a restaurant owner of the first surge of severe pain from a ruptured disc. 'There was virtually no position for comfort, and only the slightest relief from pain while lying on my back with my knees bent.'

This description could just as easily have come from any of the other 64 US survey participants who suffered a ruptured disc. Readers who are familiar with the agony of disc pain will certainly empathize.

The pain and incapacitation caused by a ruptured disc are well established. So is the frequency of the disorder: in the UK survey, nearly a quarter of the respondents (543 people) had been diagnosed with a ruptured disc. But concrete and accurate information about how to recover from a ruptured disc has not been available, obscured as it has been by a storm of conflicting opinions and data.

In particular, US survey participants found themselves searching, often in desperation, for answers to the following crucial questions:

- How can I resume everyday activities as quickly, safely and productively as possible?
- What are the alternatives to surgery?
- To what extent can I treat myself?

- Which of the many different kinds of practitioners are best for ruptured disc sufferers?
- What steps can I take to prevent further injury?

Most survey participants were not able to get adequate answers to these or other more specific questions when they needed them. Usually they had to learn the hard way – from unhappy experiences, through trial and error.

Thanks, however, to what these individuals eventually learned – and shared with me – the information that follows can provide the clarity you need to take charge of, and resolve, your own case.

I have divided this chapter into two sections: acute and chronic pain from a ruptured disc.

Acute Pain: How to Relieve It

Using Painkillers

Most ruptured disc patients do get some relief from strong painkillers such as Oxycodone or morphine. Medication of this potency is potentially addictive, but survey results indicate that the advantages far outweigh the risks. If you can take the medication orally, then you can use it by yourself at home. If intramuscular injections or intravenous drips are called for, however, your doctor will probably want you to go to a hospital. Remember, though, if good nursing service is available to you, any kind of pain medication can be administered at home. The most commonly prescribed analgesics – aspirin or paracetamol with codeine – may not be strong enough alone to counter acute, severe ruptured disc pain.

Surgery: Should You or Shouldn't You?

Most back problems cannot be resolved by surgery. But if you're one of the thousands of back sufferers every year who receives at least a tentative or best-guess diagnosis of a ruptured disc, you will need to consider the decision with as much background information as possible.

For starters, you should know that a diagnosis of a ruptured disc – based on a manual examination, with or without scans or X-rays – is not definitive. Among the US survey participants, for example, 98 received a preliminary diagnosis of a ruptured disc, but only 65 of these underwent either further tests to confirm the diagnosis or disc surgery, or both. The comments in this chapter are partly based on the experiences of these 65 individuals. Among them, 33 had surgery and 32 did not.

Those who decided against surgery had these outcomes after an average of six years:

- 52 per cent were virtually pain-free
- 27 per cent were functional but limited in activities such as sitting, housework, gardening, lifting and athletics
- 21 per cent were more disabled than functional

Now look at the outcomes for the surgery cases that were evaluated an average of five years after hospitalization:

- 33 per cent were virtually pain-free
- 30 per cent were functional but limited
- 37 per cent were more disabled than functional

On a scale of 0 (pain-free) to 10 (disabled), US survey participants who had surgery had an average pain rating of 5.0, five years after surgery. On the same scale, non-surgery patients had a lower average pain rating of 3.9. Both groups had identical diagnoses based on comparable tests.

The UK survey results for disc surgery were rather more positive. They were as follows:

Number of patients who rated disc surgery in the UK survey	207
Provided dramatic long-term help	37%
Provided moderate long-term help	24%
Provided temporary relief	20%
Ineffective	9%
Made patient feel worse	10%

These statistics should help you make an informed decision about whether or not to have surgery to correct a ruptured disc.

But statistics never tell the whole story. Insights, attitudes and feelings also have a lot to do with decision making. That's why I think you'll be interested in the anecdotes that follow. They let you listen to others in your situation – to know how they felt while grappling with different options, and how they feel now in retrospect.

Some Ruptured Disc Patients View Surgery as a Cure

Doctors themselves hardly ever refer to surgery as a cure. No matter how optimistic a surgeon might be, he knows he can't restore your back to its original condition. He also knows that surgery cannot create the kind of fitness you need to prevent further injury to your back. Yet, with some individuals, for reasons no one can pinpoint, surgery does seem to 'cure' ruptured discs.

Take the case of a domestic appliance store-owner. She couldn't be more pleased with the results of her laminectomy (surgery that removes the gel portion of a disc as well as a small amount of bone that blocks access to this disc). Twenty years ago, as a young woman, she bent over one morning and collapsed on the floor in pain. The next day she was hospitalized. The following day she underwent surgery. Two months later she went back to her job. Now, looking back at her rush to the operating table, she says, 'I don't know why people are afraid of back surgery. It literally cured me. I'm overweight, I don't exercise, and I haven't had a single ache or pain for twenty years.'

Is this survey participant a rare exception? Possibly, but she's not alone. Judging from the US survey data, about one in twenty ruptured disc patients makes a complete and permanent recovery from surgery, even when he or she goes back to doing the very same things that caused problems in the first place.

An artist in the US survey did almost as well as the domestic appliance retailer. 'A laminectomy caused instant relief,' she told us. 'I sit and paint all day, and I have had very little pain for the past five years. I was taught exercises but I don't do them.'

Will lack of fitness catch up with this survey participant? Possibly not. But keep this in mind: for every one individual who resumed full activity after surgery – without making any effort at rehabilitation – there are nineteen others who were much worse off because they didn't work hard to put their backs in good shape.

For Most People, Surgery is Just One Step Towards Recovery

Here is a more typical experience. A self-employed businessman struggled through episodes of incapacitating pain from a ruptured disc for ten years before he had a laminectomy. 'The blinding pain in my buttock and leg vanished almost immediately after surgery,' he said. 'My back hurt some, it was kind of sore all over, but I thought it was mostly from the surgical procedure itself.'

What were the next several weeks like?

'When I got home ten days after surgery,' he continued, 'I felt pretty good. Then, about a month later, when my activity increased, I started to get muscle spasms. The pain was moderate, but it really frightened me. Oh, no, here we go again, I thought. My surgeon told me that some spasming after back surgery was normal and that I shouldn't try to do so much yet. When I went back for a two-month post-operative check-up, I asked about back exercises and was given a pamphlet containing some. The exercises didn't help. There was still some pain from spasming, and I lived in constant fear of re-injuring myself and not being able to make a living. I decided to join the YMCA and take their back exercise programme. That worked for me and I've been pretty much unlimited in my activities ever since.'

I had one more question for this survey participant: did he think, in retrospect, that a laminectomy had been his best bet?

'Yes,' he answered, 'I felt that surgery would correct the problem, once and for all, and I was right.'

Some 30 Per Cent of Individuals Can Carry On – but with Difficulty

A public parks worker keeps at his job in spite of chronic back pain since a laminectomy five years ago. 'My pain continues to interfere with my job performance,' he commented. 'But I don't complain and I do work, even though I could be put on disability.'

An electrician also reported that there is never an absence of pain after disc surgery. 'All that my laminectomy did was get rid of the pain and tingling in my legs for a while. Other people I've talked to say the exact same thing. First the sciatica vanishes and you're really pleased. Then you realize that your back pain hasn't subsided at all. Then some leg pain comes back, and even when it's not there, the back pain is. I work because there's no alternative. It's unbelievable to me that nothing else can be done and that I'm stuck with being limited, having to lie down every day after I get home from work, for the rest of my life. Maybe other areas of medicine have become advanced, like heart operations and transplants, but not back medicine. I don't mean to trot out the cliché about "If they can send a man to the moon, how come they can't fix your back?" But is an artificial disc really implausible?'

More Than One-Third of US Disc Surgery Patients Have Remained Disabled

'The surgery seemed to relieve pain and pressure for a few weeks,' a housewife said, 'but it has left me mostly disabled. I wish that an exercise programme had been emphasized more.' Five years after surgery, this woman is still struggling to be able to function even modestly as a mother and wife. Her experience typifies the disastrous long-term outcome of more than one-third of people in the US survey who had surgery for a ruptured disc.

Another young housewife talked about the incapacitation she has lived with: 'When you start thinking about back surgery, doctors don't tell you, but I know for a fact, that one operation can lead to the need for another. I have been unable to work six of the last twelve years. A partial discectomy just relieved the pain for a couple of weeks. Then I had microsurgery, which was supposed to remove the rest of the disc material that hadn't been taken out during the first operation. The microsurgery didn't work. Then, a while later, an orthopaedic surgeon removed two ruptured discs and fused my vertebrae. This last operation helped the most, but I continue to have back pain, sciatica and muscle spasms.'

One-Third of Non-Surgery Patients Would Have Had Surgery if They Had Followed Their Doctors' Advice

Eleven out of thirty-two US survey participants decided against their doctors' recommendations of surgery. Here are a few of their stories.

A farmer with a ruptured disc had compelling reasons for not following his doctor's recommendation to have surgery. 'I needed to plant my crops or risk losing everything. So I rested a bit and planted in spite of the pain. Then things improved, so I never did need surgery.'

'"You need surgery," an orthopaedic surgeon told me after giving me a diagnosis of ruptured disc,' an executive reported. 'I mentally wasn't ready to have my back opened up so I rested for two weeks and then gradually started to exercise. My pain has now dropped enough to let me function, though with limitations.'

'You won't believe what an orthopaedic surgeon told me twenty years ago,' a commercial artist remarked. 'The doctor said that it might take months, or even years, but that sooner or later I would crawl into his office on my hands and knees, begging to be operated on. I've had episodes of pain that keep me from working a few weeks every year. So, even now, more than twenty years later, I'm still not sure I made the right choice about not having surgery. But can you believe that doctor's incredible attitude?'

A Few Survey Participants Avoided Surgery with Their Surgeons' Encouragement

A periodontist said, 'My neurosurgeon felt that surgery should not be done at all because pain persists in 80 per cent of cases. I was happy to hear this. However, all he offered was a corset and Ascriptin [aspirin]. Then I saw a physiatrist who referred me to a physiotherapist and I am gradually improving without surgery.'

'I was glad I found an orthopaedic surgeon who believed that surgery was an absolutely last resort,' said a writer. 'He believed in movement and exercise, once I could leave bed, and this helped a lot, too.'

A lecturer also appreciated his orthopaedic surgeon's caution about surgery. 'It took me almost a year to get back to "normal". Maybe surgery would have speeded up my recovery, but I doubt it. I attribute my progress to increasing daily activities and to working with a physical therapist [physiotherapist] on an exercise programme.'

Beware of Some Manipulation Treatments for Acute, Ruptured Disc Pain

No discussion of how to recover from the initial, incapacitating phase of ruptured disc pain would be complete without special mention of the role of manipulation. Half the US survey participants with ruptured discs sought help from chiropractors. Unfortunately, the results from spinal manipulation for people in severe pain were too often injurious. In addition, some conditions were misdiagnosed and opportunities for effective treatment were lost.

Keep in mind that the statistics below apply only to US chiropractors who treated ruptured disc pain during the initial phase, when patients were partially or totally disabled with sciatica.

Number of people treated in US survey	24
Provided temporary relief	5 (21%)
Ineffective	12 (50%)
Patient felt worse	7 (29%)

Here are some of the stories behind these numbers.

A dentist said, 'The chiropractor made my problem worse. At the time I was treated by him, pain was severe in my lower back and right buttock. During the process of manipulation, the condition became worse, with sciatica pain radiating down my leg into my foot.'

'I already had a diagnosis of a ruptured disc when I saw a chiropractor,' a company owner reported. 'Relatives and friends had convinced me that I should stay away from doctors and also not waste my time lying around in bed. I was limping badly with sciatica and could barely make it under my own power to the chiropractor's table. After my spine had been adjusted, the pain was worse to the extent that I had to be carried out. If I hadn't been overwhelmed by the pain, I think I would have tried to kill the guy.'

A lawyer said, 'I had a series of treatments from a chiropractor for my ruptured disc. The pain got progressively more severe during the treatments until I stopped them. It is aggravating, and it also seems unprofessional, that a ruptured disc is not seen as a ruptured disc by chiropractors, or at least not by my chiropractor. Misalignment was the diagnosis. I think if I had walked in without a head, I would have been told that the top of my spine was misaligned.'

Coping with Chronic Disc Pain: How to Manage It

Special Exercises are Called For

The exercise needs of people who have ruptured discs – compared with people who have low back pain without disc pathology – are different. And in order to maximize your chances for a complete and lasting recovery, it is important that you know about the differences and act on them. Here are highlights of what we will discuss further in this chapter about exercise:

Back exercises are not always the answer, but some form of exercise is essential. In the US survey, fewer ruptured disc patients than low back sufferers followed a regular exercise routine – 51 per cent compared with 72 per cent. One key reason for this disparity was that 15 per cent of ruptured disc patients injured themselves with exercise, while only 3 per cent of low back sufferers were harmed by it. The point is not to avoid back exercises, but to know which exercises to do and when to do them.

Ruptured disc patients need more exercises aimed at building abdominal strength. Although both strengthening and stretching were important to survey participants recuperating from ruptured discs, most felt that strengthening their abdominal muscles took priority. Low back pain sufferers, on the other hand, put greater emphasis on stretching lower back muscles.

There are two key 'non-back' exercises for chronic ruptured disc pain. In the US survey, fully one-third of ruptured disc patients acclaimed swimming and walking as 100 per cent effective for improving their condition in the long run. Only 5 per cent of low back sufferers performed these exercises regularly. In the UK survey, about a third of all respondents also gained dramatic or moderate long-term relief from swimming and walking.

Movement of Some Kind is Absolutely Essential

Learning how to perform movements that enhance flexibility and strength as well as reduce stress – as soon as possible and as much as possible after acute pain ebbs – is critical to recovery and renewed fitness for practically everyone who has had a ruptured disc. Why practically everyone? No one knows. As mentioned earlier, about one in twenty US survey participants who had a ruptured disc, and who were in bad physical shape to start with, got well and stayed well for more than five years without doing anything about fitness. But this is the exception that proves the rule. The odds are overwhelming that if you don't start a fitness programme as soon as possible, you are likely to remain considerably limited.

Practitioner-Caused Injuries from Back Exercises

'My internist [specialist in internal medicine] told me to do three exercises – sit-ups, single-leg raises, and double-leg raises,' said an assistant TV producer. 'This was after a diagnosis of ruptured disc and three weeks of bed rest. The doctor probably wouldn't have said anything about exercise. But friends had told me so much about the importance of exercise that I asked him to suggest a programme. I did five repetitions of each exercise and the pain immediately afterwards was great. These exercises set me back two weeks. A month later, I went to an orthopaedist and he assigned me to a physical therapist [physiotherapist] who provided me with exercises that helped a great deal. They weren't difficult and I felt at first that was a bad thing. But I could do them and they helped. I still do them ten years later.'

Specific Exercise Suggestions

Full bent-knee sit-ups are not recommended by most US survey participants. And straight-leg sit-ups are taboo. See Chapter 8 for instructions on how to do the modified bent-knee sit-ups recommended by a majority of survey participants. (You may find that full bent-knee sit-ups are feasible for you after at least a month on the modified version.)

Single and double-leg raises are not recommended by most US survey participants with disc problems. In fact, judging from the comments I received, it seems safe to say that the excessive pressure exerted on discs by double-leg raises should be enough to have the exercise outlawed for these back sufferers.

The value of single-leg raises is more debatable. About one-third of survey participants who had surgery for ruptured discs felt that this exercise (described opposite) helped prevent excessive post-operative scarring and subsequent limitations. And these individuals had much better outcomes than their counterparts who underwent surgery but didn't do single-leg raises.

On the other hand, a majority of ruptured disc sufferers who did not have surgery considered single-leg raises potentially harmful. In conclusion, I would suggest that you do the more conservative hamstring stretch described in Chapter 8. If you have had disc surgery, I further suggest that you be willing to try single-leg raises cautiously – if they are prescribed by a competent exercise expert as part of your rehabilitation or maintenance programme.

How to Do a Single-Leg Raise

Lie on your back. Keep one leg bent and extend your other leg flat on the floor. Lock the knee of your extended leg and raise the leg slowly until your foot is about 60 cm (2 feet) off the floor. If you stop the upward motion at this point, you will minimize the pressure on your discs. Holding your leg here – at about a 30-degree angle – for 3 seconds is a good exercise for strengthening your hips. (By the end of the first week, build up to five repetitions with each leg. Then build up to ten repetitions by the end of the second week.)

If you continue raising your leg towards 90 degrees, you will be strengthening your hips and stretching your hamstring muscles. This is the exercise that was recommended, and done successfully after surgery, by one-third of the US survey participants covered in this chapter.

Note: Not many back practitioners recommend stretching your hamstrings by bending over and touching your toes. But you may be told to do this by some specialists. You'll also find this exercise in a number of bestselling exercise books. My advice: don't do it. It simply isn't worth the risk of injury. 'I was in an exercise class touching the floor with the palms of my hands when I heard a "pop",' a business manager wrote. 'I had ruptured my disc and could not straighten up. I wound up in bed. The right exercises are crucial.'

Everyone Can Exercise His or Her Back . . . Even without Doing Back Exercises

An insurance executive summed up the thinking of 22 of 65 ruptured disc patients in the US survey: 'I feel that walking and swimming are more constructive than regular back exercises. They are more relaxing and they keep me in top shape.'

Many survey participants who do back exercises regularly concur. Said a chemist, 'Back exercises help, but walking and swimming are even more essential to maintaining my mobility.'

And survey participants who were in too much pain to do back exercises felt the same way. One retiree said, 'The only exercises I can do without experiencing pain are walking and swimming. Back exercises aggravate my problem (pressure on a nerve from scar tissue). The only thing approaching a back exercise that works for me is lying on the floor with my lower legs draped on a couch. This procedure done a couple of times every day relaxes my back muscles and eases the pain.'

One word of warning about swimming: the kicking leg action of breaststroke may be difficult for people with back pain. But if this is the stroke you prefer, you can easily modify it by doing the breaststroke arm action with a gentle 'crawl' leg action, as if you were doing front crawl.

Should Every Ruptured Disc Sufferer Do Back Exercises?

Yes, in theory. No, in reality. A social worker said, 'After surgery I was given instructions on exercise and scheduled for a few more appointments for instruction after that. Then I was on my own, but I was never able to be free from strain when I exercised. Even though the exercises were taught to me, their risks, benefits and alternatives were never explained. I was simply told that there should not be as much pain as there was.'

A psychologist noted, 'I find that back exercises increase my pain each time I have tried them over the past twenty-five years.'

On the positive side, about 60 per cent of US survey participants with ruptured discs did back exercises regularly and successfully. The following comments illustrate their range of positive feelings.

An author: 'I do my back exercises faithfully twice a day and believe that they help slowly and undramatically.'

A college teacher: 'Sit up! Sit up! Sit-ups help the most for recovery, although it took me a year after I started to exercise for my back to become reasonably normal. Most people don't realize how sophisticated the back structure is and that strengthening the abdominal muscles is essential.' This professor noted that a year and a half after surgery, he could barely walk. No exercises had been recommended by the operating neurosurgeon. Exercises he learned from a physiotherapist gradually brought him back to normal functioning.

A periodontist: 'Daily calisthenics – progressively increasing the workout – is the best way to prevent a recurrence of ruptured disc pain. The most important thing is to strengthen the abdominal musculature so that it can help support the upper body. Also, do flexibility exercises to stretch large muscle groups such as the glutei [in the buttocks] and hamstrings. Sit-ups are best for abdominal muscles. Back sufferers only delude themselves if they remain ignorant of the value of exercise and if they do not become aware of what they – and not someone else – can do to relieve their problems.' This survey participant learned the general principles of exercise, as well as specific exercise routines, from a physiatrist and physiotherapist. He then went on to shape his own daily routine.

Even if You Haven't Been Able to Do Back Exercises Yet, There May Still Be Hope

If you have not been able to do back exercises because of chronic pain from a ruptured disc, don't give up yet. Several US survey participants with ruptured discs, who were initially discouraged or negative about back exercise, eventually found it to be of great value. Some weren't aware of the potential benefits of exercise. Others were told never to exercise. Still others were given the wrong exercises, or were not taught how to exercise, or tried to exercise too soon after the onset of ruptured disc pain. Here are some of their comments:

A management consultant: 'I can function as long as I am faithful (absolutely) to the exercises prescribed by my practitioner. I do them for about 45 minutes each morning and evening.'

A lawyer: 'Go very slow at first and then build up the number of repetitions. I started off at the so-called recommended number of exercises and repetitions, and it cost me another week in bed.'

A truck driver: 'I recommend heat first, then exercises to strengthen abdominal muscles, which relieve pressure on the lower back.'

And a pharmacist who had trouble exercising at first: 'Exercise does not relieve pain, but I push the exercises somewhat in order to keep supple. I also don't do the exercises that everyone else does. My programme is prescribed for me, and it works for me.'

If you aren't doing back exercises, the programme in Chapter 8 may put you on track. These movements are gentle and easy to individualize. If, for any reason, you find the exercises hard to do, stop immediately. If this happens, or if you are not satisfied with your progress, or if you have been advised not to exercise, you could try consulting a physiotherapist, sports medicine specialist, kinesiologist, yoga teacher or physical fitness instructor.

Other Approaches to Chronic Disc Pain

Two chronically disabled ruptured disc patients in the US survey sought medically supervised gravity inversion, with fair to good results. (The treatment is described in Chapter 5.) It is admittedly difficult to find a medical doctor to oversee this approach to relieving back pain, because gravity inversion has not been widely accepted by the medical profession. Chiropractors and physical fitness instructors, however, are making increased use of the technique. You can also attempt to use gravity inversion on your own if you are relatively pain-free.

Spinal fusion, an extreme measure that permanently joins together spinal vertebrae and limits your movement, is a last-ditch measure that fails as often as it succeeds. However, I mention it because three US survey participants found that this surgery restored them to the mainstream of life after all other appropriate measures, including excellent rehabilitation programmes, had failed. They report that getting opinions from at least two surgeons is essential, and they recommend an orthopaedic surgeon rather than a neurosurgeon.

Bear in mind that some UK surgeons often do spinal fusions only at one level on the spine, as this removes movement in that segment. However, this in turn puts an additional burden on the neighbouring segments of the spine and could lead to more rapid degeneration in these sections.

Chapter 10
How to Get Rid of a Pain in the Neck

*Differences between neck pain and other kinds of back pain • Onset
• Diagnosis • Acute, severe neck pain: Staying active • Best sleep positions
• Ice • Self-massage techniques • Prescription drug pitfalls • Manipulation
• Cervical collars • Practitioners to see for neck pain • Chronic neck pain:
Physical, emotional and attitudinal changes • Stress management • Neck
posture • Neck exercises • Integrating neck and shoulder exercises into basic
back regime • Tips on avoiding neck pain while talking on the telephone,
reading, watching television, driving*

'What we have here is low back pain that has travelled north,'
said a doctor to a warehouse foreman who couldn't move his
neck without feeling severe pain.

'There may be some truth in what you say,' replied the survey
participant, who had never suffered low back pain. 'But what
should I do about it?'

'A good question,' the doctor said, reaching for his prescription pad.

It is a good question. The answer, according to US survey participants, has almost nothing to do with viewing neck pain as a bad
back problem that just happened to land higher up on the spine.
There are similarities, of course, between neck pain and low back
pain. But mostly there are differences — major differences in self-
help therapies (including the kinds of exercises to do), in practitioner effectiveness, and in the success rates of a wide variety of
treatments.

Who Can Be Helped By the Information in this Chapter?
About half the US survey's 492 participants had neck pain at one
time or another: a stiff neck when they woke up, a painful neck
after painting a ceiling, a 'crook' in the neck after holding the

telephone in an awkward position during a long conversation. If you are like these people, the first half of this chapter should prove helpful. The second half of the chapter is designed for – and based exclusively on the experiences of – chronic neck pain sufferers, people who have neck discomfort all the time, or who suffer activity-limiting episodes of neck pain.

One-third of the thirty-six chronic neck sufferers in the US survey injured their necks in accidents. And they usually suffered years of pain before learning how to improve their conditions.

'My problems stem from a minor car accident at which time I was rear-ended while stationary in my vehicle,' a human resources director told us. What happened to her reflects the experiences of many people with neck pain: 'I felt fine at first, but the next morning I could barely move my neck.' After trying manipulation, physical therapy, prescription drugs and acupuncture – and after 'a period of being totally immobile due to the most excruciating pain I have ever felt,' this survey participant found the help she needed.

A construction worker's injury also typifies the traumatic origins of most neck pain. 'I was hurt on a construction job and was in the hospital forty-one days,' the worker wrote. 'I saw many doctors. Most had different opinions on the extent of damage done to my back. All I know is that I have suffered severe pain.'

Another one-third of survey participants attributed the onset of neck pain to emotional stress. For example, a television personality suffered neck pain while two members of her immediate family were gravely ill. A teacher linked her neck pain to working with highly disturbed and disabled children. An executive experienced severe neck pain while going through a painful divorce.

The remaining survey participants in this chapter just 'found' themselves with neck pain one day. Some had had the pain for years, but at a nuisance level. Others found that it seemingly struck full blown out of the blue.

'I woke one morning and, for no apparent reason, could not raise my head or move it from left to right,' said a family therapist. Other participants who echoed her words endured pain for months or years before obtaining relief.

Don't Let Them Play Diagnostic Games with Your Neck

It is essential for your peace of mind and your bank account to know that you are not likely to get a highly specific diagnosis for neck pain. In fact, nine times out of ten you will not get the same diagnosis from two different practitioners.

Fortunately, though, this has little bearing on what you can do to improve your condition. Fortunately, too, there is widespread agreement among neck pain sufferers as to which self-help and professional treatments are best at reducing neck pain.

All this having been said, it is still useful to know about the kinds of diagnoses you are likely to receive from various practitioners. At the very least, this knowledge can keep you off the treatment treadmill.

If you see a medical doctor for neck pain, you will probably be told you have cervical strain, muscle strain, cervical derangement or a pinched nerve. If your pain started straight after an accident, whiplash will probably also be mentioned. Just what in your neck is strained, deranged, pinched or whiplashed? And to what extent? With implications for what treatment? It is a rare doctor who can answer these questions.

If you see a chiropractor for neck pain, your diagnosis will probably be misalignment, vertebrae displacement or subluxation. To the uncommon extent that chiropractors agree with doctors, they may both attribute your pain to a pinched nerve. Congenital birth defects such as incompletely formed vertebrae are also popular diagnoses among chiropractors. And no matter what diagnosis you get from a chiropractor, it is likely to be 'pointed out' to you on your X-rays.

Of course, there are cases where the need for a specific diagnosis is critically important. This is especially true if you are a neck pain sufferer with a 'treatment-specific' problem, such as a ruptured cervical disc, fractured cervical vertebra, infection, arthritis or tumour. Of the 36 US survey participants whose experiences are recounted in this chapter, 1 had a fractured cervical vertebra, 2 had ruptured cervical discs and 1 had a benign tumour; the remaining survey participants had more general diagnoses.

How to Relieve Acute, Severe Neck Pain

Avoid Bed Rest, Except When Disabling Accidents Require It
The only neck pain sufferers in this chapter who benefited from bed rest were those involved in disabling accidents. These ranged from car and truck accidents to falling off trampolines and ladders. Most other neck pain sufferers reported that bed rest made them feel worse.

Here, for example, a chemist details his experience with neck pain and bed rest:

'I woke up one morning with an incredibly stiff neck. I had had this kind of pain before from time to time in the morning, although not as intensely, but it had always lessened once I started moving. My neck would bother me some that day and the next day, but that would be it. This time the pain was unbelievable. It took me fifteen minutes to reach out a few feet to the phone on the night table. When I reached my family doctor, he suggested that I rest in bed for two days and then come see him. It didn't work. The longer I lay in one position the stiffer my neck got, so that when I finally wanted to move even a bit, it was all but impossible. I was miserable but better off sitting and walking around. Not much better. But it beat lying there.'

Sleep in a Pain-Preventing Position
The best sleep position is on your back, according to survey participants. The foetal position is next best. Lying on your stomach is the worst position, as it puts the most pressure on your neck. It also strains the rest of your spine.

Use the Right Pillow
A relatively flat pillow is the first choice of survey participants who lie on their backs or sides. A plump pillow raises the head higher than the spine and tends to strain the neck.

If you're accustomed to sleeping on your stomach, make an all-out effort to change this habit. If you cannot, at least avoid using a pillow. Elevating your head while lying on your stomach is bad for your entire spine.

Several orthopaedically designed neck pillows are available (see Product Suppliers, under Useful Addresses, p. 463). However, no

US survey participant felt that using a special pillow helped much to relieve pain or prevent further problems.

Meanwhile, UK respondents reacted rather more positively. The UK survey results were as follows:

Number of patients who rated special pillows in UK survey	464
Provided dramatic long-term relief	12%
Provided moderate long-term relief	20%
Provided temporary relief	39%
Ineffective	23%
Made patient feel worse	6%

You can also try making your own 'butterfly pillow' by tying a bandage or stocking round the middle of a large pillow, or by placing two medium pillows diagonally, slightly overlapping each other, to form a V-shape. Place your head and neck in the 'V'.

Any pillow you use should be positioned under your head and neck, but not under your shoulders. If the pillow is just under your head, your neck won't be supported. If the pillow is under your shoulders, neither your neck nor your head will be adequately supported.

Use Ice Rather than Heat

Ten US survey participants used ice for neck pain and all of them reported good, if temporary, results. Six of these people turned to cold therapy after heat therapy failed to help them. Only ten of twenty neck sufferers who used heat found that it provided relief. Apparently, heat is less effective for neck pain than for back pain. And cold therapy should be tried by more neck sufferers.

Unless your medical condition dictates otherwise, you should try cold treatments for the first 48 hours after the onset of neck strain. You can assume that ice will outperform heat for easing spasming and contracted muscles in your neck and shoulders. It is particularly effective for people with nerve root irritation and any marked inflammation or recent injury. (See pp. 76–8 and 255–6 for details on self-help cold therapy.)

After the first two days, experiment with both ice and heat. Wet heat is the best bet for neck pain – a shower, steam, hot towels and heat pads. Any of these will give better results than a conventional heating pad. (Also, there is no indication that deeper forms of heat, such as ultrasound, are more effective than wet heat.)

Try Self-Massage for Neck Pain

Nine neck pain sufferers in the US survey had success with self-massage.

There is no single magical technique to use. But there are some useful guidelines to follow:

1. Lie in a foetal position with a small pillow under your head and neck and another pillow between your knees. This is a more relaxing position than standing, sitting or lying on your back.
2. Begin by lying on your left side, using your left hand to apply oil or lotion to the right side of your neck, the back of your neck, and your right shoulder.
3. Start the massage directly below your right ear. Apply gentle to moderate pressure with your fingertips, making small circular motions as you work your way down to your shoulder.
4. Go slowly. Relax.
5. Repeat this procedure until you have done as much of your neck and shoulder as you can.
6. Turn onto your right side and complete the massage with your right hand.

In the UK survey, a number of participants had tried self-help treatment using massage/vibrating cushions and found them particularly helpful for temporary pain relief:

Number of patients who rated massage/ vibrating cushions in UK survey	488
Provided dramatic long-term relief	5%
Provided moderate long-term relief	12%
Provided temporary relief	63%
Ineffective	15%
Made patient feel worse	5%

Prescription Medication Can Have Disadvantages

Of the thirteen US neck pain sufferers who took pain medication, nine took prescription painkillers and got no relief at all. Two adverse reactions were reported – dizziness and headaches – from prescription drugs.

There *are* painkillers strong enough to provide some relief for most kinds of severe pain, including debilitating neck pain. But the medications prescribed for survey participants with neck pain, including aspirin with codeine and paracetamol with codeine, didn't work. To make matters worse, some survey participants tried to carry on all their regular activities while taking these pre-scription analgesics – and were disturbed to find their level of alertness slowed down by the medication. According to these participants, aspirin is the best painkiller to take if you want to function and get some pain relief.

Not one of the four US survey participants who took pre-scription muscle relaxants for neck pain got relief. The same is true of the three neck pain sufferers who took prescription anti-inflammatory drugs.

Consider Trying Manipulation, the Most Common Treatment for Acute Neck Pain

Manipulation works relatively well. In the UK, manipulation is offered by some physiotherapists and a minority of GPs, as well as chiropractors and osteopaths. In the US survey, thirty chiro-practors and five osteopaths used manipulation of the neck to help promote recovery from neck pain. Some 60 per cent of these practitioners were able to offer real help. And about 25 per cent of those survey participants who were helped reported that their problems were substantially improved for years, not just for days or weeks.

'I went to a chiropractor, and his manipulation treatments helped tremendously,' said a rugby player who once had severe neck pain. 'I still go every once in a while when I feel it's needed, and the result is that I feel great!'

A warehouse supervisor noted, 'Manipulation helped my neck pain when it was so bad it was painful to breathe.'

The US survey revealed other important conclusions about neck manipulation:

- Manipulation alone is not a complete answer for a majority of patients. However, it is reported to be more effective for neck pain than for back pain, and it gives most neck sufferers enough relief to further their recovery.

- There is some risk of injury or pain. About one in seven survey participants who had neck adjustments said they had been 'injured' or made to feel worse by these treatments. They complained of increased pain for a few days, although they reported no lasting damage. 'I hate the feeling of my neck being "cracked" and I thought it just made the pain worse,' was a typical comment from these participants.

- About one-third of survey participants who were helped by neck manipulation reported temporary, minor aches from the treatment for 24 to 48 hours, followed by relief. 'Sometimes a treatment hurts, maybe for a while, but by the next day I feel great,' a broadcaster said. And a manufacturer's sales representative also felt that some aches were a small price to pay for excellent results: 'No treatments really injured me, although all chiropractic treatments left me stiff for a day or so.'

- Gentle manipulation works best. Most survey participants who had neck manipulation felt strongly about this. In fact, most survey participants who received neck manipulation went to two or more chiropractors before obtaining good results. The most effective of these chiropractors manipulated in a relatively gentle manner, usually after promoting relaxation with heat and massage. Word of mouth appears to be the only way to find this kind of practitioner.

'Gentle manipulation helps the most,' concluded a caterer. 'Anything else is too nerve-racking. You can't call and ask, "Are you gentle?" But I regret having seen chiropractors who used rougher techniques.'

An importer who suffered terrible neck pain and headaches despite more than two years under orthopaedic surgeons' care, found relief after treatment by chiropractors. 'Look for a chiropractor who will take his time,' he advised. 'That is the key because it does take more time to adjust your neck in a non-stressful way.'

Avoid Cervical Collars

You've probably seen someone at one time or another wearing an awkward, bulky-looking collar around his or her neck. If you currently have acute and severe neck pain yourself, this recollection may immediately prompt you to ask, 'Would a cervical collar help me?'

The answer is: probably not. Medical research offers no conclusive indication that the average neck pain sufferer would benefit from wearing a cervical collar. And of the five US survey participants who wore collars for pinched-nerve neck pain, only one found it helpful.

If the point of wearing a collar is to keep you out of physically stressful positions – dropping your chin towards your chest when reading, for example – you would probably be better off learning to hold your neck properly without an aid. Eventually you will have to learn to do this on your own anyway.

If, on the other hand, there is a compelling medical reason for immobilizing your neck – the risk of permanent nerve damage, for example – then you will need to wear a cervical collar. After you remove it, however, you must still work to restore lost muscle strength and flexibility. The exercises in this chapter will help you achieve that goal.

What You Should Know about the Most Widely Seen Practitioners for Neck Pain

Twenty-six out of thirty-six US survey participants covered in this chapter saw orthopaedic surgeons for neck pain – and only three of these individuals got any help at all – either temporary or long-term. Of the remaining twenty-three cases, not one reported getting any kind of positive or useful advice or treatment.

'Orthopaedic surgeons will say almost anything to get rid of a chronic neck sufferer,' said a typist. 'Their knowledge about muscle strain, necks, or chronic pain is close to nil . . .'

An editor also found a lack of skill and constructive attitude: 'The orthopaedic surgeon was very offhand about my injury. He called it mild whiplash and said it would improve by itself within a few months. But it turned out that the pain was very intense for a year.'

In case after case, orthopaedic surgeons' negative attitudes toward chronic neck pain precluded any effort on their part to help, unless obvious pathology, malformation or injury was present. Said a management consultant, 'The orthopaedic surgeon acted as though I was there just for the insurance claim.'

A musician wrote, 'The orthopaedic surgeons acted as if I were faking my pain. They said they saw nothing at all.'

There are a few positive points to be made. Two survey participants with ruptured cervical discs got excellent results from surgery performed by orthopaedic surgeons. And one survey participant felt relieved of stress after an orthopaedic surgeon conducted a thorough examination that ruled out any serious medical problem. However, there is no escaping the reality that, for nine out of ten US survey respondents, orthopaedic surgeons were not helpful for neck pain.

Holistic Chiropractic Care Was Sometimes Helpful

The results of chiropractic care for low back pain weren't especially impressive, falling far short of physical medicine and other disciplines for relieving back pain. Too often, chiropractic care left low back sufferers dissatisfied because (1) improvement was short-lived; (2) patients were in constant need of additional treatments – with no end in sight; and (3) the vast majority of patients were not helped to reach what presumably was their ultimate goal: self-sufficiency, or knowing how to take care of themselves in the long run.

However, these disadvantages did not apply to total chiropractic care (as opposed to manipulation alone) for neck pain. Here, results were generally more lasting. Most patients completed their treatments in less than eight weeks. And nearly half of all patients learned how to prevent pain from recurring.

Massage Therapists Are Remarkably Effective at Providing Substantive, Temporary Relief

Seventeen of nineteen US survey participants reported a 90 per cent chance of getting badly needed relief for neck pain from Swedish massage. Most individuals who received Swedish massage for neck pain got one or two full days of relief. This contrasts sharply with the effect of Swedish massage on low back pain – where a lower percentage of people were helped and where only a few hours' relief was the norm. And neck pain sufferers, who are dealt additional pain all too often by a variety of practitioners, reported 'no harm done' even when the massage brought no relief.

Shiatsu, or acupressure massage, was tried by four survey participants with neck pain. And the results, though statistically insignificant, were promising. Three of the four got enough temporary relief to further their progress, and the other reported dramatic, long-term relief after five treatments.

In the UK, massage may be available on the NHS, via your GP or physiotherapist. If not, self-massage for neck pain is one solution (see p. 196). Alternatively, you could try contacting the British Massage Therapy Council (see Useful Addresses, p. 463), to locate a reputable local practitioner.

In addition, survey participants strongly recommend that you do some comparison shopping among massage therapists. Prices vary widely. A higher price often means a more expensive environment rather than a higher-quality massage.

Here are additional suggestions from survey participants:

- Have a full body massage. A complete massage, with special attention to your neck, is more relaxing and beneficial than a neck massage alone.
- Find a massage therapist you like and respect. Then stay with that person for a series of massages. It takes time even for a skilled practitioner to know your body and your needs.
- Consider trying Shiatsu therapy (see p. 92). It is highly effective for relieving low back pain, and it seems promising for neck pain sufferers as well. One note of caution: reject any Shiatsu therapist who is applying too much pressure. Some discomfort from Shiatsu therapy is normal, but your judgement about pain tolerance is superior to any practitioner's.

How to Banish Chronic Neck Pain

Try to Integrate Different Therapies
No matter where your back hurts, it takes more than one kind of therapy – making more than one change in your life – to free

yourself of pain. This is especially true of neck pain, where no single approach to healing provided long-term help for the majority of neck pain sufferers in the US survey. Chronic neck pain sufferers who did away with disabling pain included at least two, and often all three, of the following changes in their lives:

1. Physical change – posture and exercise
2. Emotional change – relaxation through exercise or stress-reduction techniques
3. Attitudinal change – a different philosophy about everyday activities

Survey participants reiterate that change in any one of these areas is unlikely to control chronic neck pain – that the 'single magic step' to relief is more myth than reality. But positive steps in all three areas will give you an excellent chance for a total recovery.

Reduce Stress – A Greater Factor in Neck Pain than in Any Other Kind of Back Pain

'Does your back get worse when you are under stress?'

I asked this question of every US survey participant. And 83 per cent of neck pain sufferers answered, 'Yes.'

Not only is this statistic a full one-third higher than the average for all back sufferers, but neck pain sufferers were also more vocal about the pain-causing role of stress and the consequent need to change their lives in order to reduce stress and promote recovery.

A children's author said, 'All the physical therapy [physiotherapy] and neck and back exercises and everything else you can think of did not get rid of my neck pain, because it failed to touch the basis of the pain – stress. In spite of all my good intentions, I sit over the typewriter, tense up, become absorbed in my work, and by the time I realize it, my neck is in grim shape. What worked for me – in addition to everything else I was doing – was taking breaks every hour and jogging (which I love) in the middle of the day to prevent the build-up of accumulated tension.'

'What helped me the most was learning to relax,' a clerk typist wrote. 'Other things helped – professional massage therapy, my own exercises, and not sleeping on my stomach. But the biggest improvement came after I found a way to leave my troubles behind by joining a health club. There, I could really relax.'

'The worst neck pain I ever experienced occurred when two members of my immediate family were gravely ill and I was functioning under the assumption that I did not need to slow down under stress,' an assistant professor commented. She added, 'A psychotherapist explored the emotional stress of these crises with me, and that helped. On the other hand, an ortho-paedic surgeon discouraged my thinking about psychosomatic factors. He seemed to want to convince me that a medical injury in childhood accounted for my problem.'

This latter point – the inability or refusal of some doctors to talk about stress – fuelled the anxiety felt by many neck pain sufferers. It also tended to delay their seeking ways to control stress. In answer to another survey question about stress, US neck pain sufferers reported that only five of forty-six medical doctors 'mentioned stress in a constructive way'.

An office manager underscored this point when she reported, 'I have seen many physicians. Their attitude is that I am a healthy-looking and athletic young woman, so I can't have back or neck problems. It is all in my head. I therefore suffer from "neurosis". (This word is mine; doctors dare not actually say neurotic. They just hint at it.)'

And an electrical engineer explained, 'It isn't a question of wanting your hand held or having a daddy figure tell you that everything will be okay. It's a matter of respect for another person's pain. Anyone who can lift your spirits can also help you to mobilize your own resources against pain. But this seems to be too much to ask of a doctor. At least it was more than I got from the doctors I saw for chronic neck pain!'

Because of the high incidence of stress among neck pain sufferers, it is important to keep three points in mind:

First, if and when a medical doctor talks to you about stress, what he or she says may not be accurate.

Second, there is a small but significant chance that a serious medical condition is causing your neck pain and that this condi-tion will be overlooked because your pain will be dismissed as stress-caused. So if you have doubts about your medical problem not having been taken seriously, dispel these doubts by getting a thorough check-up – more than a quick look and another X-ray to add to the pile – including a CT scan or whatever else is needed to provide an answer.

Third, you will need to take decisive steps to manage your stress.

A slight majority of neck pain sufferers were able to manage stress by themselves, simply by doing something pleasurable and athletic. They joined a health club. They walked, swam or jogged. They took up Tai Chi or modern dance.

Other survey participants got short-term professional help. One learned visualization techniques from a mental health counsellor. Another learned yoga from an instructor. Two survey participants underwent psychotherapy. Still another got instruction in meditation.

Since stress management is a burgeoning and chaotic industry these days, this final comment, from a horticulturist, provides some much-needed perspective: 'Yes, I think that stress aggravates my neck pain. And, yes, I have learned to control it with a three-mile walk every day, come rain or shine. But I feel humble about this. I don't think that anyone, professional or otherwise, should get too preachy about stress. It is an area where there are more unknowns than knowns. The existence of stress is sometimes an excuse to treat back and neck sufferers poorly, or not treat them at all. On the other hand, the individual with an ulcer or heart condition caused by stress will be taken seriously because his problem is now a disease that can be seen and treated. My advice is to do something nice for yourself every day, some kind of exercise that will restore you, please you and put you in control. In other words, don't let about a million stress experts out there drive you crazy.'

Improve Your Neck Posture – An Effective but Seldom-Used Way to Ease Chronic Pain

With all the talk about the need for good posture to reduce back pain, correct alignment at the top of the spine got little attention from most survey participants. But take a moment now to consider your neck posture because those few survey participants who improved theirs, no matter how slightly, reaped great dividends in comfort.

'I looked in the mirror one day and realized I always cocked my head to one side, and that was the beginning of the end of twenty years of neck pain,' an assembly line worker said.

And a court stenographer found that the key to alleviating neck pain as well as low back pain was to follow a physiotherapist's advice to 'keep your chin in line with the rest of your body instead of jutting out in front.'

Here are two specific suggestions from survey participants for facilitating good neck posture:

1. Manoeuvre your way into correct posture. Try to make yourself a couple of centimetres taller for an instant by stretching your neck and head skywards. Now relax and let your chin tuck in slightly, instead of jutting or drooping. Doing this a few times during the day is a good way to position your neck correctly.
2. Use the ball-on-flagpole concept. Another good way to check and correct your neck posture is to visualize a ball (your head) perched on top of a flagpole (your spine). Keeping this image in mind will help you to maintain good neck posture and avoid future episodes of neck pain.

Neck Exercises – Often Overlooked but Effective and Helpful

Only 35 per cent of US survey participants with neck pain did exercises to improve neck fitness. And only about half of neck pain sufferers were even aware that exercise could add strength and flexibility to their neck muscles.

But neck exercises *do* help. Of the seventeen survey participants who did neck exercises, four had temporary relief, seven reported moderate long-term improvement, and three showed dramatic long-term improvement.

These results don't match the gains from doing exercises for low back pain, but they are impressive, nevertheless, since 59 per cent of survey participants with neck pain who exercised showed some long-term improvement. When you consider that there was no difference in success between survey participants who learned neck exercises on their own and survey participants who got professional instruction, you may decide to include the easy-to-learn neck exercises explained on the next page in your daily routine.

Before you try them, however, keep the following general rules in mind:

Neck exercises are best combined with low back exercises. Most survey participants with neck pain also had low back pain or occasional low back discomfort. And they found it helpful to combine neck exercises with back exercises in a regular routine. Later in this chapter, I will suggest how this can be done.

Neck exercises are as important for promoting relaxation as for building fitness. Most neck exercises are designed as much to relieve tension as they are to stretch and strengthen muscles. A few should be incorporated into your exercise routine, but the rest may be done as your stress or discomfort dictates – while at work, during a break, on waking, before bedtime – any time.

Neck exercises can be learned in minutes. You may recall from the chapter on low back pain that survey participants with activity-limiting pain maximized their progress with the help of professional exercise instruction. This is usually not the case with neck pain sufferers. You can quickly learn most neck exercises on your own.

Try the following neck and shoulder exercises along with the low back exercises in Chapter 8. The best place in the low back routine to add the following neck exercises is straight after Exercise 3 on pp. 169–70. Or you can add them to any back exercise routine after doing a few warm-up stretches.

Shoulder stretch
Lie in the Basic Position (on your back, knees bent, feet flat on the floor, arms at your sides). Raise one arm and lower it to the floor behind your head, stretching but not straining to extend the arm fully. Relax for a second. Repeat this exercise with your other arm. Alternate arms and do five repetitions with each.

Shoulder shrug
While in the Basic Position, count slowly to five while shrugging your shoulders towards your ears. Lower your shoulders and relax for a second. Repeat five times.

Neck roll

Start from the Basic Position, but with your chin tucked in a couple of centimetres towards your chest. Turn your head towards one shoulder. When you feel resistance, hold it there for three seconds. Return to the Basic Position and relax for a second, then turn your head towards the other shoulder. Do five repetitions.

Comment: These exercises are intended to relax you and keep your neck muscles stretched and flexible. A few survey participants asked if they could do these exercises when they had some discomfort. We put the question to other survey participants, who said yes. In fact, they tended to do these exercises more when they had discomfort. Keep in mind, of course, that no exercise should be done if it turns mild discomfort into pain.

You can do the following neck and shoulder exercises at work and on the go.

Note: All exercises in this section should be done from a sitting position to reduce the risk of losing your balance.

Warning: Do not attempt these exercises if you have dizziness, double vision or difficulty in breathing or swallowing. These could be symptoms of vertebral basilar artery insufficiency (VBI). This condition affects the blood supply to the brain. If this blood supply is affected by stretching or turning exercises it could result in a life-threatening stroke.

Bending

Tilt your head towards one shoulder. After you feel resistance, pause for three seconds. Return to the straight-ahead position and relax. Now tilt your head towards your other shoulder. Continue to alternate and do five repetitions on each side. Take care not to raise your shoulder to meet your ear. Many people cheat on this exercise!

Standing shoulder roll

The objective here is to move both your shoulders in a small circular motion at the same time. Simply shrug your shoulders up, roll them forward as if you were trying to make a circle, then return them to a normal position. Relax. Repeat three times. You can vary this exercise by shrugging and rolling one shoulder at a time, backwards or forwards.

Range of motion movement

If you tend not to move around much while working, and you feel your neck tightening up, here are four easy movements you can do while sitting: turn your head as far as you can to the left, then as far as you can to the right. Lower your head towards your chest, then raise it until you are looking straight up.

Dos and Don'ts That Can Benefit You Every Hour of Every Day

Don't talk your way into neck pain

Survey participants with neck pain were unanimous in pointing out that the telephone is not 'user friendly'. To put this another way, if you bend someone's ear on the phone, you are likely to bend your own neck out of shape. Indeed, long telephone conversations gave more survey participants a pain in the neck than did any other daily activity.

What to do? Don't cradle the phone between your head and shoulder. This position puts tremendous and continuous strain on your neck muscles. If you must keep your hands free while you're talking on the telephone, get a speaker-phone. A wide range of speaker-phone equipment is available from telephone and electronic appliance retailers, and on the Internet. (Cradle-shaped objects that attach to your phone make it slightly easier to hold the phone without using your hands, but they don't prevent neck pain.) It is also advisable to use the telephone in your non-dominant hand in order to leave your dominant hand free for writing and other activities.

Finally, if you're talking for more than 10 minutes, switch the telephone to your other ear. This may feel awkward at first, but will save your neck a lot of grief.

Do learn how to read without straining your neck

Reading is the next biggest source of trouble for neck pain sufferers. 'I start off in a straight-backed chair at a desk. I hold the book on the desk. And I vow to keep my head straight, instead of bending my neck towards the book. Then, I become absorbed in the reading, and before I know it, the book is in my lap and my chin is almost in my lap, too.' So said an executive search consultant who finds, as do many other survey participants, that exaggerating the downward tilt of the chin while reading causes and aggravates neck pain.

The best solution, of course, is to will yourself not to read or do paperwork with your chin on your chest. Another solution, if willpower alone won't suffice, is to buy a book holder from an office equipment supplier and prop it on your desk.

'Getting nice and comfortable and reading in bed' is virtually impossible if you have neck pain. It is absolutely impossible if you have neck pain and low back pain. Avoid putting reading material on your abdomen and straining your neck downward to see it. Likewise, avoid holding reading material over your head while you're lying down; the strain on your shoulders will affect your neck and your back. (Reading while lying down and looking up can also cause eyestrain.)

Don't strain your neck watching TV

Improper neck position while watching television is another common cause of neck strain. So sit in a good chair and keep your television at or near eye level. If you must watch TV in bed, the least stressful way is to lie on your side with a pillow under your neck. (A rule of thumb: if you would not be able to sleep comfortably in the position you're lying in to watch TV, you're lying in the wrong position.)

You definitely shouldn't lie in bed or on a sofa in a position that requires you to look down to watch TV. You shouldn't have to peer over your feet, or anything else, to see the screen.

Do relax your neck and shoulders while driving

Driving long distances, especially during bad weather or in heavy traffic, can cause a troublesome neck to flare up. Using a headrest is essential (especially as it could save your life if you have an accident). It is also important to take an adequate number of breaks – preferably every half an hour – and do some of the neck and shoulder exercises explained in the preceding section.

Chapter 11
How to Relieve Osteoarthritis-Based Back Pain

Diagnostic terms • Medical specialists who can help • Medical practitioners with less to offer • Guidelines for getting the most out of medical care • Non-medical practitioners • Prescribed and recommended treatments • Self-care • Tips from survey participants

Osteoarthritis back sufferers have a lot of questions. Do doctors take osteoarthritis of the spine seriously? Should you see a doctor? If so, what kind of doctor? And for what kind of help? This chapter provides answers, not from practitioners but from other, clearer voices – osteoarthritis back sufferers themselves.

Please note: The information and tips in this chapter apply only to individuals with osteoarthritis, and not to those with any other forms, such as rheumatoid arthritis or ankylosing spondylitis.

Taken as a group, the forty-seven US survey participants with osteoarthritis can answer your questions, bolster your spirits, and alert you to specific, practical techniques for shaking free of the pain and restrictions you encounter daily.

Here are a few of the questions they've answered:

1. How effective are various non-medical practitioners in helping osteoarthritis back sufferers? And how do they compare with medical specialists?
2. Which of many treatments touted as curative actually help back sufferers with osteoarthritis? Which have no effect? Which make matters worse? And which are at least worth a try?
3. What about diet and nutritional remedies? Do they have any value?

4. To what extent can exercise affect the outcome of spinal arthritis cases?
5. Should you ignore healthcare professionals and treat yourself?

Do You Have Osteoarthritis Back Pain by Another Name?

Osteoarthritis was the diagnostic term applied most commonly to survey participants who had a wear-and-tear disorder of the joints in their spines. But even medical doctors didn't use the same terminology to describe the same condition. Hence you may have osteoarthritis-based back pain if you were given any of the following diagnoses: degenerative arthritis . . . degenerative joint disease . . . degenerative disc disease . . . spondylitis (which literally means inflammation of the spine, although some doctors use the term to describe a bacterial infection of the spine) . . . spondylolysis (or defective vertebra) . . . degenerative hydrotrophic spondylitis . . . or bone spurs.

If you're thinking that this amounts to another confusing and unfunny back-pain name game, you're right. It's hardly funny and it is confusing, but don't let it throw you. Although you can't cure osteoarthritis, you can reduce or eliminate its symptoms and its physical limitations. Read on.

Professional Care: Can a Medical Doctor Help You?

Most kinds of medical doctors cannot help you, according to US survey participants. Only a few kinds of medical specialists can. Three out of four medical doctors seen by survey participants reportedly failed to provide them with any degree of long-term help. The major reason was ineffectual treatment consisting almost exclusively of medication, which by itself did relatively little to curb osteoarthritis pain.

These doctors did not prescribe physiotherapy. Most didn't even mention the need for movement, exercise, weight control or corrective daily habits and activities. They presumably knew these factors were important − usually essential − to a successful outcome, but they chose to start and end their treatment with medication.

It can be misleading, of course, to talk about medical doctors in general. So let's look at how well the most frequently seen doctors actually did, with an eye towards specific recommendations for you.

Medical Doctors Who Work with Physiotherapists: A Winning Formula

The odds of your controlling the symptoms of osteoarthritis, and living without limitations, increase dramatically if you see a medical doctor who either assumes the role of a physiotherapist or refers you to a physiotherapist. In fact, you have a 90 per cent chance of getting long-term help from physiotherapy under medical supervision.

Physiotherapy, which uses natural means of healing to help you move more freely – and which depends a great deal on good rapport between practitioner and patient – was the key to success for the majority of spinal arthritis sufferers in the US survey.

Rheumatologists: The Best Medical Doctors for Osteoarthritis Sufferers

The rheumatologist, who specializes in arthritis and related diseases, can provide you with a complete recovery programme, from a specific diagnosis (and a better explanation of that diagnosis than you would get from other medical doctors) to the information you need to be your own doctor as much as possible.

Of the eight US survey participants with osteoarthritis who saw rheumatologists, five got moderate long-term help and one got temporary relief.

Orthopaedic Surgeons: Better than GPs but Not Especially Helpful

The orthopaedic surgeon's record of success with osteoarthritis sufferers is better than his record with all other categories of back pain. Yet, according to the US survey, the chances are only about three in ten that you will receive long-term help from an orthopaedic surgeon for spinal arthritis.

Of the fifty-nine orthopaedic surgeons who treated osteoarthritis sufferers in the US survey, thirteen helped bring about moderate long-term improvement and four helped patients achieve dramatic long-term improvement.

The difference between effective and ineffective orthopaedic surgeons in treating osteoarthritis usually depends on the individual doctor's willingness to apply his knowledge. Chronic back problems such as osteoarthritis take real effort on the part of both the patient and the practitioner. And the outcome of any case depends largely on what you come away with from the doctor's office, not what is 'done' to you during your visit.

GPs, Family Doctors and Junior Doctors: A Lack of Interest and Knowledge

'Take two aspirin and call me' might not be bad initial advice from a general practitioner who tells you that you have osteoarthritis-based back pain. Aspirin and other anti-inflammatory drugs are, at best, merely a starting point for treating osteoarthritis. Yet, in the US survey, a full 80 per cent of doctors limited their treatment solely to medication. Sometimes these doctors mentioned the need to lose weight, reduce stress or increase exercise activities. However, no therapy other than medication was specified.

Of the thirty-four GPs who treated osteoarthritis sufferers in the US survey, five provided moderate long-term relief and two provided dramatic long-term relief.

The failure of some general practitioners even to make an appropriate referral makes it more likely that some patients, out of sheer frustration, will eventually seek help from so-called 'quacks'.

Conclusions about Medical Doctors

- If your family doctor can't give you the help you need, and he or she may not be able to, ask to be referred to a rheumatologist or pain management clinic. See Chapter 3 for further information about rheumatologists and pain management clinics.
- Be sceptical about suggestions that pills or surgery are the only answers. They seldom are. At least get a second opinion from a rheumatolgist about the need for medication or surgery. No one should limit his or her recovery programme to medication or surgery alone.
- Try not to let the gloom-and-doom attitude of some medical doctors ('I can only promise you a continuation of pain because

there is no cure for osteoarthritis') make you sink into despair. There are almost always ways to live a full life in spite of severe spinal osteoarthritis. The answer is appropriate information. And this information is available.

• You can probably enhance any doctor's course of treatment by looking over the self-help approaches presented later in this chapter. They represent the most popular suggestions made by osteoarthritis-based back sufferers who learned how to overcome disabling pain.

Non-Medical Practitioners

Chiropractors: Less Effective than Medical Doctors

According to US survey participants, chiropractic treatments for osteoarthritis-based back pain were usually a waste of time and money. Of the twenty-seven chiropractors who treated osteo-arthritis back sufferers, only four provided moderate long-term relief and none provided dramatic long-term relief. The four chiropractors who helped did not rely exclusively on manipula-tion. They offered counsel about exercise and lifestyle, and this advice was the key to whatever success the patients achieved.

Eight of twenty-seven chiropractors provided survey partici-pants with temporary relief through manipulation or, more com-monly, through a combination of manipulation and other treatments such as massage, ultrasound and electric stimulation. But the duration of this relief was brief – often just a matter of hours, and not enough to help survey participants make long-term gains.

A newspaper columnist expressed the feelings of many US survey participants about chiropractic care for osteoarthritis: 'The chiropractor seemed to help a bit, but I needed to learn to deal with the problem myself, as my back would slip out after I left the office.'

Physiotherapists: A Superior Record for Helping Osteoarthritis Sufferers

Physiotherapy for osteoarthritis-based back pain is given consid-erable emphasis in medical textbooks. However, some medical doctors don't make appropriate referrals to physiotherapists.

Of the fifteen physiotherapists who treated survey participants with osteoarthritis-based back pain, fourteen succeeded in improving the long-term quality of the patients' lives. Individualization was crucial, especially in areas of movement and exercise, as well as in teaching patients to make adjustments in the way they went about their everyday activities.

Who Else Can Help?

Nine yoga instructors and physical fitness instructors treated osteoarthritis sufferers in the US survey – and all nine helped these individuals to get better and stay better.

When you consider the high success rate of these yoga and physical fitness practitioners in helping low back sufferers – and their skill in teaching movements that foster fluidity and fitness – it becomes even more apparent that they can offer excellent opportunities for improvement.

Two participants gained similar help from Tai Chi instruction.

Prescribed and Recommended Treatments for Osteoarthritis-Based Back Pain

Anti-Inflammatory Drugs Often Don't Work Well

Although 'arthritis' means joint inflammation, most medical authorities agree that the typical osteoarthritis sufferer does not have inflammation. Nevertheless, doctors often prescribe anti-inflammatory drugs for osteoarthritis, as well as for other kinds of non-inflammation back conditions, including low back pain.

Half the US survey participants mentioned in this chapter took prescription anti-inflammatory drugs such as Motrin and Indomethacin. Here are the results:

Number of people treated in US survey	22
Provided temporary relief	7 (32%)
Ineffective	11 (50%)
Made patient feel worse	4 (18%)

These ratings are comparable to those in Chapter 5, for all participants in the US survey who took prescription anti-inflammatory medication. In the UK survey, 80 per cent of the

837 participants who took prescription anti-inflammatories for all types of back pain gained some degree of relief, though for 50 per cent the relief was only temporary.

Aspirin, which has both anti-inflammatory and analgesic value, was taken by thirteen US survey participants with osteoarthritis – and provided relief in ten cases (77 per cent). This parallels the 78 per cent relief rate reported by all US survey participants who took aspirin for back pain.

Tips on How to Take Aspirin

Aspirin is the only medication that relieved pain for a majority of participants in the US survey. Its use is so widespread that Americans consume about 50 billion tablets of this 'miracle drug' every year. However, the unpleasant side-effects of long-term aspirin use include: bleeding in the stomach, stomach upsets, heartburn, ulcers and tinnitus (ringing in the ears). Assuming that you may want to take aspirin on occasion, but find that it upsets your stomach, here are some tips from survey participants about ways to reduce discomfort from this medication:

- Take aspirin that has been buffered with an antacid. (This may reduce stomach upsets but probably won't protect you against ulcers in the long term.) Ask your pharmacist to recommend a good brand.
- Take aspirin with an over-the-counter antacid.
- Ask your healthcare practitioner about enteric-coated aspirin. The coating lets the aspirin pass through your stomach and into your small intestine, where it dissolves and is absorbed into your bloodstream.
- Take aspirin while sitting or standing rather than lying down. Remain upright for about 2 minutes. An upright position speeds the tablet's journey through the oesophagus, thereby preventing irritation of this organ.

Prescription Analgesics Get Results but Have Their Drawbacks

Prescription analgesics (painkillers) are more effective for osteoarthritis than for other kinds of back pain. Twenty-five US survey participants in this chapter took prescription painkillers – including paracetamol, Equagesic, codeine, and Tylex-codeine combinations. Here are the results:

Number of people treated in US survey	25
Provided temporary relief	12 (48%)
Ineffective	11 (44%)
Made patient feel worse	2 (8%)

Any drug with codeine in it is potentially addictive. So it is important to note that only three of twenty-five US survey participants took analgesics for more than a month at a time. Nausea and constipation were the two main side-effects.

Constipation can be eased by eating more fruit, vegetables, pulses and wholegrain foods, such as brown bread, brown rice and wholewheat pasta. It's also worth trying over-the-counter preparations such as lactulose (a sugar solution that softens stools).

Muscle-Relaxant Pills May Not Help

According to US survey participants, muscle relaxants don't seem to have much value for osteoarthritis-based back pain – or for any other kind of common back ailment for that matter.

Twelve of this chapter's survey participants took prescription muscle-relaxant pills, including Robaxin and Parafon Forte. The results are comparable to those reported by all ninety-five survey participants who took this type of medication:

Number of spinal osteoarthritis sufferers who took muscle relaxants in the US survey	12
Provided temporary relief	4 (33%)
Ineffective	8 (67%)
Made patient feel worse	0

More positively, in the UK survey, 82 per cent of the 413 participants who took prescription muscle relaxants for all types of back pain gained some degree of help. However, as with anti-inflammatories, about half of these respondents only gained temporary relief.

Massage Gets Few Raves from Survey Participants

In every category of back pain covered thus far, Swedish massage was effective at least for its relaxation value. And Shiatsu therapy got outstanding ratings for short-term relief, with some promise of lasting results. However, there is no indication that any form of massage is worthwhile for helping spinal osteoarthritis pain.

Of the eight US survey participants with this problem who tried Swedish massage, only two felt slight relief. And in no case was pain markedly eased.

None of the five who tried acupressure and other forms of massage, such as polarity and connective tissue massage, reported any gains whatsoever.

Surgery May Not Be Worth the Risks

As anyone reading this chapter knows, osteoarthritis is hardly the 'minor aches and pains' ailment some people believe it to be. Several US survey participants with osteoarthritis had disc degeneration, bone spurs and other arthritis-related problems that put pressure on nerve roots – resulting in pain, disability and questions about surgery.

The pros and cons of having ruptured disc surgery are relatively clear-cut (see Chapters 5 and 9). But the advantages and drawbacks of surgery for nerve compression caused by degenerative discs and bone spurs are far less obvious.

Five osteoarthritis sufferers in the US survey had surgery. There was one striking success which transformed a patient's life, one case where the patient became worse as a result of surgery, and three cases where the survey participants themselves weren't sure whether surgery had done them any good.

Let's look at the two extremes:

Case 1

Osteoarthritis of the spine had increasingly disabled a 39-year-old man who worked as a truck driver and loader. Over a period of years, he had been treated by a general practitioner, a physiotherapist and a chiropractor. An orthopaedic surgeon then pinpointed his problem as degenerative arthritis, with a bone spur and segments of broken disc causing excruciating sciatica pain. The orthopaedic surgeon referred the patient to a neurosurgeon, who corrected the problem by surgically removing the bone spur and shattered disc.

'The neurosurgeon was my salvation,' the truck driver said. 'The operation provided me with the first relief from years of agonizing and sometimes paralysing pain. I can only recommend seeing the appropriate specialists who can correct the problem, rather than waste time, money, and prolong the agony like I did.'

Happily, judging from research published in medical journals, this success is not a rare, isolated instance. Numerous similar cases have been reported.

Case 2

A 58-year-old housewife had essentially the same diagnosis as the truck driver mentioned above – disc degeneration as well as bone spurs that were putting pressure on her sciatic nerve. After seeing orthopaedic surgeons, a neurologist, a rheumatologist and a chiropractor – and becoming increasingly incapacitated with pain – she agreed to have exploratory surgery to see if the nerve pressure could be relieved.

The surgery wasn't successful. There was no relief. In fact, the pain seemed worse after surgery. 'I suffered terribly after surgery,' this woman said. 'I have been on strong pain medication and a tranquillizer for the past five years. I have bought everything on the market trying to get rid of pain. I still suffer each day when I walk, sit, or stand.'

So, what are the conclusions about the role of surgery in helping spinal osteoarthritis?

- *Nerve root pressure occasionally requires surgery.* Crippling sciatica, caused by pressure from a bone spur, does not always respond to medication and physiotherapy.
- *Rates of success are arguable.* Differences in the kinds of surgery for osteoarthritis, and in the reported outcomes of these cases, make it impossible to give a rule of thumb about the chances of a successful recovery.

There is no question that osteoarthritis of the spine can cause severe impairment of normal functioning. But if the treatments and approaches discussed in this chapter are applied when symptoms first appear – and if activity and exercise are emphasized – there is rarely a need for surgery.

Self-Care

Exercise, Though Not a Panacea, Is Essential

'I can't emphasize enough how important exercise is to anyone with osteoarthritis of the spine,' an assistant museum curator said.

A retired florist wrote: 'Exercise does not make me feel better per se, but I believe that it prevents further deterioration and it also helps me to live as actively as possible.'

And Stephanie, a UK survey respondent, commented: 'Personally I think self-help is the only thing that got me through my back pain. I focused on strengthening my core stability and improving my flexibility – even when it was agony doing any exercise at all.'

The facts: two out of three US survey participants with osteoarthritis did back exercises regularly, and were helped by them. More important, four out of five survey participants with osteoarthritis did some form of exercise on a regular basis – with excellent results.

Unlike low back sufferers, osteoarthritis-based back sufferers who performed back exercises did not have a lower pain rating than those who shunned exercise. Nevertheless, there is widespread agreement among spinal arthritis sufferers that back exercise helps them function better.

You should certainly do gentle stretching exercises. Survey participants found them essential for continued flexibility. And stretching exercises are important because many osteoarthritis deformities can be avoided or reduced by gently and regularly stretching each movable joint to its full range of motion.

The exercise routine outlined in Chapter 8 should suit your needs.

However, osteoarthritis sufferers in the US survey advised doing just one set of ten modified bent-knee sit-ups.

What Other Kinds of Exercises Should You Do?

You should walk. Walking at least 1.6 km (1 mile) a day helped eight out of eight survey participants make long-term progress.

You should swim. Five survey participants in this chapter swam at least 15 minutes every other day. And all five were convinced that swimming, a non-weight-bearing exercise, was the ideal therapy for osteoarthritis sufferers.

Two UK survey participants made the following comments:

'I am recently retired and, along with the osteoarthritis, am struggling with coming to terms with my change of life. A daily power type walk or cycle helps to keep me positive – having achieved something – when the temptation would be to sit back and succumb to "woe is me". It's not always easy but the reward is good.'

'Several years of twice-weekly front crawl seem to have strengthened my back sufficiently to avoid problems and allow me to lead a pain-free life. I also strongly recommend the exercises contained in a book called *Treat Your Own Back* [see Further Reading, p. 471] for coping when pain returns.'

Dr James F. Fries, author of *Arthritis: A Comprehensive Guide*, points out that activities such as walking and swimming increase strength in the bones and ligaments around worn joints. Dr Fries also believes that activity helps cartilage (which has no blood supply) to obtain the nourishment it needs to prevent deterioration.

Other activities that osteoarthritis back sufferers may find beneficial include dancing (on a sprung floor), aquaerobics (ask at your local swimming pool), hydrotherapy (see p. 432) and Tai Chi (see p. 53).

Note: If you haven't had a thorough examination, the extent of your joint damage should be evaluated before you start any exercise programme. And if your condition is severe, you should try to have an exercise programme prescribed for you by a physiotherapist.

Nutrition and Vitamins: Cures or Quackery?

Twelve US survey participants with back pain from osteoarthritis were promised an end to their symptoms if they ingested – or stopped ingesting – certain foods, supplements or vitamins.

All of these promised cures came from books, magazine articles, friends or relatives. No practitioners were involved in 'total cure' promises, although five chiropractors made dietary recommendations in their attempts to help osteoarthritis sufferers.

Only one survey participant with osteoarthritis-based back pain felt that a change in diet (taking a calcium supplement) had helped. Six participants were uncertain of the results, but reasoned that they were not doing themselves any harm (see Chapter 5 for specifics). Nutrition and vitamin supplements may have a positive role to play, but there is no proof of this at present. Megadoses of nutritional supplements may have harmful effects and should therefore be avoided. And there is evidence from the US survey that fad 'arthritis diets' fraudulently raise hopes. Moreover, false promises about diets convinced a few survey participants that they no longer had to work at keeping fit or at controlling their symptoms.

Tips from Survey Participants

These tips are listed according to frequency of mention by US osteoarthritis sufferers. The most popular tips for all back sufferers are presented in Chapters 13 and 14.

Know Yourself Well

- Stay in touch with how you feel. Don't take your 'mental temperature' all the time, and ignore minor aches and pains when you can. But slow down when you must.
- Find a middle ground between being Superman or Wonder Woman (doing everything yourself, no matter what the price) and being an invalid (letting every twinge stop you in your tracks).
- Maintain a realistically positive attitude.
- Develop the capacity to distract yourself so that you can keep your mind off your pain until the pain really needs to be dealt with.
- Experiment with ways to better yourself mentally, spiritually and physically to any degree possible . . . and try never to feel sorry for yourself.
- Work hard at making progress. And never give up!

Keep Active

- Warm up, start slowly, avoid sudden movements, and keep moving as much as possible throughout the day.
- Do daily back exercises that emphasize flexibility (see Chapter 8).
- Walk at least 1.6 km (1 mile) every day, bicycle at least 5 km (3 miles) every day, or swim a minimum of 15 consecutive minutes three times a week.
- Keep active even while resting and relaxing by turning often to prevent stiffening.

Keep Warm

- Wear several layers of clothing during cold weather. Layers tend to keep you warmer, and you can always take off a layer or two if you're too warm.
- Use a space heater in the room where you spend most of your time. (To be on the safe side, and to conserve energy, turn off the heater when you leave the room and when you go to sleep.)
- Use an electric blanket over your mattress before you get into bed.
- Use flannel sheets. They really do feel warmer than ordinary sheets.

Use Heat Therapeutically

- Two warm baths a day – one in the morning to get started and one before bedtime to relax and loosen up – are of great value. Use warm rather than hot water, and soak for about 20 minutes. Long, hot soaks can tire, rather than relax, your muscles. (For tips on how to position yourself comfortably in the bath, see Chapter 13.)
- Use a heating pad. Some survey participants used heating pads for hours at a time, but most recommended no more than 30 minutes every 2 hours. If you are using a heating pad more than this, try reducing the amount of time. You may get more relief and have less fatigue.

- Don't spend a lot of money on heat-producing devices. None surpasses the warm bath or heating pad for effectiveness or affordability.

Get Enough Sleep and Rest

'My arthritis feels worse when I don't get enough sleep' and 'Make sure you get enough rest' typify comments made by about half the survey participants covered in this chapter. In short, both exercise and rest are important. The resting position suggested the most is lying on a mat on the floor with a small pillow under your head and neck and two pillows under your knees. However, this should only be used in the short term, as – if used for long periods – it could result in shortening of the hamstrings, affecting your pelvic tilt. Sleeping positions are discussed in Chapter 7.

Keep Your Weight Down

Being overweight puts a strain on anyone's back. But spinal osteoarthritis sufferers mention the need to stay trim far more than any other group of back sufferers. Since the pain in your back is caused in large part by damage to weight-bearing joints, it makes sense that carrying less weight around could help your condition in the long run.

Look for Ways to Reduce Stress

Stress, according to survey participants, affects spinal osteoarthritis more than any other category of back pain except neck pain. Negative feelings about having a chronic disease associated with old age (although osteoarthritis is by no means limited to old age) are one factor. Having a disease for which there is no cure is another. 'I concentrate on taking each day in a calmer way,' commented a wife and mother. 'I try to get away now and then and ease up on worries and stress,' said a shopkeeper. In general, most survey participants with osteoarthritis reduced stress simply by adding a few breaks to their daily routines. For tips on how to reduce stress, see 'stress reduction techniques' in the Index.

Ask Questions about Any Medication Prescribed for You

'If an anti-inflammatory drug makes you feel worse, or has destructive long-term effects – and your doctor did not warn you about these possible effects – you are as much to blame as your doctor if you didn't ask questions or become informed on your own,' observed an airline executive on the need to question any and all medication, be it prescription or over-the-counter.

Some medicines can have serious side-effects.

'After taking arthritis drugs for twenty-five years, I now have other critical medical problems, probably as a result of taking all these drugs,' commented a nurse. She added, 'I think it's high time that people stopped acting like children and started asking questions. I don't think that anyone should take any drug without first having information in writing about it and understanding what they need to know. Your doctor should provide this information. If you can't learn what you want from him, ask your druggist [pharmacist]. If that fails, check one of the consumer guides on prescription drugs. If you still can't find out, don't take the drug.'

Try Using Rub-on Balms or Liniments
Nine US survey participants used rub-on balms or liniments on their backs once or twice a day and got minor but welcome relief from pain.

There are no magic potions. All liniments produce a warm or glowing sensation that masks pain for a short time. Liniments also increase the flow of blood to the affected area and this seems to help. 'Just the feeling of touch and warmth that you get from using a liniment makes you feel good,' said an assistant chef. 'Any other benefits are a bonus.'

Deep Heat was by far the most popular liniment among survey participants. However, liniments are only likely to be helpful if you have specific, superficial areas of discomfort. They are less useful for more widespread symptoms.

Try Heel Cushions
Four US survey participants with spinal osteoarthritis were helped by heel cushions. They used ready-made products available at chemists – Dr Scholl to name one. These people felt that heel cushions helped lessen the jarring effect on their spines when walking.

Have an Active Sex Life

A drug company salesperson spoke for many spinal osteoarthritis sufferers about the benefits of regular sexual activity: 'The "old person" image associated with osteoarthritis is depressing enough. If this is accompanied by a reduction or absence of sexual activity, the negative psychological factors you suffer will probably literally make you feel like you're in more pain.'

'Aches and pains, if they're not severe, shouldn't stop anyone from having sex,' he continued. 'You need it to feel whole, to have a better sense about yourself. Stay within your limitations, and the gentle rocking motions of sex will do wonders for your body and your mind.'

Two Special Pleas from Survey Participants

If You Need Professional Care, Insist on Being a Partner in That Care

If you can talk to your healthcare practitioner, and can feel like an equal in making choices about your case, you have the best possible chance of keeping osteoarthritis from limiting your activities.

'The role of interpersonal relationships between doctor and patient is more important than the medical society realizes,' noted an editorial researcher. 'The practice of medicine is impersonal, and that single factor has much to do with why people are not "learning to live with arthritis".'

Survey participants make it clear that if osteoarthritis were treatable primarily by medical means – medication and surgery, for example – rapport between patient and doctor would be a nice fringe benefit, but one that patients could do without. This is not the case, however.

'We are people, not just cases,' a farmer with spinal osteoarthritis said. 'We need things that doctors often choose not to give: physiotherapy, emotional therapy and just the hope and optimism you feel when someone cares about you. On the other hand, maybe it would be more realistic to try to "solve" this problem by changing our expectations of doctors. Let's just expect them to deal with technical matters and let's realize that most of us need other kinds of help, much of which we ourselves can provide.'

Avoid the 'I Give Up' Syndrome

Based on the US survey data, I estimate that one in five spinal osteoarthritis sufferers has, for the most part, given up. The reliance of these people on medicines that fail them – and their discouragement when so-called miracle remedies don't work – leaves them feeling defeated. Here are some conclusions:

A housewife: 'I am 64 years old and can't expect any change.'

A retired person: 'Nothing can be done to help me, except maybe one thing. I have in my possession a diet, which cures people of arthritis. Maybe some day I can afford to buy all the things in this diet. It's my only hope.'

A night watchman: 'There is no cure for arthritis at this time, so I suppose there's nothing I can do.'

It is easy for well-wishers to say, 'Don't give up.' But it is also a fact, documented in this chapter and in other research, that osteoarthritis sufferers can do much to combat this degenerative disorder.

Chapter 12

Advice from Survey Participants about Sciatica, Scoliosis, Spondylolisthesis

Sciatica: Case histories of five participants with non-specific sciatica • Best practitioners • Value and risk of exercise • Other treatments (prescription drugs, ice, acupuncture, gravity inversion exercise, DMSO) • Scoliosis: Chiropractic's role • Orthopaedic surgeons • Results of working with yoga instructors, physiotherapists, dance teachers, Tai Chi instructors, naturopaths • Back exercises • Tips from survey participants • Spondylolisthesis: Diagnosis • Treatment • Case history details of seven survey participants (age at diagnosis, current age, occupation, practitioners seen, treatments tried, treatment results, comments, helpful hints, emotional factors, outcome)

The three categories of back pain covered in this chapter have little in common medically. What links them is the lack of reliable information about treatment – an even greater vacuum, judging from the comments of US survey participants, than exists for other categories of back pain.

For example, sciatica is often caused by a prolapsed or herniated disc (see 'About Your Back', p. xvii). However, none of the sciatica sufferers in this section was able to learn, with any degree of certainty, the cause of their pain. All found the search for help slow and frustrating, often waiting years to discover a pain-relieving approach.

People suffering from scoliosis (lateral or sideways curvature of the spine) have an equally difficult time finding information about how to relieve their pain, although they have little problem in getting a precise diagnosis. Why is there a lack of helpful advice? A car mechanic spoke for many scoliosis sufferers when he said, 'There is a great deal that can be done. But the attitude of many doctors seems to be that nothing can be done unless you want to risk surgery. As for chiropractors, too many promise more than they can deliver.'

People suffering from spondylolisthesis (a forward or backward shift of a lumbar vertebra upon the segment below) also encountered a lot of blank gazes and shrugs of the shoulders when seeking advice. 'If you don't want surgery, then don't complain' was a comment heard by one survey participant.

This chapter helps to fill the information gap about treating sciatica, scoliosis and spondylolisthesis. In some instances, I do not have the statistically significant data needed to provide you with definite conclusions. However, even in these cases, you are likely to find value in the insights and suggestions of people with problems like yours.

Sciatica

Sciatica is a knife-like pain running down your buttocks, down the back of your thigh, continuing into your calf, sometimes into your foot – and, at its worst, into every waking second of your day. Caused by pressure on your sciatic nerve where it emerges from your spinal column, sciatica can be crippling.

However, if you have pain in your leg, you may not necessarily have true sciatica. Appropriate treatment varies, depending on whether or not there is inflammation of the nerve root (see 'About Your Back', p. xvii). For this reason, it is important to get an accurate diagnosis as early as possible, but this is not always easy.

Let's start by looking at five brief but representative cases of non-specific sciatica, then proceed to suggestions and insights gleaned from these and other cases.

Case 1: 25 Years on the Treatment Treadmill without Results

For 25 years, a 56-year-old saleswoman has struggled through painful and disabling episodes of sciatica – without ever finding a way to break this cycle. She has been treated by many practitioners, including an orthopaedic surgeon (diagnosis: arthritis and calcification of the spine), a physiotherapist (diagnosis:

neuritis and sciatica), a chiropractor (diagnosis: pinched nerve and spinal curvature) and a GP (diagnosis: neurotic). Cortisone made her feel depressed. Motrin, a prescription anti-inflammatory drug, gave her gastro-intestinal problems. Chiropractic manipulation was 'helpful but short-term'. This survey participant regularly practises yoga, which she taught herself from a book. No exercise programme has ever been prescribed or recommended for her.

Conclusion: Although the self-taught yoga therapy helps a bit, no treatment has brought about substantial long-term gains.

Case 2: Individualized Exercise Therapy Restores Full Activity

A 61-year-old writer had chronic back pain for more than two decades. The pain was manageable, but then it became crippling when accompanied by 'pins and needles and agonizing pain in my legs and sharp muscle spasms in my back'. Feeling no better after treatments from two orthopaedic surgeons and a neuro-surgeon – all of whom felt that he needed surgery for degenerative discs – the patient sought help from a physiatrist. 'He recommended a course of treatment which included electric muscle stimulation, a trigger point injection and an exercise programme. The exercise programme really did the trick. I suggest that most sciatica sufferers get into the hands of a good physiatrist and physiotherapist. I believe I would still have a severe problem if it were not for the wonderful treatment I received.'

Conclusion: 'After eight years I have very little pain, often none at all. It is necessary to do recommended exercises.'

Case 3: Disabled by Inappropriate Exercises . . . Then Helped by the Right Ones

The orthopaedic surgeon who first saw this 28-year-old artist told him his problem was 'psychosomatic'. A second orthopaedic surgeon said there was 'nothing to worry about'. A third orthopaedic surgeon told the patient he had a ruptured disc. 'A prescription of "back arches" (lying on my stomach and raising my chest and legs) from this orthopaedic surgeon seemed to lead from mild lower back and leg sensations to such pain that I literally could not walk.' Finally, pelvic tilts, mild stretching exercises and swimming brought about slow but major improvement.

Conclusion: 'One must learn one's own exercise needs and limitations and individualize a programme accordingly. What aggravates my problem does not bother my friends who have comparable back pain. My pain often increases when I push exercise too far.'

Case 4: The Patient's Own Good Judgement Proves Crucial

Four orthopaedic surgeons attributed this 35-year-old law student's sciatica to a 'minor but inoperable disc protrusion in the lumbar region.' Not one of the doctors, however, recommended a comprehensive recovery programme. The patient then went to a private sports rehabilitation clinic, where he was advised to take two aspirin a day. The aspirin was useless. However, the patient did eventually recover. He attributes his success to: (1) swimming 1.2 km (¾ mile) per week ('Swimming is the only safe form of exercise I can indulge in. When I miss more than two or three days, my back tightens up noticeably.'); (2) a series of stretching exercises prescribed by a chiropractor; (3) a change of attitude ('In general I try to take things a little easier. I slow down or rest when I am fatigued, and spend more time standing or walking rather than sitting for long periods of time.').

Conclusion: Professional input helped a bit, but in the final analysis, the patient used his own judgement to shape an exercise programme and a lifestyle that ensured long-term progress.

Case 5: Individualized Rehabilitation Comes to the Rescue

A 31-year-old restaurant worker with sciatica saw a group of doctors at a major medical college. A neurologist there diagnosed her problem as 'perhaps disc' and an orthopaedic surgeon called it 'muscle sprain'. Treatment consisted of some muscle-relaxant pills. According to this survey participant: 'The neurologist and the orthopaedic surgeon sent me back and forth, suggesting the need for time, surgery, etc.' The patient later saw a chiropractor, who reported 'a misaligned vertebra putting pressure on a nerve root and disc.' Massage, whirlpool and electric muscle stimulation helped in the short run. An individualized exercise programme, prescribed by the chiropractor, finally turned things around for this woman. Her severe pain is gone; she experiences only occasional discomfort.

Conclusion: Once pain subsides, a comprehensive and appropriate exercise programme for each individual is the key to success.

Three Important Conclusions

1. The dismissal by some doctors of sciatica as something caused by a ruptured disc – and treatable solely by surgery – leaves sciatica sufferers in the lurch. If a disc problem isn't found, some doctors may label the patient neurotic. The label seems unfair. Slightly more than one-third of all participants in the US survey had some sciatica at some point. And the majority of these individuals did not have a confirmed diagnosis involving a disc problem.
2. Exercise therapy – the right exercises at the right time – is crucial. The rate of injury from inappropriate exercise is higher for sciatica than for any other kind of back pain.
3. The 'pill-and-surgery' approach was unconstructive and frustrating for most survey participants with sciatica. Moreover, it caused people who were already in great pain to feel helpless and demoralized. But there are practitioners with a positive attitude about sciatica – and the skills to justify this attitude.

Who Can Help You?

The cases presented touched on the negatives of being treated for sciatica by most medical doctors. The following comment from a nurse offers a summary: 'I don't know why I have sciatica. Spina bifida (a congenital defect of the spinal column), pinched nerve, muscle strain and stress are but a few of the diagnoses I've received. What I haven't received is useful information.'

In providing long-term help to six of eleven sciatica sufferers in the US survey, the physiotherapist stands out among nonmedical doctors. The Shiatsu therapist trained in exercise therapy may also be a good bet, promoting lasting recovery for three of six survey participants with sciatica.

To the modest extent that they are expert in the exercise rehabilitation process, chiropractors can help promote long-term
results. Chiropractors helped thirteen out of forty-five (29 per
cent) of the US survey's sciatica sufferers to improve substantially. In addition, twenty-one of forty-five sciatica sufferers got
temporary relief through chiropractic care.

The Value of Exercise

Back exercises are essential. But you need good professional
advice about which exercises are appropriate and which should
be avoided at this stage.

It should encourage you to know that case after case of disabling sciatica improved when individualized exercise therapy
was used as the major treatment after acute pain had eased.
Virtually all these cases entailed guidance from an exercise
expert, an individualized programme, a conservative and progressive exercise sequence that avoided single-leg raises (at least
at first), double-leg raises, other straight-leg exercises, and full
bent-knee sit-ups.

Almost without exception, self-taught exercises are not as
therapeutic as those worked out by you and an exercise expert. A
physiotherapist is your best bet. See pp. 71–2 for a list of other
qualified exercise trainers.

A pianist who had sciatic nerve pain since the age of 15
made this point about professional exercise instruction: 'I had
tried back exercises on my own. They had worked, but not that
well. The set of exercises I learned from a chiropractor are
much more extensive and effective. The right exercises are the
only sure way to help sciatica, except for ways to reduce stress.
The chiropractor also urged me to ease up on jogging and to
swim more.'

A drummer agreed: 'Nothing really worked except the back
exercises prescribed by a physiotherapist.'

Exercises you see in the mass media are not for sciatica
sufferers. 'I do the exercises I see on TV,' said a housewife, 'but
they make me worse. Some mornings I can hardly lift my legs.'
A survey participant living on benefits added, 'I try to pick out
exercises from magazine articles. But I keep being re-injured and
it seems that nothing can help me.'

Survey participants agreed that the exercises outlined in Chapter 8 make up the kind of safe-not-sorry exercise programme that can help a sciatica sufferer make meaningful progress in a few months' time.

Also, as noted in the case histories earlier in this chapter, swimming and walking are both highly recommended.

Other Treatment Approaches

- Medication can be helpful for mild or moderate sciatica. Start by trying over-the-counter aspirin or paracetamol. If these don't work, get a prescription for a strong analgesic to dull severe pain. Note: If sciatica is secondary to inflammation of nerve roots, a non-steroidal anti-inflammatory drug, such as Ibuprofen or Indomethacin, may be essential.
- Ice eased pain for eight of ten US sciatica sufferers. (See pp. 76–8 for tips on using ice to treat back pain.)
- Acupuncture helped two of four US sciatica sufferers. In one case cited earlier, ten treatments resolved more than two decades of intense pain.
- Gravity inversion exercise helped the three sciatica sufferers who tried it. (See pp. 82–5 for details, including a warning about unsupervised treatment for any painful back ailment.)
- DMSO helped all three sciatica sufferers who used it. (See pp. 78–80 for further information.)

Scoliosis

The information in this section focuses on practical approaches and therapies you can use to reduce or do away with back pain caused by scoliosis, a lateral (sideways) curvature of the spine that usually becomes apparent during pre-adolescence or adolescence. The emphasis is on self-care. I do not have enough research data to pursue topics such as diagnostic testing, surgical implants and the desirability of surgery, corrective braces or electric stimulation. Only two of the thirty-one US survey participants in this section had surgery and only four used braces.

Scoliosis sufferers covered in this section had moderate to severe curvatures that were diagnosed by more than one practitioner as the cause of their back pain. Participants with minor scoliosis, which seemed not to be the cause of back pain, are not included here.

The question asked most frequently by survey participants with scoliosis was, 'Do you know what kind of practitioner can help?' I will begin by discussing the relative efficacy of widely seen practitioners, then explore professional treatments and self-help therapies.

Do Chiropractors Relieve Scoliosis Pain?

Please note that I am not addressing the question of whether chiropractors can correct scoliosis. They cannot, although some chiropractors promised to cure or correct scoliosis in a few survey participants.

Number of people treated in US survey	31
Provided dramatic long-term help	3 (10%)
Provided moderate long-term help	5 (16%)
Provided temporary help	9 (29%)
Ineffective	11 (35%)
Made patient feel worse	3 (10%)

Judging from these survey results, chiropractors do provide some measure of relief 55 per cent of the time, but the relief is mostly short-lived. Chiropractic manipulation, used alone, helped thirteen of twenty-seven patients in the short run. What helped in the long run was exercise therapy.

'My chiropractor says that manipulation will prevent scoliosis from worsening in the long run,' said a tennis instructor. 'But I have not found chiropractic manipulation to help.'

'Chiropractic manipulation did nothing over the long run,' said a student.

A fast-food restaurant employee concluded: 'Manipulation gave very little help in the long run. Besides, the chiropractor proposed a long-range manipulation treatment at high cost, so I did not continue.'

What level of temporary relief does chiropractic manipulation provide?

'A competent chiropractor can always get my back properly adjusted,' said a microfilm technician. 'Generally, one treatment a month is sufficient, although I have had periods where I needed an adjustment every day or so.'

'The spinal adjustments helped a lot at first, but it seemed that I became dependent on the chiropractor,' said a steel industry worker. 'I got immediate relief but always began hurting again in a few days. Then it seemed that I hurt all the time anyway.'

Do Orthopaedic Surgeons Help?
According to the adult, non-surgical case respondents covered in the US survey, orthopaedic surgeons were less effective than chiropractors. And the exercises they prescribed caused setbacks in three cases. However, it should be noted that orthopaedic surgeons are usually the practitioners who undertake corrective surgery in the worst cases of scoliosis in children and young people. And in the UK there are some orthopaedic surgeons who specialize in this field.

Number of people treated in US survey	23
Provided dramatic long-term help	2 (9%)
Provided moderate long-term help	1 (4%)
Provided temporary help	2 (9%)
Ineffective	15 (65%)
Made patient feel worse*	3 (13%)

* These people were injured by prescribed back exercises.

Is Any Practitioner Worth Seeing?
Yes.

After unproductive years of seeing 'mainstream' practitioners, twenty-two of thirty-one US scoliosis sufferers in this section got long-term relief by receiving treatments from these practitioners.

Practitioner	Number of scoliosis patients treated	Number who achieved long-term improvement
Yoga instructor	8	8 (100%)
Physiotherapist	7	4 (57%)
Dance teacher	3	3 (100%)
Tai Chi instructor	2	2 (100%)
Naturopath	2	2 (100%)

All these practitioners taught scoliosis sufferers gradual and graceful movements. And all kept morale high through heartening interpersonal skills.

Back Exercises and Scoliosis

Traditional back exercises seem to pose a greater than usual risk of injury to individuals with scoliosis. Of the twenty-two US scoliosis sufferers who did back exercises regularly, six were injured by these exercises.

'The back exercises taught to me by an orthopaedic surgeon were difficult for me to keep up,' said a photographer. 'They have caused recurrences of injury.'

An editor who learned exercises from a popular back book commented, 'I am still unsure about the advisability of back exercise. I don't know if stretching helps or hurts, although the books say that flexibility is important, and that is probably true. But stretching seems to be hard to do gently and correctly (for me anyway). I tend to overdo and my body reacts with a sore back.'

A housewife expressed a more positive, more popular attitude about back exercises: 'Back exercises are valuable, but they don't seem to work as well for me as for people I know who have "regular" low back pain. And they don't provide the advantages of other forms of exercise – swimming, yoga or Tai Chi.'

In contrast with other kinds of back sufferers, survey participants with scoliosis had better luck exercising without professional input. These individuals also avoided all exercises that caused them discomfort – no matter how conservative and 'universally safe' the exercises were reputed to be. Finally, most scoliosis sufferers who were successful with back exercises did other forms of exercise as well, such as swimming or cycling.

Since back exercises help more scoliosis sufferers than they injure, should you try them? I'm going to hedge by saying that if yoga appeals to you, practise yoga instead. Otherwise, try the exercises in Chapter 8. But discontinue any and all of these exercises if you feel even the slightest bit worse.

Yoga: Perhaps Every Scoliosis Sufferer Should Try It

Eight scoliosis sufferers practised yoga regularly, and all eight found it helpful – more helpful than traditional back exercises.

'Yoga has done wonders for my back and well-being,' a ceramics artist said. 'I used to be in pain almost constantly and now it is rare that my back hurts – just when I am overtired.'

'The joy of discovering yoga is indescribable,' a teacher commented. 'I have been to dozens of doctors, all the top specialists, and then some. Now even the doctors in my family are believers.'

These eight individuals got personal instruction from a professional. (See p. 112 for information on how to select a yoga instructor.)

Other Helpful Exercises

There is every indication that scoliosis sufferers who give their bodies a constructive workout every day have the least pain and lead the fullest lives. Swimming was as effective as yoga for eight survey participants. Walking and cycling each helped five scoliosis sufferers. Dance helped three. Tai Chi helped two. (Jogging also helped two, though it's not generally advisable for back pain sufferers because it usually involves some degree of jarring impact on hard or uneven ground.) Remarkably, all these activities, including yoga, helped every scoliosis sufferer in this survey – without exception. Moreover, scoliosis sufferers who had the most dramatic recoveries from severe and chronic pain participated regularly in at least two activities, such as yoga and swimming.

Tips from Survey Participants

Note: The order below reflects the frequency with which topics were mentioned.

1. 'Give your body a good physical workout every day. Be an athlete. There is no better answer for scoliosis pain.'
2. 'Rest when the pain gets bad, because this will actually allow you more total active time than if you keep going until you drop.'
3. 'Wet heat of any kind – bath, shower massage, whirlpool, jacuzzi – usually gives temporary relief.'
4. 'Avoid favouring one side by shifting your weight from one leg to the other when you're standing still, by not over-emphasizing one-sided sports like golf and by using light weights to help balance muscles.'

5. 'Even when your back hurts, and all you want to do is sit in the most comfortable chair you have, sit for only 20 minutes to half an hour and then move around for 10 minutes.'

6. 'Don't listen to predictions from doctors about whether you'll have trouble delivering babies.'

7. 'Don't agree to surgery just because you're told how much worse you'll be in ten years. No one but God knows that. And it isn't that you have to become worse.'

Spondylolisthesis

In 'spondylolisthesis', derived from the Greek words for vertebra and slip, one of your vertebrae, usually the lowest lumbar vertebra (L5), slips forward or backward slightly. This slippage exerts great strain on your back muscles. It can also cause nerve compression and sciatica.

Spondylolisthesis is easier to diagnose than to pronounce, as it is one of the few back ailments that can be spotted on conventional X-rays. It is difficult to treat, however, since the slippage of the spine plays havoc with the back muscles.

Still, there were more successes than failures – albeit very hard-earned successes – among the ten US survey participants with spondylolisthesis. These ten cases obviously cannot support definite conclusions, but the comments and suggestions have significant value. As one spondylolisthesis sufferer put it, 'I don't know of anyone with a problem like mine. I wish I did, so I at least could compare notes. I'm sure people with spondylolisthesis could learn a lot from each other.'

To enable you to hear from other spondylolisthesis sufferers, I will highlight seven of these cases.

Case 1

- Age at diagnosis: 21
- Current age: 51
- Occupation: Lawyer
- Practitioners: Chiropractor, orthopaedic surgeon, physiotherapist.
- Treatments: Manipulation, physiotherapy emphasizing exercise training, back brace, shoe lift to correct pelvic tilt, bed

board, changed daily habits – including proper lifting and sleeping in the foetal position.

- Treatment results: 'Manipulation helped very little; shoe lift helped considerably; exercise programme – prescribed by orthopaedic surgeon and taught by physiotherapist – helped dramatically.'
- Helpful hints: 'Sleep on side in foetal position on a firm mattress and bed board. Bend your knees when you sneeze. Crouch, don't bend, to pick up objects from the floor. Lift carefully with your legs and arms, not your back. Reduce weight of objects lifted or weight carried if possible. Exercise to strengthen abdomen. Lose weight.'
- Emotional factors: 'I'm a relaxed person. However, any substantial tension, rare as that is with me, seems to focus on my weak spot, i.e. lower back.'
- Outcome: 'Ninety-five-per cent cured ten years ago . . . no problem since except occasional low back twinge.'

Case 2

- Age at diagnosis: 24
- Current age: 26
- Occupation: Sales assistant
- Practitioners: Three orthopaedic surgeons, two neurosurgeons, two GPs, one chiropractor.
- Treatments: Exercise therapy, traction, ultrasound, massage, manipulation, muscle-relaxant drugs.
- Treatment results: 'Manipulation worsened my condition. Traction helped temporarily, as did ultrasound and massage. The muscle relaxants helped, but side-effects were bad so I quit taking them. Exercise, learned mostly from my own research, helped greatly.'
- Comment: 'All doctors except a GP and a neurosurgeon treated me coldly.'
- Helpful hints: 'Exercise is a must – walking, swimming and back exercises in particular. Also, 2-to-3 grams of vitamin C daily help me.'
- Emotional factors: 'Stress is a factor. In this area, though, for the most part, doctors did more harm to me than good.'

- Outcome: Functional, with pain mostly under control.

Note: Traction is not supported in the UK back pain guidelines.

Case 3

- Age at diagnosis: 21
- Current age: 61
- Occupation: Not stated
- Practitioners: Four orthopaedic surgeons, neurosurgeon, physiotherapist.
- Treatments: Physiotherapy including exercise training, prescription drugs including Indomethacin and Clinoril, surgical procedures including spinal fusions and a 'stepladder' inserted in the spine, ultrasound, TENS.
- Treatment results: 'Three spinal fusions did not work. The fourth one – involving the insertion of a "stepladder" – worked very well. None of the treatments injured me. I could not tolerate Indomethacin or Clinoril. The TENS unit works well for me.'
- Helpful hints: TENS therapy.
- Emotional factors: 'Stress affects my back.'
- Outcome: Somewhat incapacitated with persistent pain.

Case 4

- Age at diagnosis: 10
- Current age: 55
- Occupation: Unable to work; disabled by spondylolisthesis.
- Practitioners: GP, chiropractor, osteopath, orthopaedic surgeon, gynaecologist.
- Treatments: Anti-inflammatory medication, physiotherapy, exercise (walking), heat, electric muscle stimulation, massage
- Treatment results: 'What helps me the most is the heat and massage and electric stimulation from the chiropractor. I have been seeing him for eight years. The prescription drugs were not effective.'
- Comment: 'The chiropractor has helped me very much. When I first went to him I couldn't hold my head up. Now I can turn

it from side to side, and the chiropractor is keeping me walking. He calls it maintaining me.'
- Helpful hints: 'Keep moving.'
- Emotional factors: 'I was told that I was a mental case and that there was nothing wrong with me. One thing that was wrong was a large tumour that had to be removed.'
- Outcome: Poor. The patient is disabled.

Case 5

- Age at diagnosis: 22
- Current age: 28
- Occupation: Student
- Practitioners: Orthopaedic surgeon, physiotherapist, chiropractor, Alexander instructor, Feldenkrais instructor, Rolfer.
- Treatments: Manipulation, Alexander technique instruction, Feldenkrais instruction, Rolfing, physiotherapy.
- Treatment results: 'Alexander technique helped the most. Physiotherapy made no difference. Rolfing hurt me and set back my gains (in terms of pain) months from what I had achieved from the Alexander work. Needless to say, I discontinued Rolfing after two treatments.'
- Comment: 'The Alexander instructor was the only one who looked at my body as a whole. He was also the only one who gave me the responsibility of working things out myself with the proper input.'
- Helpful hints: 'Making love loosens up the hips. Try to do things an easier way, rather than straining your back when it is not necessary to.'
- Emotional factors: 'My back pain is worse when I'm under stress.'
- Outcome: Functions well with a minimum of pain.

Case 6

- Age at diagnosis: 24
- Current age: 28
- Occupation: Not stated.
- Practitioners: Five GPs, chiropractor.

- Treatments: Ice, heat, exercise, medication – Valium, paracetamol, Equagesic, Carisoma.
- Treatment results: 'The exercises and muscle relaxants were most effective. None of the other treatments mattered.'
- Comment: 'I went to four doctors complaining of back pain before one took me seriously. By that time, I was almost crawling. The doctor X-rayed my back, gave me exercises to do, and explained that the problem is progressive and that exercise minimizes or stops the progression. About six months later I went to a chiropractor who would not accept the X-rays taken by the doctor (pecuniary reasons I suspect). I didn't continue with the chiropractor.'
- Outcome: Fully active with some chronic pain.

Case 7

- Age at diagnosis: 26
- Current age: 33
- Occupation: Sales representative
- Practitioners: GP, chiropractor, yoga instructor.
- Treatments: Traction, manipulation, ultrasound, prescription muscle relaxants, yoga.
- Treatment results: 'Yoga worked best – it is tremendously effective and, in my opinion, more effective than regular back exercises. The muscle relaxants were useless. I received just the tiniest amount of assistance from the chiropractor and stopped seeing him after six visits.'
- Comment: 'In the long run, it is imperative that you see somebody who actually knows more than you do about exercise and rehabilitation. In my case I saw a yoga instructor who understood back problems. It should be obvious to all back sufferers that many doctors, and chiropractors for that matter, know less about exercise than the most well-informed back sufferers.'
- Helpful hints: 'A cautious, progressive and complete exercise programme.'
- Emotional factors: None.
- Outcome: A complete success with minor lower backache when tired.

Note: Traction is not supported in the UK back pain guidelines.

Finally, a UK survey respondent had the following very useful advice for fellow sufferers: 'Spondylolisthesis (mine is anterior slip of L5 on S1) should not be manipulated, nor should one do any exercises which involve "back extension" (bending backwards). Thus, many exercises recommended for "normal" backs should not be tackled by us!

My exercise is therefore:

- Hydrotherapy – exercises taught at the Salisbury branch of BackCare in 1990: carried out 2–3 times weekly nowadays in swimming pool (cooler temp. unfortunately) or jacuzzi.
- Gym – rower and treadmill (but not cycle because of unstable pelvis).
- Swim – on back only, because of spondylolisthesis.
- Walk – but only very fast, and for only short periods (because of spondylolithesis it is uncomfortable to stand or walk slowly).
- Core stability exercises.

When confronted with dining chairs without lumbar support – in hotels etc. – use a "Backfriend", and remain at the table for as short a time as possible.

All my own upright chairs slope back and offer lumbar support. These all relieve tremendously the likelihood of pain in my mid-back building up – but make me a social eccentric!'

Section 5
Self-Healing

The people who cope best are those who stay active and get on with their life despite the pain.

The Back Book by Roland et al, published by HMSO, 1996

Try to keep positive. It is important not to underestimate the power of human thought. Having chronic pain does not mean the end of life as you knew it. You can be in control.

Managing Back Pain, published by BackCare, 2004

Ultimately, nobody can do as much for your back condition as you can do for it.

A survey participant

Chapter 13
The 25 Most Often-Mentioned, Proven-Effective Ways to Free Yourself of Back Pain

Attitude • Lifting • Mattresses and bed boards • Sitting • Posture
• Hydrotherapy • Moist heat • Cold therapy • Self-massage • Exercise
• Breaks in routine • Walking • Carrying • Avoiding surgery • Learning
about prescribed medication • Shoes and shoe inserts • Health clubs
• Swimming • Mind-body activities • Proper eating • Weight control
• Positive reinforcement • Reverse-gravity relaxing and exercising
• Hanging from chinning bar • Miscellaneous (warm-ups in the bath,
aspirin before activity, smart dressing, avoiding constipation, liniment,
meditation, back aids)

The US questionnaire asked survey participants, 'Do you have any "helpful hints" or home remedies for other back sufferers?' The UK questionnaire also asked respondents for any advice they could give other back sufferers on coping with everyday life.

Almost everyone had something to say. Comments ranged from the important but commonplace – such as advice about lifting, posture, sitting and exercise – to the unusual but important – have your leg length measured to see if a shoe insert is needed – to the frustrated – 'Everyone gives advice, but it's impossible to know which to follow' – to the desperate – 'No, I have no advice, but I pray that you have some for me.'

Here are the 25 most popular and proven suggestions from the 492 participants in the US survey, many of them echoed by UK respondents. Interestingly, almost everyone agreed about the points covered in this chapter.

This near-unanimity is important, as it does not exist among back practitioners. Even if you have seen some of these tips covered in self-help books, you may have had trouble judging their significance – working out how much emphasis you should give them, or how you should think about them. The advice in this chapter is different. It combines the mechanics of back care – correct posture when you stand or sit, for example – with the perspective you need to make each tip work for you.

1. The Most Frequently Mentioned Helpful Hint Involves an Intangible: Attitude

Your attitude about your body is the basis for improvement. A college professor summed up the feelings of many survey participants about the importance of attitude when he said, 'In order to get rid of back pain, you have to be willing to learn and unlearn. You need to be receptive to looking at new ways to do things that have become ingrained over your entire lifetime. This is as much a matter of attitude as of mechanics, because attitude determines whether or not you will learn and apply what you need to know to reduce or eliminate back pain.

'You can have the best exercise instruction in the world,' the professor added. 'But only you can ultimately decide whether to exercise, and how much, and at what pace – and whether certain exercises just aren't right for you. You can buy yourself the best chair ever made for back sufferers, and then sit in it for three hours at a time, even though you know that taking a break every half hour is the only way to keep your back pain-free. You can consult gurus galore about stress and then blow it all simply by not being in touch with yourself, by not even being aware that you are under stress.'

The point is well made. You have to know yourself. You have to be sensitive to your condition. Then, and only then, can you learn to beat back pain. This isn't to say that self-awareness can cure you, but if you're not aware of how you feel, then you can't make decisions about what you must do to maintain back fitness.

2. When Lifting, Bend at the Knees, Not at the Waist

Survey participants were adamant about lifting properly. They talked more about this activity than about exercise, posture or any other physical aspect of promoting back fitness. Here are pointers for lifting all sorts of objects:

- Bend at the knees to pick up anything, whether it's as light as a tissue or as heavy as a baby or a potted plant.
- If it's difficult for you to squat, or to get back up, place a chair or stepladder near you and lean one hand on it for support. Keep your back straight when doing this.
- Use a mechanical 'grabber' to retrieve light objects – anything from a pen to a magazine to a small book – from the floor or high shelves. (The Easyreacher, available from some product suppliers, see Useful Addresses, p. 463, is less expensive than many other grabber devices, lightweight and durable.)
- Keep the object you're lifting as close to your body as possible.
- When lifting a heavy object, if possible, turn your back to it and extend your arms behind you.
- Instead of lifting and carrying something heavy, see whether you can slide it to its destination. If so, turn your back to the object and pull it as you would a wheelbarrow. Don't push it with your foot or leg. And don't pull it towards you while facing it.
- Ask yourself whether the object to be lifted really has to be lifted by you. If in doubt, ask for help.

See pp. 154–7 for additional information about lifting.

3. Change Your Sleeping Arrangements to Suit Your Back

You spend a third of your life in bed. So it isn't surprising that your sleeping arrangements can have a great impact on your back.

Keep in mind the following recommendations from a majority of survey participants: Even if your mattress is firm, use a plywood bed board, available from a timber merchant. Sleeping in a bed away from home is particularly troublesome. To prevent problems when you travel, take a folding bed board. You can order folding bed boards from some product suppliers (see Useful Addresses, p. 463).

Some survey participants travel with their regular bed boards loaded on top of their cars. Others reserve rooms at hotels or motels where bed boards are supplied on request. If all else fails, and you feel you're in for a bad night, slide the mattress off the bed – or ask a member of the hotel staff to do it for you – and sleep on the floor.

No matter how much support your bed gives you, though, you have to position yourself to take advantage of this support. About three-quarters of US survey participants do this by sleeping on their sides. The remainder sleep on their backs with pillows under their knees. However, this is only advisable in the short term. Sleeping in this position in the long term may lead to shortening of the hamstrings, which could affect your pelvic tilt.

See Chapter 7 for additional information on mattresses and how to get in and out of bed without aggravating your back. Several UK survey respondents found Tempur mattresses beneficial, though one felt that claims made in advertisements were rather overstated. These mattresses are available from several product suppliers (see Useful Addresses, p. 463).

4. Learn How to Sit . . . and How Much to Sit

The best sitting apparatus ever invented is a combination of a place to rest yourself and the knowledge and awareness you carry around with you. Even though you have the finest chair available, all is for naught if you don't get up and stretch instead of trying to sit through an aching back. All is for naught if you don't get up and get that footstool from across the room, sit up straight, and avoid crossing your legs. The potential for harm from bad sitting habits is tremendous.

Always sit on a firm seat. Too soft and your back will feel the strain. Too hard, like uncovered wood or metal, and you can literally get a pain in the rear.

If your chair seat is too soft, a piece of plywood covered with foam will firm it up. Or you can buy a seat cushion to keep you from sinking into soft chairs or sofas. They are obtainable from specialist medical and back shops or Internet sites (see Useful Addresses, p. 463). Use a back support. Office chairs are usually the only ones that come with built-in lumbar supports. If you use an office chair, make sure its support fits your back, for unless the back of the chair is adjustable, the lumbar support is likely to be too low for you. Also, make sure that the back of the chair does not tilt until and unless you want it to.

With most other chairs, you need to supply your own back support. Following are some of the products that meet this need. Several different manufacturers now make back support aids, so shop around for the product that matches your needs and budget. The support mentioned most frequently by UK survey participants was the Backfriend, available from several product suppliers (see Useful Addresses, p. 463). This is lightweight and easily portable and is therefore ideal for travelling in cars, buses, etc.

- Lumbar cushions were mentioned by the largest number of US survey participants. These moulded cushions are designed to fit the contours of your lumbar spine. They are usually lightweight, comfortable, have removable and/or washable covers, and can easily be taken to luncheons, meetings and shows. Various makes and models are available from medical and back shops and from Internet sites.
- 'Collapsible' cushions are available in a variety of shapes and sizes, if a cushion is needed that will fit into an attaché case or overstuffed suitcase. The better sort can be inflated with a detachable hand bulb rather than by mouth.
- If a chair has the kind of back that your back dreads – curved or without much to hold you up – then one of the many adjustable back supports may work where other cushions don't. These are designed to act as a substitute for the kind of chair back you need. Depending on the make and model, they may come with attachment straps, attachable cushions for the small of the back and shoulder area, and a choice of washable fabrics. They are usually lightweight and can be obtained from medical and back shops and Internet sites (see Useful Addresses, p. 463).

See Chapter 8 for additional information about sitting.

5. Correct Posture, Including 'Slouching', Can Ease Back Pain

If you have chronic low back pain, a slight change in the way you stand can help ease this pain. For example, a jutting bottom emphasizes the 'S' curve in your lower back. So keep your bottom tucked in a bit. Practising Exercise 2 (Pelvic Tilt) in Chapter 8 will make it easier for you to maintain this 'tucked-in' alignment.

More good advice: Tuck in your chin, tighten your abdominal muscles, and keep your knees slightly bent.

Finally, don't believe the myth that good posture means that your weight must be evenly distributed on both legs. Believing this can cause you great discomfort when you're standing in one place for a long time. Shift your weight from one foot to the other every few minutes. Some experts consider this to be 'slouching', and hence bad for you. But since your 'S' curve is less exaggerated when you stand this way, you will probably feel better.

See Chapter 7 for additional information about posture.

6. Turn Your Bath into a Pain-Relieving Hydrotherapy Centre

Being in a bath is painful for some people. If your muscles are contracted, you might find it difficult to sit up and bathe or to lean back on the hard surface and relax. Moreover, just lying in a bath can put pressure on tight muscles or inflamed nerves. But there are usually ways around all these problems. About half of the participants in the US survey got backache relief from taking baths. Their suggestions should help you find more enjoyment in the bath:

- Warm water is better than hot. Hot water is more effective as a counter-irritant – you feel the heat and not the pain – but too much heat can tire your muscles to a point that spasming starts up or increases. Also, lying in a hot bath for a long time is risky if you have high blood pressure or medical conditions that are adversely affected by excessive heat.
- A 20-minute bath is ideal, say most survey participants. Longer than this is potentially more harmful than beneficial.
- Using an extra-thick bath mat and filling the bath as high as possible will reduce pressure on inflamed muscles and nerves.
- Instead of reclining with your legs fully extended, lean your back against one end of the bath, raise your knees, and keep your feet flat.

- Tuck a folded hand towel between the small of your back and the end of the bath. Just this much support can greatly increase your comfort.
- To avoid stiffness from being in one position too long, prop your feet on the sides or edges of the bath from time to time.
- A small, inflatable bath pillow that attaches to the bath with suction cups will allow you to lean back more comfortably and avoid straining your neck and upper back. Medical and back shops and mail order suppliers sell them (see Useful Addresses, p. 463).
- A body-length inflatable cushion that attaches with suction cups is a good bet if you can't tolerate pressure on your hips, buttocks or back.

7. Apply Moist Heat While in Bed
It's not always convenient or desirable to get into a bath to soothe your aching muscles with moist heat. So here are some alternatives:

- Apply a hot, wet towel to your back. One way is to soak a towel in hot water, wring it out, wrap it in another towel, and apply it to your back. The effect is likely to feel wonderful but short-lived – only about 3 minutes – and become annoyingly cold shortly thereafter.
- Use a heat pack but first wrap it in six layers of towel in order to avoid the risk of a thermal burn. Also, take care not to lie on a heat pack as this can also lead to burning. The wrapped pack should be laid on your skin instead.

See additional information about heat therapy in Chapter 5.

8. Use Cold Therapy to Reduce Muscle Spasm
The value of cold therapy for many back sufferers, contrary to popular wisdom, is not limited to the first 24 to 48 hours after injury. In fact, cold therapy remained more effective than heat therapy over long periods of time for US survey participants with neck pain, sciatica and severe muscle spasms.

- Large freezer bags filled with ice were the top choice among survey participants who used cold therapy. Zip-lock bags all but assure that icy water won't leak out. Rather than empty the bag after your treatment, try laying it flat in the freezer for reuse. (The rubber-screw-top ice bags available at chemists have limited value, primarily because they are usually not large enough to cover the entire affected area.) The easiest method is to use a bag of frozen peas, as they can be moulded around the painful area.

- Note: Even though no survey participants who used ice were injured in the process, there is a risk of ice burn or even frostbite. Therefore, never apply ice directly on your skin, unless someone is continuously moving the ice from one area to another. If you're using ice cubes, put them in an ice bag or plastic bag and place a thin towel (a damp tea towel works well) between the bag and your skin. If your skin turns red, discontinue use.

- Instant cold packs are especially useful when you don't have quick access to a freezer – on car rides or camping trips, for example. These gel packs turn cold in seconds when you squeeze and shake them. Reusable cold packs are available from many chemists.

See additional information about cold therapy in Chapter 5.

9. Use Self-Massage to Ease Pain and Promote Relaxation

Rubbing away pain on a daily basis with self-massage is a popular remedy among survey participants. Various self-massage techniques, as well as techniques that require a partner's help, are discussed fully in Chapters 4 and 7. The two most effective involve: (1) applying acupressure with the ball of the thumb to areas of pain caused by muscle spasm; and (2) ice massage, using either a paper cup filled with ice or a 'friction mitten' available at surgical supply stores.

In addition, fifteen US survey participants got instant pain relief by using a wooden body roller specially designed to apply acupressure to the long muscles on either side of the spine.

Body rollers of different kinds are available at many alternative health stores. They are well worth trying, with this one note of caution: if you are in the recovery stage, do not place a roller under your middle or lower back. The pressure from it, and the degree to which it arches your spine, might be more than you can tolerate.

See additional information about massage in Chapter 5.

10. Exercise Regularly
Both US and UK survey participants all advocate regular exercise. Chapter 8 sets out a complete low back exercise programme – including how to think about exercise, how to warm up, what exercises to do, what exercises to avoid, how to know when you need professional help, and where to find this help. In Chapters 9 to 12, you'll find specific advice about exercise for pain caused by ruptured disc, neck ailments, osteoarthritis, spondylolisthesis, sciatica and scoliosis.

11. Give Yourself a Break
'Two 10-minute back breaks each day are the difference for me between progress and deterioration,' said a church choir conductor. And a majority of survey participants agree that giving your back a few respites every day is the best way to lower the stress that heightens back pain.

The most popular and helpful way to take a back break is to lie on the floor with your calves and feet propped on a chair or sofa. The effect is even better when you combine this strain-easing position with deep breathing.

See the Index for additional information about stress reduction.

12. Walk at least 1.6 km (1 mile) a Day
Walking was helpful in the long run for 98 per cent of US survey participants who made it a regular part of their routine. The activity not only added strength and flexibility to their backs but improved their muscle tone overall. Equally important, walking at least 30 minutes a day, four times a week, greatly reduced stress for these people.

Standing or walking a lot on your job 'doesn't count', according to survey participants. What *does* count is brisk, mind-clearing, arm-swinging, uninterrupted walking.

13. Carry Common Objects Comfortably
Those things you hold near to you every day as you go through your activities at work or home could be contributing to back

discomfort. A few precautions here can make a noticeable difference.

- Lighten shoulder bags and handbags. Ten women and two men in our survey got relief from back pain when they cut down their everyday load. They switched to lighter-weight handbags or shoulder bags, carried fewer objects, and shifted the handbag or shoulder bag from side to side to avoid muscle imbalance. Using a small rucksack instead of a handbag or shoulder bag may make you look less elegant, but rucksacks are the most comfortable way for some people to carry weighty necessities.
- Watch where you put your wallet. Sitting on a bulky wallet all day can literally cause or aggravate sciatica pain. The solution is not, as some survey participants quipped, to give everything in your wallet to a back specialist. Instead, keep your wallet somewhere else – in your jacket pocket, side pocket or a shoulder bag.
- Divide up your shopping. Carry your groceries in two shopping bags with handles and distribute their weight evenly. Don't clasp shopping bags to your chest or walk with them balanced on your hips. Avoid cardboard boxes. And, in general, keep the weight to a minimum. 'Buying everything you need for the week doesn't mean that you have to carry that week in one trip,' said a housewife. 'No medals are given out for wounded backs incurred while carrying an extra ten tins of dog food,' she added.
- Get yourself a wheeled trolley for bringing home your shopping.
- Put your laundry on wheels, too. You can buy a wheeled laundry cart at hardware and department stores, or you can put your laundry bag in a shopping cart.

14. Avoid Surgery if Possible

Many participants in the US survey believed that back surgery was often recommended without good reason. Of every four participants who were advised to have disc surgery, only one elected to have it. See Chapter 9 for steps you can take to avoid surgery.

15. Learn More about Medicines before Taking Them

All medicines have risks and side-effects that your doctor may not always explain to you. So you should carefully consider which medicines you decide to take on a regular basis, and whether or not their benefits outweigh the side-effects they sometimes cause. Judging from the experiences of UK survey participants, the most important point is to match the strength of the analgesic to the level of pain, thus enabling you to avoid using stronger painkillers, which are likely to cause more side-effects. However, you should also use medication early on, before high pain levels set in. (This will help you avoid taking large quantities of painkillers later on, when the increased pain has already started and it is too late for the medication to reduce it significantly.)

16. Treat Your Feet Well and Your Back May Thank You for It

More than a dozen US survey participants reported major relief from back pain when they switched from relatively high-heeled shoes (clogs, boots or women's high-heeled court shoes) to shoes with heels only a little higher than the soles.

Another ten survey participants were helped by heel lifts, heel cushions, arch supports and prescribed shoe inserts (orthotics).

A wide range of custom shoe insoles are available, made from highly shock-absorbent materials. These lessen the impact on your spine of walking or running. Ask at chemists, specialist sports and supply shops, or check the Internet. Start by using your inserts for half an hour the first day and use your new footwear half an hour more each succeeding day.

17. Join a Health Club

'It's not that I can exercise any better at the club, at least in terms of doing back exercises,' said a lawyer. 'But the camaraderie, the whirlpool, and the change of environment are good for me. I'm as stress-free as I can be after a workout at the club, and the same is not true after a workout at home.'

Almost 12 per cent of participants in the US survey joined health clubs. Most initially doubted they could find the time for this activity, but they viewed the time spent working out as essential to their physical and emotional well-being.

18. Enjoy the Healthiest Exercise Ever Invented

'If someone announced the invention of an activity that was non-weight-bearing, had great aerobic value, and stretched and strengthened virtually every muscle in your body, everyone would want to join in and it would make jogging seem like a medical disaster by comparison,' said the owner of an excavating company who eliminated his back pain by adding swimming to his back exercise routine.

There was not a single naysayer about swimming in either survey. There were, however, these cautionary notes: avoid the breaststroke and butterfly unless your back pain is unquestionably a thing of the past. (Even then, you might have difficulty with these strokes.) Also, avoid the overhand crawl until you're pain-free. Then work at it gradually. The sidestroke is easiest on your back; the backstroke is next best if you keep your arms close to your sides and use a short fluttering stroke.

19. Participate in a Mind-Body Activity

Some 10 per cent of US survey participants had a remarkable degree of success with yoga, and, to a slightly lesser extent, with modern dance and Tai Chi.

These three very different activities have one thing in common: they help the whole person. They increase back fitness while they bolster spirits and reduce stress.

Although some survey participants taught themselves yoga, modern dance or Tai Chi, professional instruction invariably made the experience more beneficial.

20. Eat Properly

Dietary habits that were viewed just a few years ago as the offbeat fetishes of health-food fanatics are now increasingly accepted by back sufferers, the general public and even the medical establishment: go light on junk foods and processed foods. Eat more fruit, vegetables and wholegrains. Cut down on animal fats. Reduce your intake of caffeine, sugar and alcohol. Substitute poultry and fish for beef.

What does this advice about nutrition have to do with your back? No one knows for sure. But, as a computer industry worker said, 'Eating properly makes you feel better about yourself and that just might help your back.'

It certainly can't hurt.

21. Lose Weight

'I think losing weight helped me some,' said a railroad employee who shed 11 kg (25 lb) in an effort to curb back pain. 'But,' she added, 'losing weight seemingly should have done more than it did. I keep thinking of all the thin people with back pain, and all the fat people whose backs never bother them, and I wonder if losing weight matters.'

Carrying less weight around can't hurt your back. And according to survey participants, it is likely to help a bit.

Be careful though. The process of losing weight can hurt your back. Three survey participants who were overweight, and who tried to lose weight, were injured while doing exercises from trendy diet and fitness books. These exercises are not meant to be rehabilitative, and their adverse effects actually discouraged some back sufferers from learning more appropriate exercise routines.

22. Make a Positive Reinforcement Tape

At a time when you're feeling fit and optimistic about your back, make a tape of all the things you should think and do daily to keep your back in good shape. Then play the tape on days when you need positive feedback and reinforcement.

23. Try Reverse-Gravity Relaxing and Exercising

Advertisements for back-care products sometimes exaggerate dramatically. But, according to US survey participants, reverse-gravity equipment is even better for your back than it claims to be. Exercising or just relaxing while hanging upside down or tilted towards the inverted position may ease pain appreciably.

Proprietary inversion devices can be expensive and take up a lot of room. Even a compact unit may need 0.4 square metres (4 square feet) or more of floor space. Those who have neither the money nor the room for a full system may be interested in a doorway chinning bar and inversion boots combination. Inversion racks and a choice of inversion boots can be browsed and ordered online from several product suppliers (see Useful Addresses, p. 463). Alternatively, ask at a medical or back shop.

See additional information and cautions about gravity inversion in Chapter 5.

24. Hanging from a Chinning Bar Can Increase Your Mobility and Flexibility

A few osteoarthritis back sufferers and low back sufferers found that 1 or 2 minutes of hanging – gripping a chinning bar and suspending themselves with their feet off the ground – reduced low back pain. Chinning bars are available from several product suppliers (see Useful Addresses, p. 463).

Non-inverted hanging has the potential to stretch out and relax the muscles and ligaments that support your spine. If you want to try it, follow these tips from back sufferers:

- Make certain that the bar is secure. If the frame of your doorway is not in the best shape, don't even try to install a chinning bar there.
- Position the bar so that you can just reach it on your tiptoes. Lower than this and you'll have to tuck your knees under you, a more awkward way to hold yourself up.
- Start by hanging for only 10 to 20 seconds. Even if you feel terrific, go slowly. Increase your hanging time by 10 seconds a day until you can hang for 1 to 2 minutes, twice a day.
- If you feel more than a little achy 18 to 24 hours after hanging, then this probably isn't for you and isn't worth trying again even when your aches have gone away.

25. Miscellaneous Tips Mentioned by Three or More Survey Participants

- If you have a very tight lower back, do slow, gentle shoulder shrugs and knee-to-chest stretches while reclining in a warm bath. (A body-length inflatable cushion makes it easier to do these warm-ups.) Then do your regular back exercise routine immediately after the bath.
- Before attempting unusually strenuous activity (anything

from tennis to snow shovelling) take two aspirin. The anti-inflammatory and analgesic properties of this drug may subdue aches before they can start up.

- Be a smart dresser. Wear an extra layer of clothing that you can take off if you're too warm. Bring along a jacket, sweater or fleece to put on after athletic activities. Getting chilled may never give you a cold, but it can play havoc with muscle spasms.
- Avoid constipation by drinking enough water and including enough bulk and fibre in your diet.
- Use a liniment (such as Deep Heat) to temporarily take your mind off aches and pains.
- Meditate. Even if you don't learn meditation from a professional, you will find it relaxing to take time every day to free your mind of all thoughts and concerns.
- If you don't own a firm mattress, a bed board, a straight-backed chair, a back cushion and a footrest, you should invest in these items. If your doctor prescribes them, the cost may be tax-deductible.

Chapter 14
Helping Your Back: Tips for Performing 25 Common Activities

Making love • Making the bed • Staying warm • Getting enough rest
• Reading at bedtime • Organizing wardrobes for easy dressing • Using
the toilet • Bathing • Cleaning the bathroom • Washing dishes • Dining
• Washing floors • Sweeping • Reaching high shelves • Sitting • Vacuuming
• Dusting and window washing • Moving furniture • Painting • Shovelling
snow • Raking leaves • Splitting and carrying firewood • Lifting and hauling
debris • Gardening • Sitting at a sports stadium, Beach or picnic

If you lived in Sweden and had a chronic back problem, a physiotherapist might spend an entire day and evening with you just to observe how your activities affect your back. Wherever you went, whatever you did, the therapist would be there. Then he or she would compile detailed recommendations about what you should and shouldn't do to help your back around the clock.

In the USA, backs tend to be observed by X-rays rather than eyes. Back sufferers usually have to compress their medical histories into a few minutes of hurried conversation. Back practitioners rarely if ever get to see their back patients in action – sleeping, walking, working at the office, watching TV, eating, making the bed, driving, playing tennis, gardening and picking up the baby. As a result, the real culprits behind back problems are seldom seen, discussed, pinpointed or – most important – eliminated.

What should you do? Become your own back doctor. How? By making use of the most potent diagnostic skill of all: direct observation. Watch yourself from morning till night. Track yourself from room to room, place to place, activity to activity. That's what this chapter helps you to do. While reading it, you may want to make some notes about specific changes you can make to help yourself.

Of course, there is no quiz or test at the end of this chapter. But do try to think of the material as a test of how serious you are about self-care, about taking responsibility for yourself to the greatest possible extent, about changing your life to reflect the proven principles of good back care recommended by survey participants and discussed throughout this book.

More than 95 per cent of participants in the US survey who got dramatically better – and who no longer have back pain – literally had to change their lives to achieve this new level of back fitness. The following suggestions and guidelines are based on advice from about a hundred US survey participants. The tips are organized according to the places in and around your house where you may need specific information. I begin in the bedroom with positions for sex, because survey participants mentioned these more than any other topic covered in this chapter.

The Bedroom

Note: For tips about sleeping positions, watching TV in bed, and manoeuvring your way into and out of bed, see Chapters 9 and 12.

1. Making Love

'To the extent that the body is not flexible, the mind has to be,' commented a commercial artist who couldn't work for six months because of a ruptured disc. 'You can almost always find a way to have sex if your attitude about it is flexible and if you realize that your mind is the key to sexual pleasure. Some sex of any kind is better than deprivation, which can cause depression and bring about a heightened sense of pain.'

Most back books make much ado about the physical aspects of sex, including how a wide variety of intercourse positions can restore your sex life. Here are the three positions for intercourse recommended most by survey participants:

Face to face

Lying on your side with your knees bent, facing your partner, is the least risky sexual intercourse position for a back sufferer.

Since the position is also a natural one for non-sexual intimacy, it avoids the need, as one survey participant put it, 'to make a big deal about rearranging yourself in order to have sex.'

Front to back

Lying front to back, nestled like spoons, with the man behind the woman, is another safe position for sexual intercourse. Many couples feel that this position also facilitates penetration.

Modified missionary

If you are comfortable lying on your back with your knees elevated – and if your partner is strong enough to keep most of his or her weight off you – then this is also a safe position for sexual intercourse.

If the woman is the back sufferer, she assumes the bottom position, and places a small pillow under her head and neck and two plump pillows under her knees. Her partner lies on top if he can support most of his own weight. The easiest way for the man to do this is to get into what looks like a push-up position, with his hands placed on either side of the woman's shoulders.

If the man is the back sufferer, he lies on his back and his partner lowers herself on him in a seated position, with her knees and legs bearing most of her weight. If the woman cannot bear most of the weight herself, this position should be avoided.

Although these sexual intercourse positions topped the list of suggestions by survey participants who had an active sex life despite back pain, many survey participants declined to recommend specific positions. They felt it best to talk in terms of what you should not do and leave the rest up to individual preferences and limitations. 'As long as I don't arch my back excessively during sex, I'm fine,' said an accountant. 'I would only suggest that back sufferers do whatever they feel like doing, and know they can do, at any given time.'

A marine biologist said, 'The fear of injury during sex had a disastrous effect on my sex life for years. The solution is not to read a manual about sex, or try to hide from it, but to talk about it openly with your partner. And once you've discussed what you can't do, talk a lot about all the wonderful pleasures you can have. Then stop talking and start doing.'

'Keep in mind that intercourse is not the only option,' noted a physics teacher. 'Masturbation, whether alone or mutual, is a healthy option. So is oral sex, which can be done comfortably in the foetal position.'

And a federal employee concluded. 'The rocking motion of gentle sex is the best therapy ever invented for a back sufferer's body and mind.'

2. Making the Bed

Bend your knees instead of bending at the waist to reach the bed. Get into a kneeling position and stay there as you make your way around the bed. Work slowly and keep repositioning yourself to avoid overstretching your back.

Unless your bed rolls effortlessly, it's best to keep it free-standing, away from the walls. Otherwise you'll be forced either to reach too far in smoothing sheets and blankets, or to move the whole bed each time you want to straighten it.

Don't make the bed at all if you're in severe pain. And don't bother turning over your mattress every few months unless you have someone there to help you.

3. Staying Warm in Bed

Survey participants with muscle spasms or osteoarthritis-based back pain are quick to feel the painful effects of a chilly night. Appropriate sleepwear, blankets and room temperature are usually enough to avoid problems. But if you can't get comfortable, back-care products are available that may generate more warmth under and around your body, such as mattress pads, both electric and non-electric.

4. Getting Enough Rest

Nearly all back sufferers report increased back pain when they get less sleep than usual. On days when you don't get enough rest, you can protect your back simply by easing up on strenuous activities that tend to cause you problems. Also, survey participants note a tendency to 'slump' into poor posture when tired, and need to watch extra carefully how they stand and sit.

5. Reading at Bedtime

Reading in bed is one pastime most survey participants have had to learn to live without. If you like to read just before going to sleep, they advise, get a good chair for your bedroom. It is all but impossible to read in bed without hurting your back. And if you need a little extra push to make this change, remember that most sleep experts say that reading or working in bed is a major cause of insomnia.

6. Organizing Your Wardrobe

If you're recovering from a bad back, have someone help you rearrange your wardrobe so that you can reach the things you need without effort. For example, instead of keeping your shoes at the bottom of your wardrobe, put them in a shoe bag on the door.

If it is a strain to reach for objects on a high shelf, move them to a more accessible spot or leave a small footstool in or near your wardrobe.

It may be worth purchasing a 'gripper' device such as an Easyreacher (available from several product suppliers, see Useful Addresses, p. 463). This can extend your arm's reach by over 60 cm (2 feet). It will help you retrieve objects from the floor or high shelves without the need to arch your back, bend or stoop.

The Bathroom

Note: See Chapter 13 for suggestions on how to turn your bath into a therapy centre for relieving back pain.

7. Using the Toilet

Toilet seats are rather devilish devices for back sufferers. They are awkward to get down to, unsupportive to sit on, and difficult to get up from. But just as there are easier ways to get into bed, so there are ways to take the strain off a painful back when using the toilet.

For example, until you are free of disabling pain, rails on both sides of the toilet can be helpful. They are safe and simple to install, and are reasonably inexpensive.

Another way to ease the pain of getting on and off the toilet is to raise the seat itself, and there are at least two ways to get around the discomfort of not having your back supported on the toilet. One is to wear a lumbar support belt whenever you use the toilet. Another option is to wedge a lumbar cushion between your back and the back of the toilet.

8. Bathing

When you're recovering from a back injury, getting into and out of the bath can also be a problem. Bath safety rails are available and are not too difficult to fit.

9. Cleaning the Bathroom

To avoid back strain when you clean the bath or toilet, kneel rather than bend over. Instead of stretching across the bath with a sponge, use a scrubber with a long handle.

The Kitchen

10. Washing the Dishes

Leaning over the sink to do the dishes is difficult for most people and especially so for back sufferers. And dishwashers don't completely solve the problem. However, here are some helpful suggestions:

- Turn your body to one side before you stretch to reach the taps. It's easier to lean sideways.
- Stand right up against the sink counter. Standing even a few centimetres away from the sink can vastly increase the amount of back pain you feel. (A plastic apron will keep you drier and more comfortable than distance from the sink.)
- Lift whatever you're washing out of the sink and hold it close to your body as you clean it. (A mat on the floor will keep the lino dry.)
- Put your washing-up bowl on the draining board to give additional height.
- Shift your weight from one foot to the other every few minutes.
- Support one foot on a footstool or open the cupboard under the sink and rest one foot on the ledge.
- Soak whatever pots and pans may take long to clean – and go back to them later.

- The minute your back feels tired, switch to a less stressful chore, or simply take a break.

11. Sitting at the Table

If you are uncomfortable sitting at the table, especially during long meals, follow survey participants' advice about straight-backed chairs, back cushions and footrests (see pp. 158–64 and 252–3).

12. Washing the Floor

Use a sponge mop that can be squeezed dry with a lever high up on the handle. These are available in most supermarkets and hardware stores.

Think about your posture as you work. Keep your abdominal muscles tightened and your spine leaning forward only slightly. You may find you can stand straighter if you hold the mop with one hand instead of two.

13. Sweeping

The really tricky part here is collecting what you have swept while remaining upright. You can do this with a long-handled dustpan.

14. Reaching Food on High Shelves

Standing on your tiptoes and reaching as far as you can to get boxes and jars down from shelves can aggravate pain in your back. One solution is to use a footstool. Human nature being what it is, this tends to work only if you keep the footstool right where you work – and keep plants and other decorative objects off it.

Another solution, especially if you're too uncomfortable to climb steps, is a 'gripper' device such as the Easyreacher (available from several product suppliers, see Useful Addresses, p. 463).

The Living Room

15. Sitting

If you have lovely looking but unbearably soft chairs and sofas in your living room, try concealing a 1 cm (½ inch) piece of plywood under their cushions to provide more support. Even then you should still keep a good straight-backed chair – or at least a firm reclining chair for yourself – in the living room.

If you don't usually sit in the living room – and you don't have a good sitting arrangement for yourself there – make one up before friends come.

A printer explained why: 'My wife and I like our living room to look nice, and frankly, a straight-backed chair doesn't fit into our decor. Of course, my back is more important than appearances. But I have found that if I don't get a chair, back support and footstool set up before company comes over, I'm not likely to do it at all. This may sound silly, but it embarrasses me to bring in "special provisions" for my back. It means having to talk about my back, and few subjects are as boring to me and to my company. However, if one of the wooden kitchen chairs is already in place in the living room, with a nice footstool as well as the plain black lumbar cushion that I have, then I'll sit the way I should and not have any problem the next day.

'To help my back and my wife,' the printer continued, 'I'm the one who asks people if they want more of anything. This is an unobtrusive way for me to take a break from sitting. People who don't know me that well may think I'm a good host or a liberated husband. But the point is that I've been a good host for ten years and I haven't had a backache after a party for ten years. I would like to address a final comment to your male readers. I don't lift the groceries out of the car. My wife does. If that sounds bad, so be it. The truth is that some men would rather wind up in traction than harm their macho image.'

16. Vacuuming
Enough vacuuming will give almost anyone a backache. And judging from the comments of survey participants, it is clear that the people who suffer the most back pain from vacuuming are those who are compulsive about this chore. If this description fits you, try to change your attitude about routine chores by following these suggestions from survey participants:

• Don't vacuum when you're in pain. 'Resist, relax, take a bath – stop being so compulsive,' said one housewife.

- Invest in a vacuum cleaner that you can push with minimal exertion and bending. Work with one hand at a time, if you can. You'll feel better with one hand at your side.
- Don't vacuum for more than 15 minutes at a stretch. And stop sooner than that if your back feels fatigued.

17. Dusting and Window Washing
The strain of dusting or cleaning high places can often be reduced simply by using a longer cleaning tool, especially one that combines a duster/squeegee on the head. Long-reach window washers are also available.

18. Moving Furniture
When you want to redecorate your living room, or any other room for that matter, don't try to push furniture around. Buy a small dolly mover and wheel it to and fro.

19. Painting
There's no easy answer to the many problems your back can encounter while painting, but here are some helpful suggestions from survey participants:

- Stand as close as possible to what you're painting. Your posture will be better and your arms will remain relatively close to your body.
- When you're painting walls, position yourself so that your arms are at a level between your chest and waist.
- Use whatever apparatus will get the job done fast – brush, roller or paint gun. Rollers are usually best. Brushes can take too long, and paint guns are too heavy to hold for any appreciable time.
- Know your limits. The rest of the wall does not have to be completed immediately if finishing it will finish you.
- Hire someone to do the ceilings. If you can't, find a friend with a strong back. Failing that, look down every few minutes, take a 1-minute break every 5 minutes, take a 10-minute break every half-hour, and do the standing neck and upper-shoulder exercises described in Chapter 10.

Outdoors

20. Shovelling Snow and
21. Raking Leaves

According to estimates based on the US survey data, these two seasonal activities cause several million people a year to seek professional treatment for their backs. The strain of raking and snow shovelling comes from excessive forward leaning and arm extension. In this awkward and unsupported position, your back is extremely vulnerable.

One obvious but usually impractical solution is to avoid these tasks altogether, either by neglecting them or hiring someone else to do them. You could also invest in blowers, tractors and other expensive outdoor equipment.

However, there are rakes and shovels with a gooseneck bend design that allows you to stand up straighter and shift some of the lifting oomph from your back to your arms.

For either raking or shovelling, you'll be warmer and more comfortable if you dress in layers. You can always remove outer clothing to avoid getting overheated. Several survey participants recommended wearing a long undershirt made of a 'wick-through' fabric that keeps moisture away from the skin and thus helps prevent chills and spasms. Cotton may feel best next to your skin when dry, but it loses most of its insulating properties – not to mention its nice feel –when it gets wet.

When you shovel, remember to:

- bend your legs and not your back
- keep the shovel as close to your body as possible
- keep the size of each load modest.

For raking:

- keep your knees slightly bent
- position one foot in front of the other
- avoid excessive leaning
- kneel or squat – don't stoop – whether you're lifting one leaf or one million.

When you rake leaves into piles, never attempt to move an entire pile with your rake. Use a long-handled scoop or 'claws' to pick up leaves, grass cuttings, pine needles and rubbish spills.

To carry bags of leaves, take two small bags of equal weight at a time, leaving your arms at your sides. Holding a large bag out in front of you can really harm your back.

If you have to carry autumn leaves any distance, a cart built for this purpose will save you wear and tear.

22. Splitting and Carrying Firewood

Chopping wood is a wonderful activity that can benefit many back sufferers. 'It's a great outlet for stress,' said a bank manager, 'and far better than jogging to let out aggression.'

'Chopping wood is great for getting the kinks out and maintaining muscle tone,' said a chemical factory worker. 'You're outside and doing something vigorous and constructive.'

But there's a darker side to the story for back sufferers, because for every survey participant who extolled chopping wood, another reported an injury from it.

Here are some suggestions to help you enjoy yourself safely:

- Find an axe with a weight you can mange. A heavier axe may save you swings, but your back will feel better wielding a lighter weight through more swings of the axe.
- Keep your knees bent and your feet shoulder-width apart.
- Avoid swinging exclusively from one side; a muscular imbalance may result that could cause or aggravate back pain.
- Stop when you're tired.

23. Picking Up and Hauling Debris

Don't try dragging rubbish or other items around yourself. Invest in a wheeled cart.

24. Gardening

'If there's a gardener someplace out there who has never clutched his sacro-iliac after being in a stooped position too long, let him come forward now,' a watercolour artist commented about the relationship between gardening and back pain.

'There are two givens about gardening,' a retiree and avid gardener said. 'Physically, it isn't good for your back. Spiritually, it is good for your back.'

And a paper products manufacturer observed, 'Only one thing motivates me to do my daily back exercises . . . and that's to keep in good enough condition to continue doing more gardening . . . which in turn continues to threaten my back with mayhem.'

Clearly, gardening is a thoroughly enjoyable activity for many. Equally clearly, it caused survey participants more back pain than any other popular pastime, including jogging and team sports.

What can be done? Quite a lot.

According to most survey participants, the paper products manufacturer quoted above had the best suggestion: exercise your back to keep it in shape for gardening. Do not follow in the footsteps of one survey participant who, speaking from his bed while recuperating from a bad episode of low back pain, said: 'Gardening is all the exercise my back needs. I may have overdone it again, but in any event, my back is always too tired after gardening to do back exercises.' (See Chapter 8 for a complete back exercise programme.)

Think of gardening activities as a way to strengthen your arms and legs – not your back. In other words, use your legs and arms to lift, carry, pull, dig and scrape – and try to give your back a free ride. Kneel and squat. Don't scoop or slouch. Don't garden with your back.

Face the fact that gardening is physically stressful – and be realistic about what you can accomplish. As mentioned above, it is theoretically possible to work in the garden without bending at the waist or working your back into a state of protest. But that's like saying you could garden without getting your hands dirty. You could – but no one does. An airline stewardess found this way out of the dilemma: 'If you like gardening as much as I do, you're going to ache the next day. I try to tell myself that my back will be okay if I treat it only half as well as I treat my plants. This basically means trying to keep my back straight. I do this by thinking about posture, as well as by using tools with long handles and keeping them close to my body. As a last resort, if my back really hurts and there is more weeding to be done, I plant myself in the garden – on my side – and get the weeds up that way. I look funny. I might even smell funny. But I'm back gardening the next day.'

Use the right tools. Long-handled 'claws', mentioned in the preceding section, are useful for more than picking up leaves. They also help you pick up weeds, stones and other objects that shouldn't be in your garden. Invest in other long-handled tools to keep you upright while you cultivate, weed and aerate your garden. Finally, the right equipment for watering your garden can help keep back problems at bay. Many devices for this purpose are available at garden centres and hardware stores – including lightweight hoses on retractable reels, inexpensive connectors for hard-to-reach outside taps and elaborately timed sprinkler systems.

25. Sitting at Outdoor Events

Many survey participants suffered more back trouble from observing sporting events than from participating in them. For example, parents who sat and watched their kids at school sports days had a tough time on 'backless' benches. Beach lovers found it more uncomfortable to read at the beach than to take a long swim. And back sufferers at picnics found it more difficult to sit unsupported than to make a long hike to the picnic grounds.

There is an obvious solution: bring along your own seating arrangements. For instance, stadium chairs (folding chairs without legs) are available from some camping and outdoor equipment shops. But most survey participants were too embarrassed to do this. Even back sufferers who were willing to bring a good folding chair to the beach wouldn't bring the same chair to a picnic or to a sports field.

But since the essence of sitting comfortably at outdoor activities is to care more about being good to your back than about what others think, prove it by bringing along whatever it takes to make yourself comfortable. This might be a favourite folding chair or an exercise or insulation mat.

Part 2
Back Pain: What Exercises Really Work

Section 6
The Magic Bullet

No-one pretends exercising is easy. Painkillers and other treatments can help to control the pain to let you get started. It does hurt at first, but one thing is sure: the longer you put off exercise the harder and more painful it will be. There is no other way. You have a straight choice: rest, or work through your pain and recovery.

The Back Book by Roland et al, published by HMSO, 1996

Chapter 15
Exercise by Prescription

Are you in bed? Right this moment, are you suffering spasms of incapacitating back pain? Wondering how long you'll have to lie there this time? Worrying about when you can get back to work?

I hope not. But if you are, or if the memory of such an incident is still all too fresh in your mind, I believe this book can give you the help you need to end your episodes of back pain once and for all.

Indeed, the long-awaited, highly touted cure for back pain – the treatment that could relieve the agonies of an estimated 80 per cent of the British public and save the country over £1.6 billion each year in direct healthcare costs – has actually been discovered. It is called exercise. And it works.

Unfortunately, few people really understand the enormous benefits to be gained from exercise, and even fewer people with back pain are therefore willing to invest any time or effort in an exercise programme specifically aimed at controlling their painful symptoms. Many of the 8 million plus British people who suffer from periodic bouts of back pain continue to think that there must be a more scientific solution to their woes. They cannot accept the fact that exercise is simply the best, most potent medicine available to treat a back problem.

This lack of knowledge about exercise is a national tragedy. The fact is, as little as 10 minutes of exercise a day for two weeks will bring about a striking degree of improvement for most people. The US survey showed that many of the most widely used treatments for back pain were either ineffective or downright dangerous. It also showed that the right exercises, performed the right way, were the only key to a pain-free back.

These recommendations, originally published in *Backache Relief*, reflected the positive experiences of many survey participants who enjoyed dramatic, long-term relief from back pain, without suffering repeat collapses. What accounted for these individuals' successful outcomes? In a word, exercise. The secret to remaining pain-free, they said, lay in learning – and sticking to – a well-designed exercise programme.

The book in your hands outlines just such a safe, sane exercise programme. It gives clear, simple instructions and step-by-step drawings to help you learn the exercise routines with ease. It will also help you devise your own individually tailored exercise programme to accomplish any or all of the following goals:

- Prevent back problems from plaguing you in the future
- Treat a disabling episode of acute pain
- Achieve lasting relief from chronic backache
- Make lifestyle changes that can put an end to back pain

The advice and suggestions about exercise in this book are based not only on survey research, but also on a continuing review of hospital studies investigating the value of exercise for back pain. Numerous studies, completed since the publication of *Backache Relief*, have added further proof that exercise can succeed in helping to alleviate back problems – even after other treatments have failed. Medical researchers all over the world now state confidently that a combination of aerobic, stretching, strengthening and endurance exercises can bring about genuine improvement for most painful back conditions. Instead of dismissing back pain as 'the price we pay for walking upright', specialists are at last coming to see back pain as the consequence of not walking upright enough – of spending too much time sitting at a desk, in front of the television or behind the wheel.

For example, a study conducted at the University of Copenhagen, divided 105 patients with chronic low back pain into three groups. One group underwent three months of intensive exercise training, which entailed thirty workout sessions. The second group attended just as many sessions in the gym, but were asked to perform only a fraction of the activity. The third group had the most sedentary time of all, performing some mild exercise at their sessions, but spending more time receiving heat treatments and massage.

As the doctors reported in 1991 in the journal *Pain*, the subjects in the active-exercise group who continued training at least once a week over the follow-up year were in the best shape, with less pain and greater mobility than they had at the study's outset. The positive result held as true for women as for men, regardless of age. The researchers also noted that the patients' pre-existing conditions had little bearing on their improvement. Indeed, even some veterans of chronic back syndromes got better as a result of the increased activity.

The programme offered in this book is neither rigorous nor difficult. Some of the exercises may seem no more strenuous to you than an everyday activity such as getting out of bed or shopping for your groceries. Yet the simple act of stretching your legs and strengthening your abdominal muscles will have profound effects on the way you look and feel. A small amount of effort will pay off in a noticeable improvement in well-being.

More validation for exercise emerged from a study at Sweden's Sahlgren Hospital. The participants there included 103 industrial workers who had been out of work for eight weeks because of low back pain. The doctors instructed half of this group in gentle, individually tailored exercises and safety tips for avoiding injury. Not surprisingly, this half ended up going back to work sooner, feeling better. Over the ensuing year, those who exercised and 'watched their backs' lost fewer work days than others who did not learn such precautions, according to the researchers' 1992 report in the journal *Physical Therapy*.

In the USA, where back pain accounts for 40 to 50 per cent of all lost work days, and as many as one-third of all workers' compensation payments, employees in all sorts of industrial and office settings could be helped by performing exercises at home and learning the back-kindest ways to go about their jobs. You will find tips of this sort in Chapters 13 and 14.

When medical studies compare exercise to no exercise, few researchers are surprised to find that the exercise effort pays off in terms of pain relief. Other studies go even further in establishing the importance of exercise – by comparing exercise to other widely used treatments for back pain. For example, Dr Richard A. Deyo of the University of Washington School of Medicine and School of Public Health has tested exercise against transcutaneous electrical nerve stimulation, called TENS. In treatment, the TENS device, about the size of a television remote control, is hooked up to the patient's back via wires and electrodes that gently and steadily jolt the areas of muscle spasm. The electric current is said to send signals to the brain that block other nerve signals carrying pain messages. It is also believed to stimulate the production of endorphins (natural pain-relieving hormones produced by the body). The device is usually used for 15 or 20 minutes, several times a day.

For his research project, Dr Deyo gave each of his subjects either a real TENS device or a sham TENS unit that gave no jolt but looked like a working machine. Since he never told patients of the differences, each expected some help to come from the little machine. At the same time, Dr Deyo also put several of the participants on a programme of stretching exercises to be performed in addition to the TENS treatments. After a month, the subjects who had exercised were better off than those who hadn't, regardless of whether they had the real or false TENS units. Only the exercise proved valuable. But the subjects didn't seem to understand the connection. Despite the improvement, most of them had given up exercising by the time they had a follow-up examination two months later – and their pain had returned.

To help you stick to your exercise programme, I've come up with ways to work it into your daily routine, so that you won't look at exercise as just another impossible demand on your time. Chapter 19 gives the details of these strategies, and Chapter 21 offers tips on sustaining your motivation to exercise even when people or problems may tempt you to give up.

Another 'treatment' long advocated as a way to beat a bad back is weight control. Doctors have suggested that dieting to lose 2–4.5 kg (5–10 lb) would reduce the strain on the back and therefore ward off future episodes of back pain. However, it seems that many doctors who gave this advice were just trying to shift the blame onto the patient instead of offering helpful exercise advice. In fact, the evidence shows that only the very obese stand to gain back pain relief from losing weight. The person who is just a few kilos or pounds above his or her ideal weight is at no greater risk for back trouble than a thin man or woman. And besides, exercise and increased activity tend to bring weight under reasonable control without the stress of dieting.

Prolonged bed rest for back pain is now recognized as the main culprit in delaying recovery and causing a host of other unwelcome problems, including bone loss, general weakness and blood clots in the legs. Despite this, a 1998 survey showed that, on average, British GPs still recommended bed rest to one in four of the people who asked them about back pain.

Even if you are staying at home because you are in too much pain to go to work, and you cannot manage to sit in a chair, you will probably do better if you spend a good part of each day standing up and resting on your feet, as opposed to staying in bed. Chapter 20 offers a few preliminary 'exercise positions' for people who have been confined to bed by intractable pain, and who are just beginning to be able to exercise.

Further endorsement for exercise activity emerged from the so-called Quebec Task Force, a large consortium of researchers and back doctors who reviewed a worldwide collection of clinical reports. They concluded that only two things truly help people with common low back pain: aerobic conditioning (exercise, that is) and education about the proper way to sit, stand, lift and carry. You will find a guide to appropriate aerobic exercises in Chapters 24 and 25. For tips on performing everyday activities, you can refer back to Chapters 13 and 14.

If you have consulted a doctor about your back pain, you may well have received some exercise advice already. If, however, your doctor has not mentioned the importance of exercise in alleviating back pain, I urge you to raise the subject yourself. Take this book along to show the doctor, and get his or her opinion on the safety of the programme for your specific condition. The exercises contained here are safe and will pass any practitioner's cautious inspection. Chapter 25 even includes exercises particularly recommended for specific back pain conditions, such as osteoarthritis-based back pain and scoliosis.

Whatever condition your back is in, you can improve your condition with exercise. Even if you have not been able to exercise in the past, and feel limited by pain now, you can find suggestions in this book that will enable you to work a helpful amount of exercise into your life.

Chapter 16
Alternatives to Exercise

Exercise is almost invariably better for your back than anything else you can put onto or into your body. Compared with all other back pain treatments, exercise makes the most sense because it is harmless, affordable and effective.

As we know, back pain afflicts an estimated 80 per cent of the British population at one time or another, and costs over £1.6 billion annually in direct healthcare expenses. There are also huge costs to the economy generally. For instance, nearly 5 million working days were lost in the UK through bad backs in 2003/2004.

If you are currently suffering from back pain, wondering what course of treatment to pursue or what kind of practitioner to consult, you no doubt have a lot of unanswered questions. Following are the questions I hear most often from people with back problems – along with answers gleaned from the US and UK surveys and my reading of the medical literature.

How Long Should I Rest in Bed?
The answer is: avoid going to bed and resting because of back pain. As soon as you can, return to normal activities and gentle exercise. If necessary, use painkillers to help you remain active. You should try to stay at work or return to work as soon as possible. The longer you stay off work, the lower your chances of returning in the long term. Bed rest is not a treatment. It just contributes to weaker muscles and stiffer joints, and so getting going after a period of bed rest can be extremely difficult. All this can be avoided by not going to bed with a bad back.

I Want to See a Doctor. Can My GP Help Me?
If your family doctor knows you and knows back pain, this may be all the help you'll ever need. If, however, your family doctor's

answer to a back problem is only to pull out a prescription pad you may need to look elsewhere.

Your family doctor may decide to refer you to a specialist, such as an orthopaedic surgeon, a rheumatologist or a neurosurgeon. Referrals make sense in medicine, so long as the family doctor is really trying to bring in an expert's opinion and assistance – and not merely dismissing you and your back pain by shipping you off to someone else.

General practitioners frequently refer their patients with back pain to an orthopaedic surgeon. Don't let the word surgeon scare you. Only about 1 to 3 per cent of all cases of back pain can be treated surgically, so the odds of your needing an operation are slim. Instead, a well-informed orthopaedic surgeon will try to diagnose your condition and prescribe the necessary exercises, or perhaps call in a physiotherapist to work with you. An orthopaedic surgeon who is less well informed – or less inclined to work with people outside the operating room – may say, 'There's nothing really wrong with you.' This throws the ball back in your court, so to speak, making you feel worse than ever. Now you not only hurt, but you've also been told that you hurt for no good reason. But don't lose hope if this happens to you! This is the time to work out a recovery plan, preferably with your family doctor's help, that involves a graduated programme of stretching exercises plus walking.

Do I Need X-Rays to Discover What's Wrong with My Back?

Probably not. The very process of having an X-ray may set you up for needless anxiety and disappointment – or worse. Since only a few back conditions show up on X-rays, most X-ray findings are negative. In other words, they don't give you any useful information.

About 80 per cent of all cases of low back pain can be traced to problems with the muscles, ligaments or discs. And none of these soft tissues show up on an X-ray image. Only bones do.

In some cases, X-rays reveal real conditions that may have nothing to do with the current source of pain. Suppose, for example, that you have mild scoliosis, which means that your spine is not perfectly straight. Somehow you have made it through life with no idea of this benign condition. Now that you find yourself in pain, however, some practitioner may be all too ready to blame your discomfort on the scoliosis. It is more likely that you have a muscle spasm or strain, unrelated to the X-ray finding.

Another common X-ray finding in practically anyone over the age of thirty-five is some degree of arthritis in the facet joints of the spine. Even if this is the case for you, the odds are still over-whelmingly in favour of your back pain being of a muscular origin – and having an exercise solution.

One real problem with X-rays is that doctors who rely on them often conclude, from reading your X-ray, that 'there's nothing really wrong with you.' But really, there is something wrong. It's just that what's wrong with you doesn't show up on the X-ray.

What about Chiropractors? Aren't They as Good as – or Better than – Medical Doctors for Treating Back Pain?

Chiropractors fared slightly better, at least in the short term, than orthopaedic surgeons in the US survey, which compared and rated more than one hundred types of practitioners and treatments. They enjoyed their greatest success, among the US participants, with acute cases of low back and neck pain. They were less helpful to people who had severe chronic pain; in fact, they often proved counter-productive, as when they attempted to treat conditions such as herniated disc, sciatica or severe arthritis pain. Likewise, they had little success in correcting scoliosis.

The hands-on manipulation for which chiropractors are famous worked best when it was done gently. Overall, chiropractic manip-ulation seemed less important, in terms of patient satisfaction, than these practitioners' holistic approach and willingness to listen. Chiropractors dispensed exercise advice as part of their treatments, which was all to the good, and sometimes they gave nutritional counsel as well as advice about lifestyle and the role of stress in aggravating back pain.

Chiropractors, like orthopaedic surgeons, base their diagnoses on X-rays, but, unlike orthopaedic surgeons, they invariably see a specific cause of pain on an X-ray. These causes are termed 'subluxations' and 'misalignments', often resulting in 'pinched nerves', which the chiropractor aims to correct through manipu-lation of the spine.

The chiropractor's real secret of success, however, is a knowledge of exercise combined with the ability to build a good rapport with patients – and encourage them to exercise.

How Can I Find Out Exactly What's Wrong with My Back?

You may not be able to find out – ever. The US survey showed that practitioners made diagnoses based on their medical speciality and frame of reference. This means that two doctors from different fields are more than likely to give you two different names for your condition, and two different explanations of what caused the problem. Or neither one will be able to pinpoint the cause of pain with any degree of specificity.

Although some episodes of back pain can be linked to strains incurred during over-exertion or in falls, at least as many bouts strike literally out of the blue. Even if you don't know exactly what the cause of your pain is, you can still get better by staying active and taking gentle daily exercise.

Do I Need Medication?

If you need painkillers, it's best to take them regularly. This should prevent the pain from getting severe, and help you to stay active. Paracetamol may be strong enough, if you take it regularly at full strength. For an adult, this is 1,000 mg (usually two 500 mg tablets), four times a day.

Some people find anti-inflammatory painkillers more effective than paracetamol. These include Ibuprofen (available over the counter or on prescription). For others, such as Diclofenac, Naproxen or Tolfenamic, you will need a prescription. Note: Anti-inflammatory painkillers are unsuitable if you suffer from asthma, high blood pressure, or severe kidney problems or heart problems.

If anti-inflammatories are not suitable for you, or do not work well, you could try a stronger painkiller such as codeine. Codeine is often taken in combination with paracetamol. Many people find that codeine makes them constipated, and it may make your back pain worse if you strain to go to the toilet. To avoid constipation, you should drink lots of water and eat plenty of fruit, vegetables and wholegrain foods.

Muscle relaxants are sometimes prescribed for a few days for tense back muscles (which can make pain worse).

How Do I Know if I Have a Slipped Disc? And What Treatment Will I Receive if I Do?

Many doctors diagnose a 'slipped' – or, more correctly, a 'herniated' or ruptured disc – by the degree and location of the patient's pain. This condition frequently causes numbness or tingling in the legs, all the way to the feet. The back, buttock and leg pain may well be excruciating.

Although herniated discs do not show up on X-rays, as explained above, they can be visualized with other imaging procedures such as CT (computed tomography) scans and MRI (magnetic resonance imaging).

The discs, twenty-three in number, are positioned between the second vertebra of the neck (the axis) and the base of the spine (the sacrum). They cushion the bones and add mechanical strength to the spine. The structure of the disc itself – soft inside, firm outside – invites comparison to a jam doughnut. An injury or deterioration can make the 'jam' bulge out into the spinal canal, where it may press on a nerve root, causing extreme pain and sometimes threatening paralysis.

In most cases, a herniated disc does not require surgery. However, because of the intense pain and the risk of neurological impairment associated with a herniated disc, you will need to seek a medical opinion. Remember, though, that many people have recovered with the aid of strong pain medication alone. (This is a situation in which such medicines are clearly indicated.)

As most herniated discs end up correcting themselves, experienced physicians reserve surgery as a last resort, to be avoided until all other, safer approaches – including 'tincture of time' in a six-week dose – have failed to deliver relief. Only about 5 to 10 per cent of people with herniated discs actually require surgery, according to studies conducted at Harvard Medical School.

Advances in surgical technique have given rise to 'scarless' disc procedures that can be performed on an outpatient basis, with tiny arthroscopic instruments and lasers. These operations tend to lead to fewer complications and faster recuperation at home than traditional disc surgery. But these approaches don't yet match the success rates of the traditional operations. And instead of simply lessening the stress of surgery for those who need it, the seemingly benign procedures are more likely to be offered to people who don't really need surgery.

Manipulation, according to the US survey results, is one treatment that can sometimes make the pain and disability of a herniated disc considerably worse.

Could My Back Pain Be Caused by Some Other Health Problem?

It could indeed, and that's why it makes sense to see a medical doctor for a thorough check-up when you have back pain. Conditions that can cause backache include arthritis, kidney disease, colitis and certain forms of cancer.

I'm a Bit Overweight. Would Dieting Help My Back Pain?

It depends on how overweight you are. Many doctors say that losing 2 to 4 kg (5 to 10 lb) by dieting will reduce the strain on your back and help you avoid future episodes of back pain. In fact, if you are only slightly overweight, dieting probably won't make much difference to your level of back pain. If you are more seriously overweight, the extra weight is bound to put more stress on your back so it may be worth trying to lose some of it. However, exercise and increased activity tend to bring weight under reasonable control – without dieting.

How Can Exercise Help My Back Pain?

Exercise stretches and strengthens the four sets of muscles that support the spine. Your abdominal muscles, for example, although they are not directly attached to the spine, form a girdle around your internal organs and contribute to good posture. The abdominals also assist the extensor muscles of the back, which flank the full length of the spine, to maintain proper alignment of the vertebrae. Your hip and buttock muscles help support and govern the position of your back while you're sitting, standing or walking. Muscle pain typically arises from weakness, spasm or loss of elasticity due to age or inactivity. All of these conditions can be remedied through exercise.

Some People Get Over Episodes of Horrible Back Pain by Trying Nutty Home Remedies, and Others Get Better Without Doing Anything at All about It. So Why Should I Bother Exercising?

It's true that many – perhaps most – episodes of intractable back pain end of their own accord, regardless of the treatments applied. The on-again, off-again nature of some back problems, in fact, has given false endorsements to many dubious types of treatment over the years, from corticosteroid injections to DMSO. Doctors and patients alike may attribute sudden improvement to whatever treatment is fashionable at the time.

Back pain can disappear, in time, with no treatment whatsoever. People who discover this fact for themselves may argue that exercise isn't worth the bother. But exercise can stave off recurring bouts of back pain, which tend to grow more debilitating with each successive onset. And back pain that goes away in response to exercise, studies show, tends to return when the exercise is stopped. In other words, your back will thank you for initiating and sticking to a safe exercise programme.

Chapter 17
A Programme for Permanent Improvement

By now you understand the value of regular exercise in preventing and treating back pain. All that's left is to devise a personally tailored programme that will fit into your life. Adopting the programme means committing yourself to performing a few stretching and strengthening exercises for 10 to 15 minutes a day – and engaging in aerobic activities for 3 to 4 hours a week. This is the biggest lifestyle change the programme demands, but, as you'll see, the reward is measured in an even bigger change in the quality of your life. If you've never exercised regularly before, get ready to feel great!

I urge you to ignore the popular image of exercise as vigorous and competitive. For back sufferers, as one of the US survey participants pointed out, 'Slower is generally better, gradual is faster, and vigorous is self-defeating.' To put it another way, 'Any pain, less gain.'

All the back exercises mentioned in this book were performed by the US survey participants, who judged them to be safe and sound. I believe you'll agree. Not every participant performed every exercise, of course – nor should you expect to do so. From the full set, I will help you select those few that best suit your needs, depending on the location, type, severity and duration of your back pain. Your exercise choices should match your level of fitness, comfort level, schedule and tastes. They must enhance your general health, too, so I urge you to check with your doctor about any special restrictions imposed by your personal medical history. Having a wide range of exercises from which to choose will not only enable you to personalize your programme, but also to change it from time to time – either to make your routine more challenging as you gain experience, or to introduce new exercises for the sake of variety.

The stretching and strengthening exercises are all explained in detail in Chapters 8, 22 and 23. The aerobic exercise options are also discussed at length, in Chapter 24, with specific suggestions for getting started. My aim in this chapter is to explain the goals of the different types of exercise, and to show how they can work together to promote back fitness.

Your programme will consist of three types of exercise:

1. Aerobic activities, such as walking and swimming, that increase your stamina and improve your cardiovascular fitness
2. Stretching exercises, such as Knee Drops, that keep your muscles flexible and help prevent spasms
3. Strengthening exercises, including Push-offs and Bent-Knee Sit-ups, that firm up the muscles you need to maintain good posture and to carry out everyday activities without putting your back at risk.

Aerobic Exercise

You will spend most of your exercise time engaged in aerobic activities. In fact, aerobic exercise demands a certain minimum time period – at least 20 minutes per session, and preferably 45 minutes to an hour, repeated three or four times a week. The sustained nature of the activity is what raises your heart rate and gets your blood pumping as you burn oxygen. These effects give aerobic exercise its other well-known name, cardiovascular activity. Indeed, the benefits of sustained activity for the heart and circulatory system have by now gained universal acceptance.

But for you, as a person with back trouble, aerobic exercise has another important role. Sustained aerobic activities nourish your spine by increasing the blood supply to the tissues. To treat your back well, whether you are trying to protect it from deterioration or help it heal after injury, you do best to pursue aerobic exercise.

The strong relationship between cardiovascular exercise and the health of the spine has implications for other lifestyle choices. You've probably heard at least a million times that smoking is bad for your heart and lungs. But the fact is, smoking damages the spine, too, through its effect on the blood circulation. Nicotine and other components of cigarette smoke compromise the micro-circulation – the network of tiny blood vessels throughout the body that feed all the tissues, including the discs. Physicians' surveys have identified cigarette smoking as one of the major risk factors for back pain. Among backache sufferers, smokers outnumber non-smokers four to one. And in follow-up studies of people who have undergone operations for the repair of herniated discs, cigarette smokers prove five times more likely to have a poor outcome than post-operative patients who don't smoke.

Alcohol, like cigarette smoke, also constricts the blood vessels and can contribute to poor circulation around the discs. Moderate drinking in social situations probably contributes very little to disc degeneration, but alcohol abuse can aggravate back pain from this source.

You may feel immediate positive effects from aerobic exercise, in addition to backache relief. These could include increased energy during your waking hours, coupled with better sleep at night. You may find that you feel calmer during your aerobic activity period, and that you look forward to this time of day, at least in part, for the stress relief it brings. Over the long term, aerobic exercise will help you shed unwanted kilos or pounds, since such activity burns body fat and calories. Provided you don't simultaneously increase your food intake, aerobic exercise will gradually whittle away your excess weight.

Aerobic exercises tend to be everyone's favorites because they are intrinsically enjoyable, or can be made that way. Many of them can be done in the company of others, and therefore provide opportunities for pleasant social contacts. Walking wins most people's vote for the best aerobic exercise, since it is safe and effective and can be done virtually any time, anywhere, indoors or out.

Stretching Exercises

Your muscles tend to tighten with disuse. If you lead a sedentary life, you can keep your muscles long and supple by intentionally stretching them with exercise. That primes them for action.

You probably already know too well what happens when you rely on overly tight muscles to help you make some sudden move: They fail you by going into spasm and slapping you with pain. Now they are in a state of painful contraction, and they may refuse to come out for a long time. The secret of successful treatment for spasm, just like the key to its prevention, lies in gentle stretching.

It's always a good idea to warm up before you stretch. Typical exercise programmes for fit people often call for 5 minutes of jogging on the spot as a warm-up. But jogging is often uncomfortable for people with back pain because it usually involves a jarring impact on the ground or another hard surface. You can therefore warm up in any number of gentler ways. Some survey participants reported taking a warm shower or bath or using a heating pad just before exercise. This enabled them to stretch more readily, get more from the therapy, and increase their rate of progress. If you choose to exercise first thing in the morning, you may get an ample warm-up by moving around in bed and then walking for a few minutes before you begin.

When you stretch, try to concentrate on stretching to the point of resistance – and then moving just a fraction beyond it. But, I implore you, don't push through pain. Over-stretching can be worse than not doing any exercise at all, since it can tear the muscle fibres or induce spasms and pain. Carefully executed back exercises can bring you noticeable improvement in just a few weeks. Please try to be patient. Remember that exercise therapy, no matter how cautious it may seem to you, is almost always better than anything you can put into or onto your body.

Although aerobic exercise can be limited to three or four days a week, stretching does the most for you when you do it every day. This is not just a physiological reality, but a mental one as well; by stretching every day, you make stretching a habit, and you are more likely to stick with it. In Chapter 21 I will discuss other strategies that can help you sustain your motivation to exercise.

You may choose to perform all your stretches at once, in a single session, or break up your exercise into two periods, one in the morning and the other at night. The twice-a-day approach works especially well for people who are recovering from an acute episode of back pain, because it helps them make speedier progress. Those who have already attained back fitness, however, and are exercising to maintain the good feeling, can do equally well with a once-a-day regime.

Each exercise session needs to have its own internal order. After your warm-ups, I suggest you begin with the easiest, gentlest movements, and progress through the more difficult stretching and strengthening exercises. Then cool down by walking at a leisurely pace for about 5 minutes.

You will notice that many of the stretching and strengthening exercises call for you to make forward-bending movements with your spine, as when you perform the Knee-to-Chest Rock. Exercise experts call this movement flexion. Hospital studies have shown that flexion exercises work quickly and effectively to increase the mobility of the lower back.

Another pro-back movement, called extension, works to lengthen the spine. You can experience this sensation when you stretch your lower back in executing the Pelvic Tilt.

None of the exercises in this book requires you to hyperextend or arch your back. In the Cat Stretch, you have the opportunity to arch your neck, but the instructions tell you to omit this step if neck arching is even the slightest bit uncomfortable. Exaggerated arching is precluded for two reasons: (1) arching the spine, I believe, puts too much pressure on the discs, and (2) arching the lower back stretches the abdominal muscles.

Regarding the latter, the abdominal muscles really don't require stretching; they have too great a tendency to stretch and sag by themselves. What you really need to do with your abdominals is build their strength by performing exercises such as the Pelvic Tilt, the Bent-Knee Sit-up and the Sit-down.

Strengthening Exercises

The exercises that build strength in your muscles usually involve working against some resistance – to make the muscles work hard so they grow big and strong. It's tempting to think that you can accomplish this goal with aerobic exercise alone, but the fact is you also need specific exercises that call for a short burst of strength from muscle contraction.

Strengthening exercises may be isotonic or isometric. The isotonic ones involve motion against resistance. For example, in a Push-off, you push the weight of your body about 30 cm (12 inches) in an effort to strengthen your shoulders and upper back. The isometric exercises involve no obvious movement, just working against resistance. For example, in the Side Press, you push against a wall to strengthen your arm. You may be working just as hard as you did in the Push-off, but only you can tell how much effort you're expending – since the wall doesn't move.

Fitness enthusiasts who exercise in gyms build strength by lifting weights. Weight-resistance work is not included here, because I feel it's unnecessary in order to address the problem of back pain. Lifting and manoeuvring the weight of your own body is sufficient, I feel, for the goals of this programme.

Many exercise instructors believe that strengthening exercises should not be done every day. In your back exercise routine, however, I want you to include them and perform them with the stretches – especially the Pelvic Tilt and Bent-Knee Sit-ups. Unlike weight-resistance exercises, these strengtheners won't tax your body and call for a day or more of rest for muscle repair and recovery between sessions. Instead, these exercises will safeguard your posture and work to reduce your pain.

Sample Exercise Programme

The following programme is suitable for a person who is reasonably fit, occasionally has back pain, but is free of neck pain.

Aerobic Activity

Walk for 20 to 40 minutes, three times a week.

Stretching

The range of repetitions listed below represents the first day of doing the exercises (the first number) and a month later (the second number).

- Knee-to-Chest, see pp. 342–4 (three to six repetitions)
- Knees-to-Chest Rock, see pp. 344–5 (two to five repetitions)
- Knee Cross, see pp. 352–3 (two to five repetitions each side)
- Cat Stretch, see pp. 354–6 (three to six repetitions)
- Knee Spread, see pp. 366–7 (two to four repetitions)
- Hamstring Stretch, see pp. 368–7 (two to five repetitions each side)
- Thigh Pull, see pp. 372–3 (two to four repetitions each side)
- Runner's Stretch, see p. 375 (two to four repetitions each side)

Strengthening

The range of repetitions listed below represents the first day of doing the exercises (the first number) and a month later (the second number).

- Pelvic Tilt, see pp. 359–60 (five to ten repetitions)
- Bent-Knee Sit-ups, see pp. 364–5 (five to ten repetitions)
- Sit-downs, see pp. 362–3 (one to five repetitions)

Chapter 18
A Special Message for People with Chronically Disabling Back Pain

If you have chronically disabling back pain, please read on.

First, let me assure you that you are not alone. Over 1 million British people are severely disabled by back pain that has resisted every treatment brought to bear. Some of these individuals have what physicians call 'Failed Back Syndrome'. This is an unfortunate euphemism for a poor surgical outcome from discectomy or another operation on the spine. The term makes it sound as though the patient's back were guilty of some kind of gross failure, when really it is the surgery or other treatments that failed to bring improvement to the person. The individual continues to suffer, but with less hope than before, and the hope diminishes as the realization grows that no help may be forthcoming from any source.

Even without surgery, some backache sufferers find themselves growing progressively worse, no matter what they do. I want to tell you about one of these people, a participant in the original US survey, who suffered the kind of anguish you may be going through.

When he filled out his survey questionnaire, Bob had seen both orthopaedic surgeons and chiropractors, as well as osteopaths, naturopaths and numerous other conventional and alternative health practitioners. No two of his twelve diagnoses were the same, so he never knew what was wrong with his back. Still, he continued to read widely about back pain, to seek professional help, and try each new seemingly sound and rational remedy.

In a page he stapled onto the survey, Bob described his predicament:

'Some doctors who know about the chronicity of my problem won't even allow me to make an appointment to see them. If they do agree to examine me, they're all but itching to get me out the door. It is assumed that I have workmen's [workers'] compensation or some other kind of insurance, which I don't, or that I'm a neurotic who enjoys the attention. Actually, I live alone, and nobody pays me any attention unless I'm up and about. Some people obviously think I'm a malingerer, even though I worked from age fourteen to forty. It's just been the past five years that I've not been able to be on my feet long enough to hold down a job. I am living off my savings, which are about depleted.'

The questionnaire explained that the information people provided would be used in a book I was writing about back pain (*Backache Relief*, Times Books 1985, NAL/Signet 1986). Bob was a little concerned about that. In a postscript he added, 'I hope that your book won't leave out people like me. I hope it won't be another simplistic *Six Minutes a Day to Relief*, full of "guaranteed safe" exercises I can't even do.'

I did not leave Bob out of my first book, and I won't leave him – or you – out of this one, either.

If you are suffering from long-standing, seemingly intractable back problems, you may require special preparations or expert exercise guidance from a trained practitioner before you can make use of the exercises described in the next few chapters. Bob, when I last heard from him, had started to find his way out of that prolonged disability, and to look forward to functioning normally once again.

What follows are some suggestions on fighting your way back from extreme disability over a long period of time.

Try Seeing a Physiatrist

Physiatrists are doctors of physical medicine and rehabilitation. These practitioners are accustomed to treating debilitating conditions, from spinal cord injuries to strokes, and are not easily frightened off by pain that has a long history. They are not trained as surgeons, although they can spot problems that do require surgical treatment, and then make appropriate referrals. Physiatrists recognize the value of exercise, and have a thorough knowledge of exercise as a prescription drug. Of all the medical specialists, the physiatrist is the most likely to be able to create an individualized exercise programme that promises gradual improvement.

Physiatrists are also likely to recommend physiotherapy. The physiotherapist will work with you on the successful execution of your exercises, as well as giving you other treatments that could include advice, manual therapy or electrotherapy.

In the UK, we do not have an equivalent of the US physiatrist. Instead, the closest practitioner is likely to be a doctor who specializes in rehabilitating those who have suffered from debilitating pain and disease, including those with chronic back pain. You can talk to your GP about whether or not you could be referred for such specialist treatment. If your condition is suitable, your GP will also refer you for physiotherapy.

Make a Plan for Achieving Progress Slowly

If your back pain has been growing worse over a period of years, you can't really expect to suddenly hit on one solution that will solve your problems overnight. Anyone who promises you that kind of outcome has to be lying.

Accept the fact that your recovery may take as long as a year, and promise yourself that by the end of the year you will have made substantial progress. And then set out to make that promise come true the way several of the US survey participants did – gradually. Very gradually.

Try to stop blaming yourself for being incapacitated. Instead of fixating on all the things you used to do that you can't do now, concentrate on what you can do – even if it's only washing the dishes or walking round the garden. Set yourself a new goal each day or week – perhaps walking a little further or doing something a little more challenging. When you reach that goal, enjoy your success, rather than belittling your achievement as small or insignificant. Long before a year is out, you'll be ready for the pre-exercise positions in Chapter 20, and then for a simple programme of gentle movements to establish a lifelong habit of taking regular exercise.

Try to Reduce the Stress of Incapacitation

Being out of work breeds its own stress. Being in pain is stressful. But stress, in turn, can often aggravate pain, setting up a vicious circle of emotional and physical anguish. If you have neck pain, you may be especially vulnerable to aggravation of pain by stress. Knowing the role stress can play for someone with long-standing backache, please consider the stress-reduction strategies in Chapter 27 as being of particular importance for you.

Make Your Environment Work for You

You may feel 'trapped' by your disability. But there may be many small changes you can make in your surroundings that will collectively contribute to an improvement in your condition. To take an obvious example, ask yourself if your mattress is really firm and comfortable. Are you supporting your body with pillows to your best advantage? If you're watching television, is the set positioned so that you can see the screen without straining your neck or body alignment? Even if you're not carrying out your normal daily activities now, check the suggestions in Chapters 13 and 14 to discover ideas about back-safe strategies for doing a variety of everyday tasks. If you follow these suggestions as you make progress, you can avoid further injury.

Remember That Your Attitude towards Your Body Is the Basis for Improvement

By celebrating each small success and making your environment as pleasant as possible, you are respecting and nurturing your body. In time, your pain will lessen and you will be able to do many more things. Believe it or not, you have an advantage over many other backache sufferers, and that is that you will never take your recovery for granted. Once you regain your ability to move, you will take such joy in movement that no one will ever have to nag you to exercise. No doubt you will look forward to that 15 or 20 minutes a day spent exercising as quality time when you are alone, quiet, in touch with yourself, meditative, knowing that you are doing something good for yourself. And because you have that attitude, you can look forward to keeping yourself well.

Section 7
The Motivation

Once people accept exercise as medicine, the hardest thing is to get them to take that medicine regularly.

Chapter 19
How to Work Exercise into Your Life

Exercise is a life-transforming tool for back sufferers that will make more of a difference to your sense of well-being than anything else – including the best food, the greatest sex, the most exhilarating fun. The only catch is that you have to do it to reap the benefits.

If you're like most busy people, you already have too much to do. There isn't room in your day for even 15 minutes of stretching and strengthening exercises, let alone the 45 minutes to an hour, three times a week, that would satisfy the aerobic exercise requirement of this programme.

I'm going to help you find the time – somehow – because, again, I am confident that exercise will prove more beneficial to you in the long run than any other approach you can try.

Let's start with the argument that you just don't have any time. What if I told you that a relatively small time commitment to exercise could buy you an insurance policy against the next time you might have to call in sick to work because 'My back has gone out again'?

If time is money, then the time you invest in exercise, which costs you nothing, saves you whatever amount of time and money you could conceivably spend on chiropractic, osteopathy, massage therapy, and so on – the next time your back muscles seize up and lay you low.

What's that? You say you're already running so flat out that you can't give yourself enough sleep at night, and so you're tired all day? That's no excuse, either. As you'll see, exercise, especially regular aerobic exercise, will change the way you feel, every minute of the day. Instead of depleting your energy, as you might suppose, exercise actually gives you more energy. Even though it burns up calories and cuts through fat on your body, it doesn't make you tired. On the contrary, exercise makes you feel more alert and alive – and because you tend to sleep better when you exercise, you're likely to find that you feel more rested even when you spend fewer hours in bed.

Maybe these arguments sound too pat. I set up a straw man, then knock it down, but meanwhile, you really are too busy to exercise. Let's try another approach. Let's look at your day and see if there's somewhere, anywhere, that we can squeeze in the requisite amount of exercise. Maybe you can do your exercises while you're looking after your children or warming food in the microwave. If you can allow for three 5-minute mini-exercise sessions spread over the course of the day, you'll benefit from even that much, I promise. So ask yourself the following questions, and maybe you'll find the answer to the problem of not having time to exercise.

If You Go Out to Work . . .

- Can you walk to work instead of driving or taking public transport?
- Do you have time to walk in your lunch hour?
- Is there a health club or a pool near your workplace where you can swim during your lunch hour?
- If you work in a building that has several floors, can you climb the steps instead of taking the lift?
- Can you interest your employer in starting a 'back school' to help your co-workers learn exercise and back-friendly work habits on the job?
- Honestly, if while sitting at your desk, you went through the whole series of neck-stretching exercises, from Left-Right to Head Pull (see pp. 378–82), would anyone think you were doing anything so terribly strange?
- Couldn't you also get away with performing most of the neck-strengthening exercises, as well as the routine for the shoulders and upper back (see pp. 384–95)?
- If you need to talk to a colleague in the building, would you consider walking there for a face-to-face conference instead of dialling his or her extension on the telephone?

If You Work at Home . . .

- Isn't it possible to lie down on the floor and stretch your back while you're taking a respite shorter than a coffee break?
- Since no one's around to watch you, can you do your neck exercises while you're on the telephone? (That way, you'll avoid doing something to hurt your neck, such as cradling the phone between your ear and your shoulder for too many minutes at a time.)
- When it's time to go to the post office, can you walk for 20 minutes?

If You Are Caring for Young Children . . .

- Wouldn't the baby love to go for a long walk in the pushchair?
- Can the baby play or sleep on a quilt on the floor while you do your routine lying down nearby?
- Why not make your exercises a family activity? Or make them into a game like 'Simon Says'?
- Can you walk briskly along with your older children while they ride their bikes?

If You Are Doing Housework . . .

- Can you find opportunities to make every chore a stretch? (This may involve putting aside some of your labour-saving devices in favour of doing things the old-fashioned way, such as hanging laundry on a line instead of putting it in the tumble-dryer.)
- If your house has more than one level, would you mind making several trips up and down for the laundry? (Taking the steps more frequently would probably be better for your back than struggling to carry a heavy load either up or down.)

If You Own Your Own Home . . .

- Can you turn autumn leaf raking, winter snow shovelling, and summer lawn care and gardening into aerobic activities? (If so, be sure to approach these activities safely, following the tips in Chapter 14.)

If You Enjoy Soaking in the Bath Every Evening . . .

- Can you execute a Pelvic Tilt (see pp. 359–60) underwater?
- How about a Bent-Knee Sit-up (see pp. 364–5)?
- Did you know that exercising in a warm bath can be especially soothing?

If All Else Fails . . .

- Would you consider carrying out your neck, upper back and standing back exercises in the shower?
- Can you find 5 minutes, three times a day, to lie down on the floor and stretch your muscles? (Look out for opportunities, such as when you're waiting for another family member to finish using the bathroom, or for the oven timer to tell you that dinner is ready, or for your favourite television programme to begin.)
- Can you find a friend who also needs to exercise, and who will keep you company while you both walk aerobically?
- With the above possibilities in mind, can you create your own opportunities to give yourself the benefit of regular exercise?

You can. Of course you can.

Chapter 20
How to Assess Your Exercise Readiness and Assemble Your Tailor-Made Programme

Now that you're motivated to exercise – aware of all the pain-relieving, mobility-increasing benefits a programme of regular exercise can bring you – you're ready to begin selecting the elements of your individually tailored exercise routine.

In this chapter, I want to help you determine your level of exercise ability, based on factors such as your age, your assessment of your own general fitness, and the duration of your back pain. Then I can make specific exercise suggestions. An 'off-the-hook' exercise programme cannot possibly suit you as well as a programme designed with your needs in mind.

The nature of your back problem also guides you in identifying the ideal exercises for you. As I said earlier, few people can give a specific name or diagnosis to their back pain. Nevertheless, certain identifiable conditions, including sciatica and osteoarthritis-induced back pain, call for particular precautions.

Let's begin with a simple self-test that will match your level of back pain and limitation with a reasonable set of exercise goals.

Self-Test of Exercise Readiness
Please circle the number that best completes each of the following statements:

Most days, I am . . .

1. inactive because of pain or chronic disability
2. inactive by choice – a 'couch potato'

3. moderately active
4. very active

When I get up in the morning, I feel . . .

1. severe pain that never seems to go away completely
2. pain that warns me to be careful
3. pain on some days, no pain on others
4. hardly any pain at all

As I go through the day, I find that I . . .

1. need most things done for me
2. need help to do some things
3. manage well on my own, if I'm careful of my back
4. can keep up a normal pace of activity, at work and/or at home, with comfort

My back pain stems from . . .

1. osteoarthritis, or herniated disc or sciatica
2. an accident that injured my back some time ago
3. muscle spasms
4. some unknown cause

Because of my back pain . . .

1. I've had surgery at least once
2. I've been confined to bed several times, and am somewhat limited in the things I can do
3. I've had to stay in bed on occasion, but between episodes of pain I get along fine
4. I may think twice before I try some new activity, but I can pretty much do what I want

My experience with exercise in general and back exercise in particular is . . .

1. non-existent
2. limited

3. moderate
4. extensive

My age is . . .

1. over sixty-five
2. mid-fifties to early sixties
3. early forties to mid-fifties
4. forty or younger

Now I'd like you to classify yourself in one of four categories, based on your responses to the above questions. If you circled all ones, for example, or mostly ones, then you are in the 'Basic Preparation' category. If your answers included more twos than ones, consider yourself in the 'Proceed with Caution' group. If you found the threes to be most descriptive of your condition, please put yourself in the 'Gentle Exercise' category. If you scored fours consistently, you are no doubt ready for the 'Regular Exercise' category.

Over time, as you make progress and change your level of flexibility and strength, you may move on through the categories at whatever pace seems right for you. There is nothing to stop a person who begins in the Basic Preparation category from becoming a Regular Exerciser. Indeed, by preparing for exercise and then proceeding with caution at first, you can expect to progress to Gentle Exercise and finally to Regular Exercise. And you needn't stop there.

The Four Categories of Exercises

Category 1: Basic Preparation

If you suffer from a case of chronically debilitating back pain, please see the special message in Chapter 18 before you read on. I have every confidence that you will be able to use the exercises in this book, but first I want to prepare you to perform them safely.

If you are just now recuperating from an acute episode of debilitating back pain, you can try the following pre-exercise positions as soon as your contracted muscles have eased enough for you to move around in bed — or be up and about for just a few minutes at a time. These are such conservative movements that they are safe to attempt before your pain lessens enough to permit other exercises. Give yourself a week or two of assuming these positions, as meaningful first steps towards full activity.

Start slowly and hopefully. There's no need to do all the positions in one session, or even all in one day at the outset. If you can be comfortable in the Basic Exercise Position for 5 minutes the first time you try it, move on to the Pelvic Lift later in the day or the next morning. Once you master the Pelvic Lift, and can assume that position for 10 minutes at a time, twice a day, you may attempt the Knee Clasp.

Basic Exercise Position

If you have been in severe pain, the muscles and ligaments in your lower back have no doubt contracted, creating an exaggerated 'S' curve there. Holding the Basic Exercise Position for several minutes will begin to correct this. You can gauge the amount of correction each time you slip your hand under the small of your back.

Starting position: Assume the foetal position, lying on your side with both knees bent. *a*

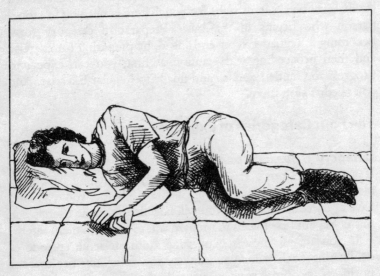

a

Steps:

1. Roll onto your back, and place your arms at your sides. *b*
2. Position your feet flat on the mattress, with your heels about 15–45 cm (6–18 inches) from your buttocks.
3. Hold this position for about 2 minutes.
4. Slip one hand, palm down, between the small of your back and your mattress. *c* (over the page)
5. Remove your hand, and lie in the Basic Exercise Position for another 2 or 3 more minutes.
6. Repeat Step 4. You'll likely find there's a bit less room for your hand, now that you've been lying flat a longer time.
7. Return to the starting position.

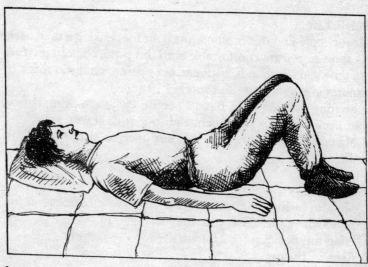

b

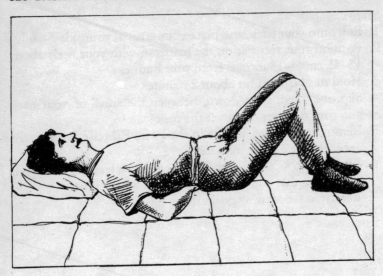

c

Pelvic Lift

Most people find this position just right for relaxing a tired back.
As soon as you are comfortable with this pose, you can increase
the time you spend in it, 1 minute per session, until you reach 10
minutes in the morning and another 10 at night.

Starting position: The Basic Exercise Position – lying flat on
your back with your knees bent and your arms at your sides.

Materials: A bath towel, folded just once, so that it is not too
bulky.

Steps:
1. Slide an inch of the folded towel under your buttocks, at the
   point where they meet your thighs.
2. Hold this position for 2 minutes.
3. Remove the towel.
4. Later in the day, repeat Steps 1–3.

Knee Clasp

These manoeuvres are starting to feel like bona fide exercises. Please remember that the point of this stretch is to let you relax in a comfortably flexed position – and not to challenge you to draw your knees towards your chest as far as you possibly can.

Starting position: The Pelvic Lift Position – lying flat on your back with knees bent, arms at your sides, and a folded towel just under your buttocks. *a*

(Turn over the page to see steps 1–7.)

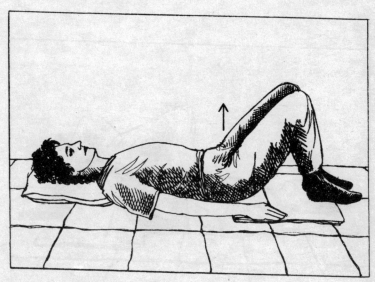

a

Steps:

1. Bring one knee up towards your chest and hold it there with your hand. **b**
2. Bring the other knee up. **c**
3. Clasp your hands together, holding your knees just below the kneecaps.
4. As gently as you can, pull your knees a few inches towards your chest. **d**
5. Hold this position for a count of six.
6. Return to the starting position.
7. Repeat Steps 1–6 six times.

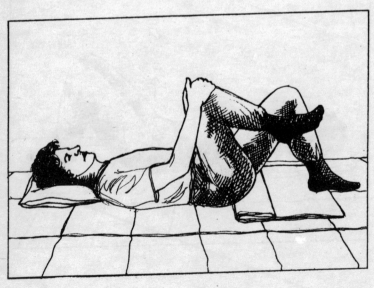

b

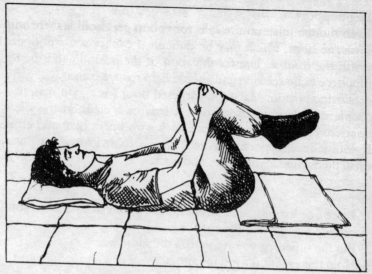

c

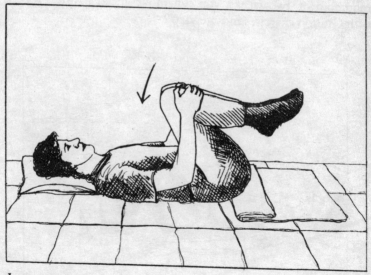

d

Leg Support

Even though this exercise calls for you to get down and then up from the floor, which may be difficult, I expect you will find it worth the trouble. The combination of the position and the leg support can be relaxing and should help reduce pain.

Starting position: Lie on a carpeted floor (or a gym mat, or a couple of folded blankets) near a sofa or a chair, in the Basic Exercise Position – flat on your back with knees bent and arms at your sides. Support your neck with a folded towel, or put a small pillow under your head and neck. *a*

Steps:
1. Raise one leg with knee bent and rest your calf and foot – but not your thigh – on the sofa or chair. *b*
2. Put the other leg up on the sofa the same way. *c*
3. Hold this position for 5 minutes.
4. One leg at a time, return to the starting position.

Once you master these preparatory exercises, which may take a minimum of two weeks, you can move ahead to the Proceed with Caution exercises in Category 2.

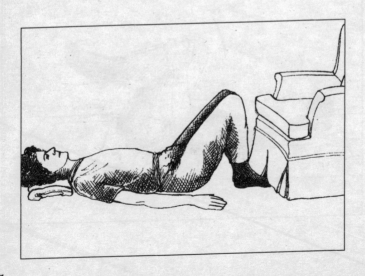

a

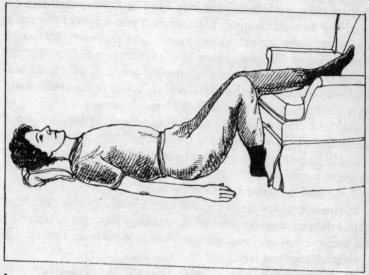

b

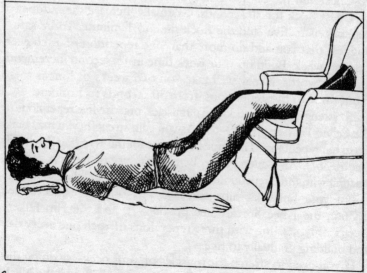

c

Category 2: Proceed with Caution

A long history of back pain may have kept you inactive for a troubling amount of time. The exercises that will help you make important gains are necessarily gentle ones that carry no risk of further injury. Because all of the exercises you may attempt under this category heading are spelled out in Chapters 22 and 23, I will list them here by name, and refer you to the appropriate page numbers, rather than reprint all the directions.

For your aerobic activity, try walking. Begin slowly, and for a maximum of 20 minutes at a time, three times a week. Allow yourself to pick up the pace and extend the time period as your progress permits. Your ultimate goal in this category will be to walk for half an hour, four times a week.

If you know how to swim, and have a pool available, you may want to alternate walking with swimming. (Please see Chapter 24 for a discussion of swimming strokes to determine one that is appropriate for you.)

To stretch your lower back, rely on the Knee-to-Chest (see p. 342–4), the Knees-to-Chest Rock (see pp. 344–5), and the Simple Knee Cross (see pp. 349–50). You may begin with three repetitions – three on each side, that is – of both the Knee-to-Chest and the Simple Knee Cross. Try to sustain the Knees-to-Chest Rock for 30 seconds. Gradually increase the number of repetitions to five, and the Rock time to 1 minute. To be safe, I suggest that you add no more than one repetition of each exercise per week. Build up your Rock time in 15-second increments. In other words, it may well take you two weeks or longer to go from three to five repetitions, from 30 seconds to 1 minute.

To strengthen your abdominal muscles, practise five repetitions of the Pelvic Tilt (see pp. 359–60). As you gain strength, you may build up to ten repetitions. The same holds true for the Standing Pelvic Tilt (see p. 361). Also attempt the Bent-Knee Sit-ups (see pp. 364–5), starting with three repetitions a day, and gradually building to ten.

For your buttocks, hips and legs, rely on The Squeeze (see p. 366), the Knee Spread (see pp. 366–7), and the Hip Hikers (see p. 371), starting with three repetitions of each one every day and building gradually to five.

If you need to stretch the muscles of your neck, try doing the Left-Right (see pp. 378–9), the Yes-No (see p. 379) and the Neck

Tilt (see p. 383). It's safe to begin with three repetitions of each, then build to five. To strengthen the muscles of your neck, I recommend the Bed Head (see p. 384), beginning with three repetitions and moving up to five.

Stretch your shoulders and upper back with the Shoulder Stretch (see p. 386) and the Shoulder Shrug (see p. 387). Start at three repetitions and progress to five at the usual pace. Strengthen the upper back area with the Side Press (see p. 395).

As you gain flexibility in this stage of your programme, keep reminding yourself of the good progress you're making. It has taken you a long time to lose and then regain your sense of well-being, so let yourself enjoy every aspect of improvement.

After several weeks of slow and steady progress have brought you to the completion of the Category 2 goals, you need not rush ahead to the next level. By all means, let your own assessment of your condition be your guide. You may want to approach Category 3 by taking just a few new exercises and incorporating them into the routine you're following now. On the other hand, you may switch to the Category 3 exercises, holding on to those elements of Category 2 that seem particularly helpful to you.

Proceed with Caution

- Knee-to-Chest (see pp. 342–4)
- Total Body Relaxation (see p. 415)
- Knee-to-Chest Rock (see pp. 344–5)
- Simple Knee Cross (see pp. 349–50)
- Pelvic Tilt (see pp. 359–60)
- Standing Pelvic Tilt (see p. 361)
- Bent-Knee Sit-ups (see pp. 364–5)
- The Squeeze (see p. 366)
- Knee Spread (see pp. 366–7)
- Hip Hikers (see p. 371)
- Left-Right (see pp. 378–9)
- Yes-No (see p. 379)
- Neck Tilt (see p. 383)
- Bed Head (see p. 384)
- Shoulder Stretch (see p. 386)
- Shoulder Shrug (see p. 387)
- Side Press (see p. 395)

Category 3: Gentle Exercise

Because you are already fairly active and relatively pain-free, you can attempt a variety of movements. I encourage you to walk for fitness, or alternate swimming with walking, so that you give yourself a 40-minute aerobic workout at least four times a week. If time allows, and as your sense of your own abilities dictates, you can do up to six sessions per week of aerobic activity, each session lasting as long as an hour. I'd like you to set the pace of this activity at a comfortable level. In other words, when you walk, walk with purpose and direction as though you have somewhere to go – but not as though you have to rush because you're late for an appointment.

Work on stretching your lower back with five repetitions of the following six exercises: Knee-to-Chest (see pp. 342–4), Double Knee-to-Chest (see p. 346), Knee Drops (see pp. 347–9), Knee Cross (see pp. 352–3), Flexibility Twist (see pp. 418–19) and Twists and Tilts (see pp. 357). If you are comfortable with these movements, you may increase the number of repetitions, one at a time, every three or four days, until you reach ten.

Strengthen your abdominal muscles with five repetitions each of the Pelvic Tilt (see pp. 359–60), the Standing Pelvic Tilt (see p. 361), and the Bent-Knee Sit-ups (see pp. 364–5). At the same pace as you increase your repetitions of stretching exercises, add repetitions of these movements, too, up to ten.

Work your buttocks, hips and legs by attempting five repetitions of these four exercises: Knee Spread (see pp. 366–7), Hamstring Stretch (see pp. 368–70), Thigh Pull (see pp. 372–3), and Runner's Stretch (see p. 375). Here, too, slowly work your way up to ten repetitions.

If you have tight neck muscles, loosen them with five daily repetitions of these two exercises: Left-Right Plus (see pp. 380–1), and Head Pull (see p. 382). Progressing gradually along with the rest of the regime, you can increase the number of repetitions to ten.

Try to strengthen your neck with three repetitions each of the Neck Push (see p. 384) and Side Neck Push (see p. 385). Work up to five repetitions of each.

For stretching your shoulders and upper back, rely on the Shoulder Shrug (see p. 387), Shoulder Roll (see pp. 388–9), and Aeroplane (see p. 392). Try beginning with three repetitions of each, then working up to five. For strengthening these same areas, begin with three repetitions each of the Push-offs (see p. 394) and the Side Press (see p. 395), then gradually work towards five repetitions.

By the time you arrive at the full recommended number of repetitions in this category, you will be enjoying a greater range of motion, and probably less anxiety about suffering a recurrence of back pain. At this point, you're ready for 'Regular Exercise', which has a little more oomph.

Gentle Exercise
- Total Body Relaxation (see p. 415)
- Knee-to-Chest (see pp. 342–4)
- Double Knee-to-Chest (see p. 346)
- Knee Drops (see pp. 347–9)
- Knee Cross (see pp. 352–3)
- Flexibility Twist (see pp. 418–19)
- Twists and Tilts (see p. 357)
- Pelvic Tilt (see pp. 359–60)
- Standing Pelvic Tilt (see p. 361)
- Bent-Knee Sit-ups (see pp. 364–5)
- Knee Spread (see pp. 366–7)
- Hamstring Stretch (see pp. 368–70)
- Thigh Pull (see pp. 372–3)
- Runner's Stretch (see p. 375)
- Left-Right Plus (see pp. 380–1)
- Head Pull (see p. 382)
- Neck Push (see p. 384)
- Side Neck Push (see p. 385)
- Shoulder Shrug (see p. 387)
- Shoulder Roll (see pp. 388–9)
- Aeroplane (see p. 392)
- Push-offs (see p. 394)
- Side Press (see p. 395)

Category 4: Regular Exercise
Since you are on your feet and free of pain most of the time, you probably perform exercises as insurance against future episodes of back pain. Good for you! Indeed, from your active vantage point, some of these exercises may look too simple. But please

don't scoff at them. They serve the important function of focusing on the very muscles and movements that ward off back troubles. Remember, you never outgrow your need for the Pelvic Tilt!

If you crave action, start pulling out the stops in your aerobic exercise. When you walk, go quickly. Swing your arms. You can even pump them to push up your heart rate and pep up your pace. Swim if you like. And try an exercise bike or ride a bike outdoors for an aerobic alternative.

In stretching your lower back, you may use any or all of the exercises in Chapter 22. Begin with five repetitions of six of them: Knee-to-Chest (see pp. 342–4), Knees-to-Chest Rock (see pp. 344–5), Knee Cross (see pp. 352–3), Cat Stretch (see pp. 354–6), Flexibility Twist (see pp. 418–9), and Twists and Tilts (see p. 357). Increase the number of repetitions every three or four days, until you are doing ten of each.

For abdominal strengthening, go for the Pelvic Tilt (see pp. 359–60), Standing Pelvic Tilt (see p. 361), Bent-Knee Sit-ups (see pp. 364–5), and Sit-downs (see pp. 362–3). Here, too, start with five repetitions of each and work up to ten.

Stretch and strengthen your buttocks, hips and legs with the Knee Spread (see pp. 366–7), Hamstring Stretch (see pp. 368–70), Hip Hikers (see p. 371), Standing Thigh Pull (see p. 374) and Runner's Stretch (see p. 375). Try five repetitions of each for starters, then work up to ten.

Neck-stretching exercises for you could include five repetitions each of Left-Right Plus (see pp. 380–1) and Head Pull (see p. 382). Work up to ten of each of these over time.

Strengthen your neck with the Bed Head (see p. 384), Neck Push (see p. 384), and Side Neck Push (see p. 385), beginning with three and working up to five repetitions of each.

To stretch your shoulders and upper back, start out with three repetitions each of the Shoulder Roll (see pp. 388–9), Roller Blades (see p. 390), Square Shoulder Stretch (see p. 391), Aeroplane (see p. 392) and Windmill (see p. 393). As you gain proficiency with these, increase the number of repetitions to five. Strengthen these areas with five Push-offs (see p. 394) and three Side Presses (see p. 395), gradually increasing to ten repetitions and five repetitions respectively. For your hamstrings, try the Sitting Stretch (see pp. 415–18).

Regular Exercise
- Total Body Relaxation (see p. 415)
- Knee-to-Chest (see pp. 342–4)
- Knees-to-Chest Rock (see pp. 344–5)
- Knee Cross (see pp. 352–3)
- Cat Stretch (see pp. 354–6)
- Flexibility Twist (see pp. 418–19)
- Twist and Tilts (see p. 357)
- Pelvic Tilt (see pp. 359–60)
- Standing Pelvic Tilt (see p. 361)
- Bent-Knee Sit-ups (see pp. 364–5)
- Sit-downs (see pp. 362–3)
- Knee Spread (see pp. 366–7)
- Hamstring Stretch (see pp. 368–70)
- Hip Hikers (see p. 371)
- Standing Thigh Pull (see p. 374)
- Runner's Stretch (see p. 375)
- Left-Right Plus (see pp. 380–1)
- Head Pull (see p. 382)
- Bed Head (see p. 384)
- Neck Push (see p. 384)
- Side Neck Push (see p. 385)
- Shoulder Roll (see pp. 388–9)
- Roller Blades (see p. 390)
- Square Shoulder Stretch (see p. 391)
- Aeroplane (see p. 392)
- Windmill (see p. 393)
- Push-offs (see p. 394)
- Side Press (see p. 395)
- Sitting Stretch (see pp. 415–18)

That's all you have to do, really, to safeguard your back through exercise. Except that you need to keep doing your exercises. And please don't forget to go about your normal activities in a back-friendly frame of mind – even when your back forgets to remind you. You're getting to the point at which you can tell people that your back *used* to be a problem.

You can use the forms over the page to record your own exercise plan, and then keep track of additions and changes.

This is a good way to mark your progress and to troubleshoot for the causes of later soreness, but if it seems like too much paperwork for you, by all means just move on to the next chapter.

Back Exercise Progress Chart

Week: Day:

Aerobic activity_____   Length of time_____

Stretching and Strengthening Exercises

Exercise	Repetitions	Notes
_____	_____	_____
_____	_____	_____
_____	_____	_____
_____	_____	_____
_____	_____	_____
_____	_____	_____
_____	_____	_____
_____	_____	_____
_____	_____	_____
_____	_____	_____
_____	_____	_____
_____	_____	_____
_____	_____	_____
_____	_____	_____

Back Exercise Progress Chart

Week: _____ Day: _____

Aerobic activity_____ Length of time_____

Stretching and Strengthening Exercises

Exercise	Repetitions	Notes
_____	_____	_____
_____	_____	_____
_____	_____	_____
_____	_____	_____
_____	_____	_____
_____	_____	_____
_____	_____	_____
_____	_____	_____
_____	_____	_____
_____	_____	_____
_____	_____	_____
_____	_____	_____
_____	_____	_____
_____	_____	_____
_____	_____	_____
_____	_____	_____
_____	_____	_____
_____	_____	_____
_____	_____	_____

Chapter 21
How to Sustain Your Motivation to Exercise

You are your own best judge of the strategies that will work to keep your motivation and your body primed to exercise. After all, who knows you better? Are you the persevering sort who feels duty-bound to stick with every new resolution? Or are you in danger of losing interest in this exercise endeavour during the several weeks it may take for you to see gratifying results? Are you a loner who will eagerly set out for an early-morning walk before going to work? Or do you prefer a social setting in which to exercise – walking with a group of friends, perhaps, or working out at a gym?

Pain and disability may be the chief motivating factors right now, but your attention to exercise is likely to relieve pain and help you become active again. Then what? Numerous studies in hospitals have shown that even when people get back on their feet because of exercise, they tend to drop the programme within a few months, perhaps out of a sense of false security. They don't think they could end up immobilized and in pain again. But, unfortunately, statistics prove them wrong. Dropping the exercise that made them well turns out to be an invitation for pain and spasm to return. And it often returns with a vengeance.

If this exercise programme is to be of any lasting benefit, I have to give you ways to sustain it indefinitely. I have to persuade you to stick with your exercise regime through good times and bad – through family crises, during illness, on holiday, while away on work trips, and regardless of any other situation that tempts you to forget about exercise for a while.

How to Reinforce Your Plan to Exercise Every Day

- Keep a record of your exercise progress – and the improvements in your condition, including increased mobility and decreased pain. That way, you'll have a written reminder of reasons to stick to the programme.

- Set aside a place for performing your exercise routine. Keep everything you need handy – a towel, a mat, a special warm-up suit, or whatever else you've decided you need. Then you can get straight to work during your allotted time. If you live in cramped accommodation and can't create a designated exercise area, then put all the items into a shopping bag and keep it close to your favourite workout spot.

- Schedule a time of day that you regularly devote to exercise. Treat that time like a business meeting or a family outing. In other words, it's important time, and other things can't be allowed to interfere with it. (On those rare occasions when you can't stick to your set time, it's much better to find another time rather than lose that day of exercise. But if you have to miss a day because of illness, it won't set back your progress.)

- Sit down and write yourself a letter in which you explain all your exercise goals and hopes for improvement. Put the letter away in a safe place. You may never need to look at it again, but if you find yourself looking for excuses to avoid exercise, take out the letter and read it.

How to Keep Your Exercise Period Free of Distractions

- Choose a time of day when you're least likely to be disturbed.
- Ignore the telephone if it rings.
- Put a note on your door telling people that you will be back soon, and that they should not bother ringing the bell.
- Play some pleasing music that will block out any extraneous, distracting sounds. The music may also help you keep count where you need to count, and move gracefully in time to the music.

How to Get Others to Help You Stick to Your Programme

- Arrange to exercise regularly with a friend or two. This puts your exercise in a social context, which may make the activity more pleasant for you. What's more, when you're tempted to skip a day, you won't want to back out and disappoint your friends, will you?

- Enlist your children's co-operation, if they are old enough to understand, by explaining that your exercise time is important to your health, and that you want them to keep themselves occupied while you work out. If they're too young for such tactics, you can try to schedule your exercise period during the times when your baby has a nap or after your toddler has gone to bed. Another possibility is to let your youngsters join in: while you stretch and strengthen, they can exercise too – practising somersaults or other gymnastics.

How to Take Your Exercise Programme on the Road

- When you plan to visit a hotel, whether for a holiday or a work trip, ask about exercise facilities. Many hotels now have equipment rooms with treadmills for walking and exercise bikes for riding. The swimming pool, assuming there is one, may give you an opportunity you don't usually have to include some swimming. Some hotels offer walking/jogging maps of the neighbourhood.
- Since your back-stretching and strengthening exercises require no special equipment, you can do those in your room at your convenience. Try to give yourself this important attention first thing in the morning, before other demands make themselves felt.
- Long plane flights make an ideal setting for a limited exercise routine – and a sorely needed one, too, if you are to avoid feeling cramped and stiff from too much sitting. Walk up and down the aisles whenever possible. Try a few neck stretches in your seat.
- If you make long road trips in your car, do stop frequently to stretch and walk. These preventive measures can keep you from arriving at your destination in pain.

How to Modify Your Exercise Programme during Illness

- Bad colds and flu will probably ground you from your aerobic exercise. But you should try to carry on with at least some of your stretching and strengthening during the brief period when you are out of action.

Section 8
The Exercises

All the step-by-step instructions are spelled out here, accompanied by line drawings to further clarify each exercise movement.

Chapter 22
Exercises for Low Back Pain

The exercises in this chapter focus on the site of most people's back pain. The word 'low' is almost superfluous, because nearly everyone who has a backache has pain in the lower back. Right at the spot where you can reach around and place a comforting hand on your back at waist height – that's where the pain often starts.

The remedy is on the other side, in the muscles that run from the ribs to the pelvis – up and down, around and through your torso. These abdominal muscles, which consist of several layers of interacting fibres, control your posture and body alignment. Weakness or injury in these muscles usually translates into back pain. It stands to reason, then, that strengthening the abdominal muscles (and thereby protecting them from injury) can help prevent acute episodes of low back pain. It's also true that gentle stretching of the lower back and strengthening of the abdominals can constitute a pain-relieving treatment for chronic low back problems.

All these exercises have been judged safe and effective for most people by the participants in the US survey and by physician exercise specialists at the New York Hospital–Cornell University Medical Centre. As with any exercise programme, be sure to check with your doctor in case you have special restrictions. The exercises are grouped according to the important exercise goals of this chapter: stretching the lower back, strengthening the abdominal muscles, and stretching and strengthening the muscles of the buttocks, hips and legs.

As you begin to exercise, listen to your body. You risk injury by pushing yourself through pain. The bodybuilder's adage 'No pain, no gain' simply doesn't apply here. In back exercise, the only important goal is normal function in everyday life. There's no one competing with you, so please don't push yourself too hard.

Start out with a maximum of three repetitions of each exercise you attempt. Advance slowly. Give yourself at least a week at each repetition level before you try to add more repetitions. And there's no point, really, in going beyond ten repetitions of any one exercise. Once you are strong and supple enough to work through ten repetitions of all the exercises in your programme with ease, you can spend that much more time out walking or investigating other activities that bring you pleasure.

To Stretch the Lower Back

Knee-to-Chest

As you lift your knee to your chest in this gentle stretch, you will feel the curve in your lower back flatten out.

Starting position: Lie on your back, knees bent and feet flat on the floor, arms relaxed at your sides.

Steps:
1. Lift your right knee towards your chest as far as you can. (For extra stretch, try pulling your knee a bit closer to your chest with your hands.) *a*
2. Lower that same knee to and through the starting position, so that your right leg is extended straight. *b*
3. Wobble your leg to relax your muscles. *c* (on p. 344)
4. Return to the starting position.
5. Repeat steps 1–4 with your left leg.

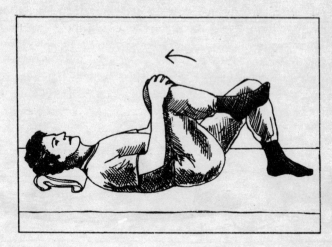

a

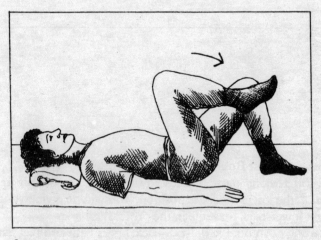

b

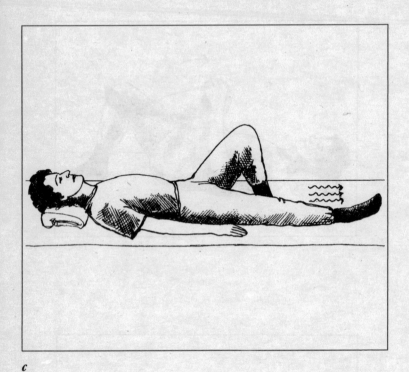

c

Knees-to-Chest Rock

This soft rocking motion takes advantage of the built-in relaxation of the knees-to-chest position. You will be giving yourself a slight lower-back massage in the process!

Starting position: Lie on your back, knees bent and feet flat on the floor, with your arms at your sides.

Steps:
1. Pull both knees to your chest, one at a time. (If you prefer, you may bring both knees up simultaneously.)
2. Hold your knees in this position. (For greatest ease, hold the backs of your thighs. If you are slightly more supple, hold your knees. To get the maximum stretch, clasp your arms around and just under both knees.)
3. Curl your head and shoulders forward, and gently rock to and fro, and from side to side in this position.

Note: Some people feel a strain in the neck while doing this exercise. If you feel just a slight strain with no pain afterwards, there should be no reason to omit this one. But if it makes you genuinely uncomfortable, ease off until you have strengthened your neck with the exercises recommended for that purpose.

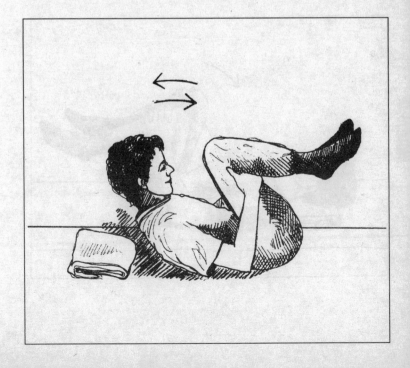

Double Knee-to-Chest

The easiest way to perform this exercise is by keeping your knees together as you pull them to your chest. With experience, and for a greater stretch, you can try holding your knees about shoulder-width apart as you raise and lower them.

Starting position: Lie on your back with your knees bent and your feet flat on the floor.

Steps:

1. Clasp your hands around your knees and pull them towards your chest.
2. Pause if you feel resistance, then try to pull gently a bit farther.
3. Hold this position for a few seconds. (For added stretch, gradually work your way up to holding this position for 25 seconds.)
4. Return to the starting position.

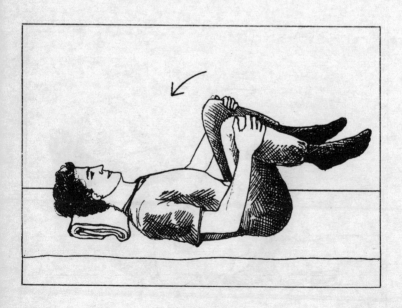

Knee Drops

Don't worry if you can't get your knees very far down when you first attempt this manoeuvre. You'll build up your ability in time.

Starting position: Lie on your back with your knees bent and your feet flat on the floor. *a*

Steps:

1. Keeping your knees together, drop them both to the right as far as you can. (Your left hip and buttock will necessarily rise off the bed or floor as your knees drop to the right, but try to keep both your shoulders on the flat surface.) *b*
2. Return to the starting position. *c*
3. Drop both knees to the left. *d*
   (Turn over the page to see Steps 2–3.)

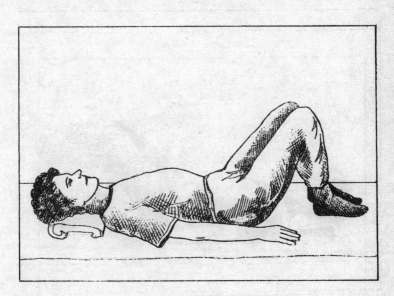

a

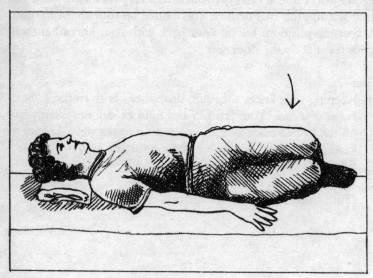

b

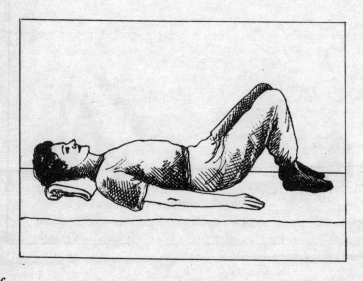

c

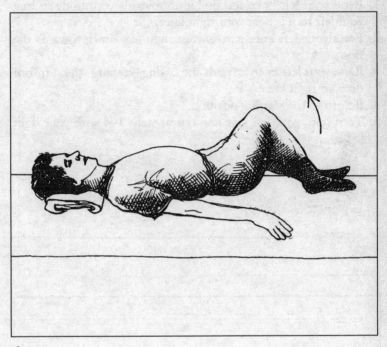

d

Simple Knee Cross

These knee movements, which resemble the slow flapping of a butterfly's wing, gently stretch the lower back and hips.

Starting position: Lie on your right side, with your legs extended. You may want to place your left hand on the floor in front of you for support.

Steps:

1. Bend your left knee and pull it up towards your body so that your left foot is near your right knee. *a*
2. Press your left knee across your right leg, down towards the floor. *b*
3. Raise your left knee towards the ceiling, keeping your left foot on your right knee. *c*
4. Return to the starting position.
5. Turn onto your left side and repeat steps 1–4 with your right leg.

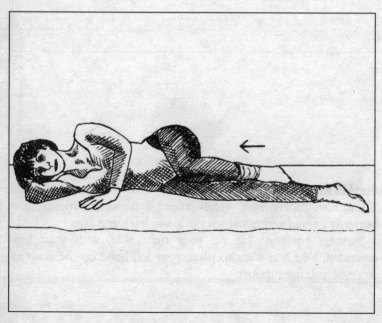

a

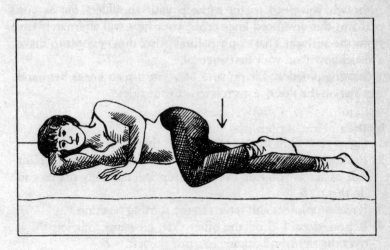

b

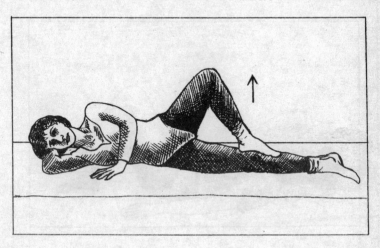

c

Knee Cross

Although you need to try to keep your shoulders flat as you perform this advanced knee cross, your hips will alternately rise from the surface. That's only natural. Also, don't expect to make a 'touchdown' on your first attempt.

Starting position: Lie on your back, with your knees bent and feet flat on the floor, arms relaxed at your sides.

Steps:
1. Cross your right thigh over your left thigh.   *a*
2. Press your legs together and tip your knees towards the right side as far as you can. (Your left hip will naturally rise as you do this.)   *b*
3. Raise your knees and return to the starting position.
4. Repeat steps 1–3 on the other side, crossing your left thigh over the right, and tipping towards the left.   *c*

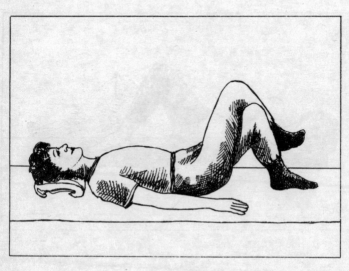

a

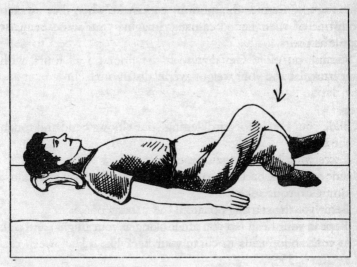

b

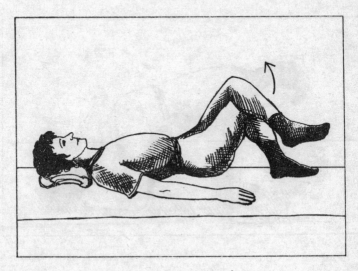

c

Cat Stretch

This exercise mimics the motions cats make when they awaken from one of their famed catnaps. Imagine your spine being as supple as theirs.

Starting position: Get down on the floor on all fours, with your back flat and your weight evenly distributed.   *a*

Steps:
1. Slide your hands forward, letting your elbows bend and touch the floor.
2. Lower your head and raise your bottom.   *b*
3. Smoothly sink back on your haunches, so that you are almost sitting on your ankles.   *c*
4. Return to the starting position.   *d*   (on p. 356)
5. Tuck in your head (so you are looking at your thighs) and pull in your abdominals to curve your back like a Halloween cat.   *e*   (on p. 356)
6. Relax your abdominal muscles and roll your head back.

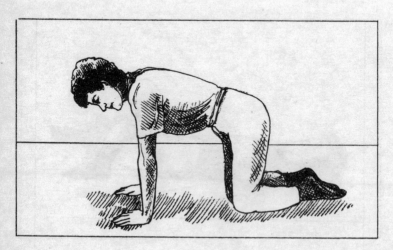

a

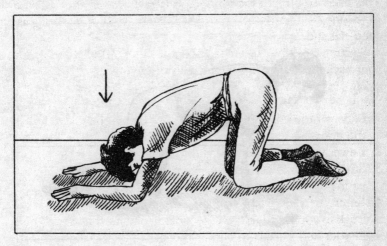

b

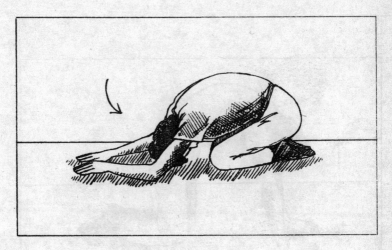

c

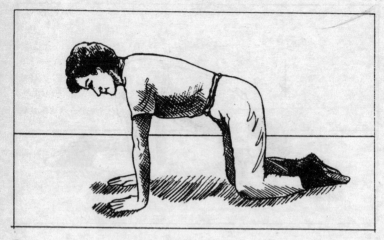

d

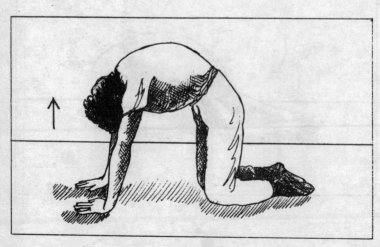

e

Twists and Tilts

Give yourself a maximum sideways stretch as you twist and turn. Fight the urge to lean forwards or backwards, or to move your lower body.

Starting position: Stand with your hands on your hips.

Steps:

1. Lean the top of your body to the right. Resist the temptation to lean forwards or backwards as you bend sideways. Also try to keep your feet, legs and hips steady. *a*
2. Straighten up slowly.
3. Repeat these motions to the left. *b*
   (Turn over the page to see Steps 4–6)

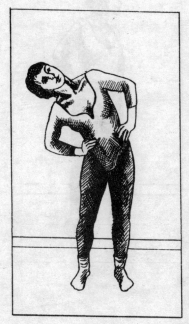

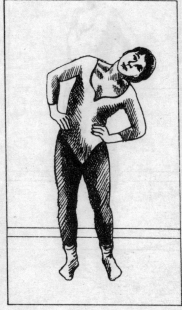

a   *b*

4. Twist the upper half of your body around to the left, as though you were trying to see behind you. *c*
5. Return to face front.
6. Repeat these motions to the right. *d*

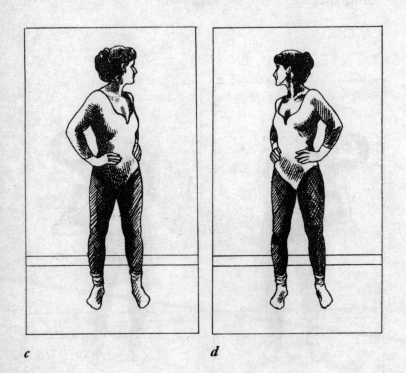

c   *d*

To Strengthen the Abdominal Muscles

Pelvic Tilt

This most basic strengthening exercise will flatten both your abdomen and the curve in your lower back.

Starting position: Lie on your back with your knees bent and your feet flat on the floor, arms relaxed at your sides. *a*

(Turn over the page to see Steps 1–3.)

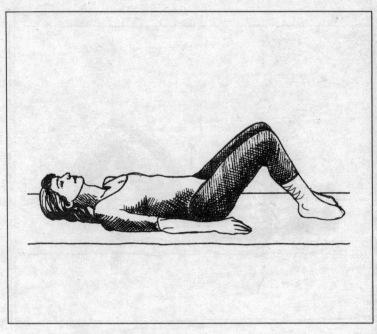

a

Steps:

1. Tighten your buttocks and pull in your abdominal muscles, so that your hips roll upward. Exhale as you do this. (Strive to work your buttocks and abdominal muscles, and resist the temptation to simply push off from the floor with your feet or hips.) *b*
2. Hold the position, but not your breath, for a few seconds.
3. Relax your muscles as you inhale and return to the starting position.

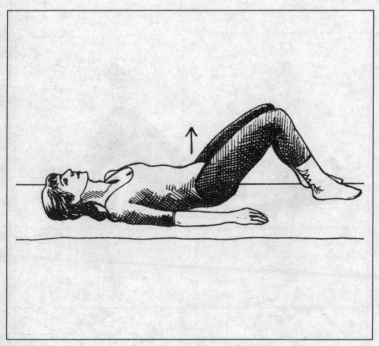

b

Standing Pelvic Tilt

A wall takes the place of the bed or floor in this upright version of the basic Pelvic Tilt.

Starting position: Stand with your back against a wall, your feet about shoulder-width apart, positioned a few centimetres away from the wall's base. *a*

Steps:
1. Exhaling, squeeze your buttocks together and pull in your gut, so that you can feel the curve in the small of your back flatten against the wall. Keep your shoulders relaxed as you do this. *b*
2. Hold the position for a few seconds as you breathe in and out normally.
3. Inhaling, relax and return to the starting position.

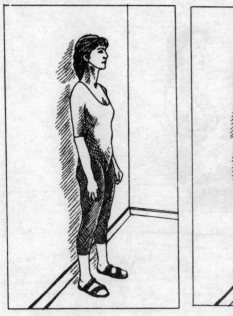
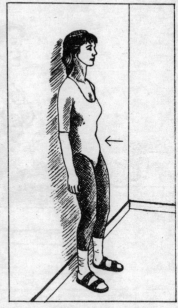

a   *b*

Sit-downs

These reverse sit-ups are a bit more challenging, so please don't attempt them until you've built up your abdominal strength. Try to maintain a 'lifted' position in your back – don't slouch and let it become too curved. Remember that the distance you move is secondary to the effort you put into strengthening your abdominal muscles.

Starting position: Sit on a bed or a bench that allows you room to lean back. Fold your arms across your chest. *a*

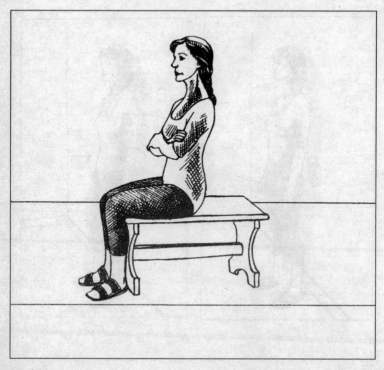

a

Steps:

1. Use your abdominal muscles to lean your body backward several centimetres – about as far as you would lift up for a sit-up. Exhale as you go. *b*
2. Hold the position, but don't hold your breath, for a count of three. Continue to exhale slowly, as this will help you control your abdominals.
3. Return to a straight sitting posture as you finish exhaling.
4. Inhale and relax your muscles.

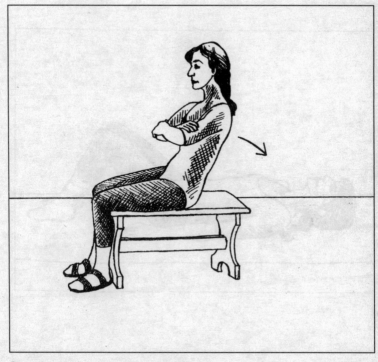

b

Bent-Knee Sit-ups

Sit-ups from a bent-knee position give just as good a workout to the abdominal muscles as the old straight-knee sit-ups you learned in school. More importantly, they are much safer for your back. Though steady breathing is important during any exercise, you'll get a real boost here if you exhale as you sit up, then inhale as you lie back down.

Starting position: Lie on your back, knees bent and feet flat on the floor, arms relaxed at your sides. *a*

Most people lead with their arms when they perform this exercise, but you can work your abdominals even harder if you fold your arms across your chest. Putting your hands behind your head can just give you a pain in the neck.

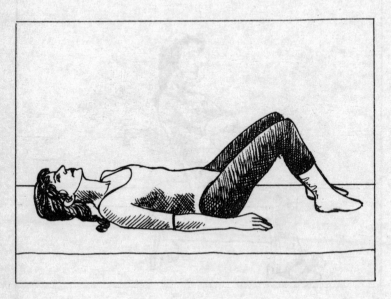

a

Steps:

1. Pull in your abdominals and raise the upper part of your body towards your knees as you exhale. (You need not rise very far – just far enough to see your navel, or to lift your shoulder blades off the floor.) *b*
2. Hold the position for a few seconds, but don't hold your breath. (Be conscious of breathing in and out.)
3. Relax your muscles slowly as you lower your head and shoulders while you inhale.

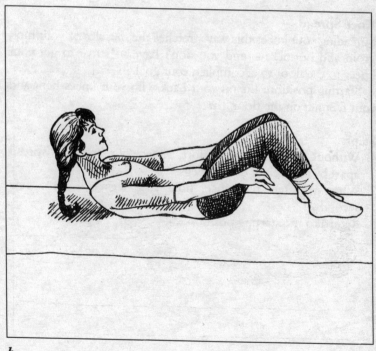

b

To Stretch and Strengthen the Buttocks, Hips and Leg Muscles

The Squeeze

Good support for the lower back rests, literally, on strong buttocks, which can be built up with this isometric exercise; nothing appears to move, but the effects can be felt.

Starting position: You may perform this exercise lying down, sitting or standing.

Steps:
1. Squeeze your buttocks together as tightly as you can.
2. Hold for a moment, then release, and relax.

Knee Spread

Spreading your knees this way stretches the muscles of your hips, groin and buttocks – and you don't have to strive to get your knees to the floor to accomplish your goal.

Starting position: Lie on your back with your knees bent and your feet flat on the floor. *a*

Steps:
1. Without expending any effort, allow your knees to spread apart by the weight of your legs. *b*
2. When you feel resistance, hold your legs still for a few seconds.
3. Return to the starting position.

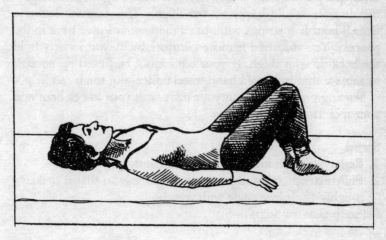

a

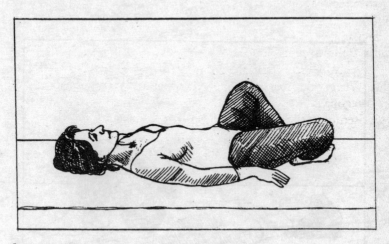

b

Hamstring Stretch

Many people who suffer low back pain have tight hamstrings – the muscles at the backs of the thighs. This exercise lets you stretch your hamstrings without straining your lower back in the process. You may find it more comfortable if you loosely hold the back of your thigh. If your hip cannot be flexed up enough to achieve this, holding a hand towel under your thigh can help.

Starting position: Lie on your back with your knees bent and your feet flat on the floor. *a*

Steps:
1. Raise your right knee towards your chest. *b*
2. Fully extend and straighten your right leg, so that it makes a roughly 45-degree angle with your body. *c*

(See p. 370 for Steps 3–5)

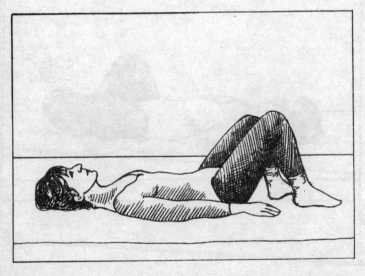

a

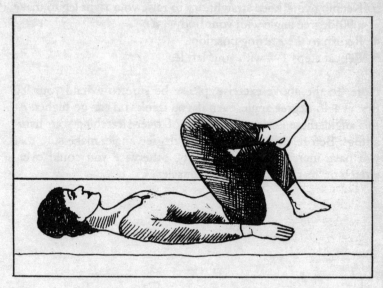

b

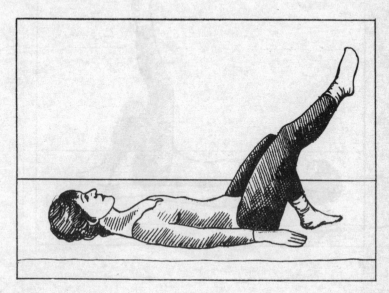

c

3. Keeping your knee straight, try to raise your right leg to make a 90-degree angle with your body. *d*
4. Return to the starting position.
5. Repeat steps 1–4 with your left leg.

Note: In the above exercise, please be sure to extend your leg first at a 45-degree angle, even if you think you can go higher. At this angle, there is virtually no risk of over-stretching your hamstrings. Before you attempt the 90-degree angle, make sure that you have increased your flexibility, otherwise you could over-stretch or 'tear' your hamstring muscle.

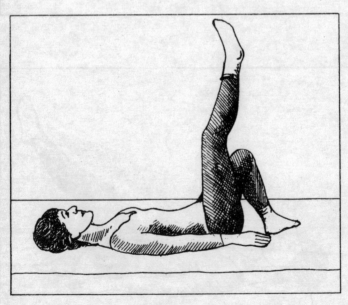

d

Hip Hikers

Keeping a full range of motion in your hips (a goal of this exercise) safeguards both your posture and your walking gait.

Starting position: Lie on your right side, with your knees straight and your right arm under your head. Prop your left hand on the floor in front of your body for support.

Steps:

1. Slowly lift your left leg as high as you can, keeping the knee straight.
2. Hold this extension for several seconds, feeling the stretch in your hip and thigh.
3. Gently lower your leg.
4. Repeat steps 1–3 twice. (This counts as three repetitions.)
5. Turn over and repeat the exercise, raising your right leg.

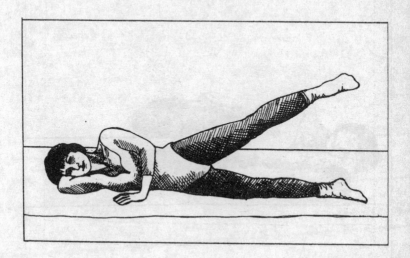

Thigh Pull

The flipside of the hamstrings are the quadriceps muscles at the front of the thighs. This exercise emphasizes body alignment as it stretches the area from hip to knee.

Starting position: Lie on your right side, your head resting on your right arm, and your left leg bent at the knee. Think of your body making a straight line from your head down the front of your thighs.

Steps:

1. With your left hand, grasp your left ankle. *a*
2. Keeping the knee bent, pull your left leg back and towards your buttocks as far as you comfortably can. Resist the temptation to arch your back.

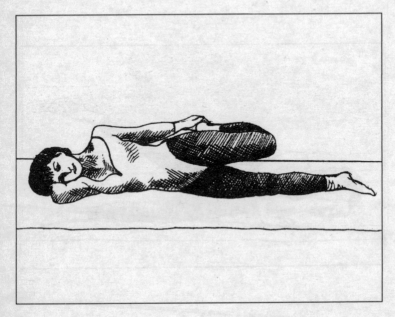

a

3. Hold this position for a few moments, feeling the stretch along the front of your thigh.
4. Return to the starting position.
5. Repeat steps 1–4 twice.
6. Turn onto your left side, and repeat the exercise with your right leg. *b*

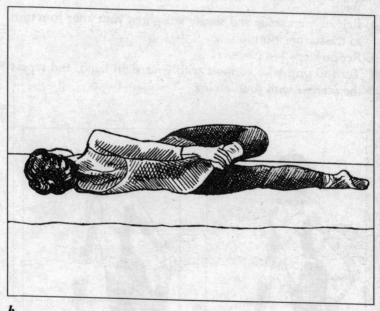

b

Standing Thigh Pull

Holding your body in a Standing Pelvic Tilt (see p. 361) while you do the following exercise will keep you properly aligned and help you avoid arching your back.

Starting position: Stand alongside a chair or other sturdy support that you can hold for balance.

Steps:

1. With your left hand on the support, bend your right knee and grasp your right ankle. *a*
2. Pull your right leg back and towards your buttocks, but not so far as to make you arch your back. *b*
3. Hold this position, feeling the stretch along the front of your thigh.
4. Release your ankle and slowly straighten your knee to return to the starting position.
5. Repeat steps 1–4 twice.
6. Turn to grip your support with your right hand, and repeat the exercise with your left leg.

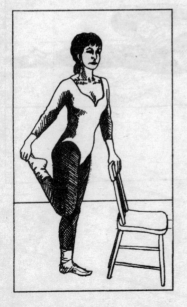 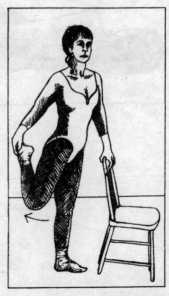

a   *b*

Runner's Stretch

Fully stretching your lower legs can improve your standing posture and smooth out your walking gait – two important factors in warding off back pain.

Starting position: Stand facing a wall, with your hands on the wall at about shoulder height, and your feet about 30 cm (12 inches) away from the wall's base.

Steps:

1. Extend your left leg about 30 cm (12 inches) behind you, keeping your left knee straight, your toes on the floor, and your heel raised slightly off the floor. You may bend the knee of your standing (right) leg. *a*
2. Try to lower your left heel to the floor, or as far as you can, feeling the stretch in your Achilles tendon. It's best not to have your legs too wide apart, as it's more important to ensure that your heel actually touches the floor. *b*
3. Hold the full stretch for a few moments.
4. Return to the starting position.
5. Repeat steps 1–4, stretching your right leg.

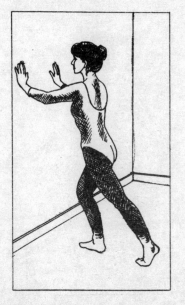 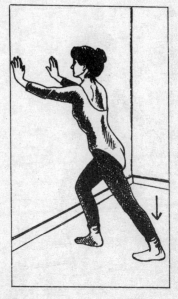

a   *b*

Chapter 23
Exercises for Upper Back and Neck Pain

Although many doctors view upper back and neck pain as 'low back pain that has migrated upward,' different treatments and exercises apply.

In the US survey, less than half of the participants with neck pain were even aware that exercise could add strength and flexibility to their neck muscles. The other half – the participants with neck pain who did perform exercises to relieve that pain – saw improvement in their symptoms. The truth is, the results from neck exercise were not as dramatic as the results of exercise for low back pain. But, based on the US survey, I believe you can greatly improve your chances of getting a dramatic benefit from neck exercise by following a few simple guidelines:

- *Combine the neck exercises in this chapter with the low back exercises in Chapter 22.* Most of those survey participants with neck pain also had some pain or discomfort in the lower back. Performing both sets of exercises in a regular routine brought the most significant improvement.
- *Perform neck exercises frequently throughout the day.* Most of the movements described below can help relieve on-the-spot tension – as well as building strength and flexibility. In other words, these exercises are 'first aid' for neck pain. Any time you feel stress and discomfort accumulating in your neck, whether you are at work or at home, try alleviating the tension with a few neck exercises. Here, slight discomfort is expected while exercising. Remember, though, to drop any exercise that – for you – turns mild discomfort to pain.
- *Maintain good posture through your neck.* A mention of posture usually makes people suck in their abdominal muscles and throw their shoulders back. Since the spine begins in the neck,

good posture also means keeping the head well aligned, as though it were a ball on top of a flagpole. To correct your neck posture, stretch your neck and head skyward for a moment – go straight up, as though your neck had grown longer – then relax and tuck in your chin, instead of letting it jut or droop. (See Chapter 14 for more suggestions on maintaining proper alignment and avoiding neck pain during everyday activities such as reading.)

To Stretch the Neck

Warning: Do not attempt these neck exercises if you have dizziness, double vision or difficulty in breathing or swallowing. These could be symptoms of vertebral basilar artery insufficiency (VBI). This condition affects the blood supply to the brain. If this blood supply is affected by stretching or turning exercises it could result in a life-threatening stroke. If you experience dizziness when you look up or rotate your head, stop these exercises immediately.

Left-Right
These slow head turns to left and right help untie the knots of tension in the neck.

Starting position: You can do this exercise lying on your back in bed, or sitting or standing, with your arms at your sides.

Steps:
1. Keeping your head level, turn it to the right as far as you can, as though to stare across your right shoulder. *a*
2. Return your head and your gaze to centre. *b*
3. Turn your head the other way to look as far left as you can.
4. Return to the starting position.

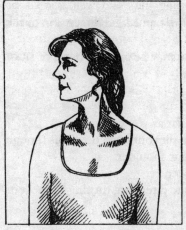

a

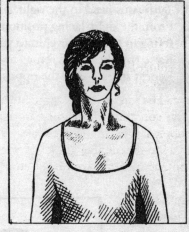

b

Yes-No
Nodding 'yes' or shaking your head 'no', the neck gets a workout
by moving the head about.
Starting position: You may sit or stand virtually anywhere.

Steps:
1. Nod your head up and down slowly, several times.
2. Turn your head from side to side, as though making a slow,
   exaggerated 'no' gesture.

Left-Right Plus

The extra chin-to-shoulder dip brings an added dimension to the side-to-side neck stretch.

Starting position: As above, you may lie on your back, or sit or stand with your arms at your sides. *a*

Steps:

1. Turn your head to the right as far as you can. *b*
2. From the right-facing position, tilt your head down, as though trying to touch your chin to your shoulder. *c*
3. Raise your head and return to centre.
4. Repeat steps 1–3 in the opposite direction, turning to the left.

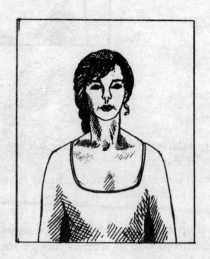

a

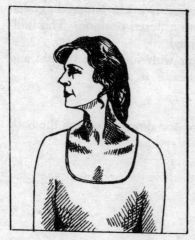

b

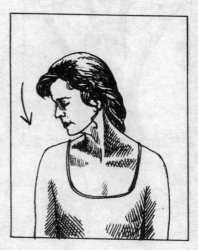

c

Head Pull

This is a gentle but effective exercise. Don't be tempted to over-press (pull the head forward into a flexed position). This additional pressure is not recommended.

Starting position: Sit in a chair with your back straight and your hands clasped behind your head. *a*

Steps:
1. Gently pull your head forward and down to stretch the back of your neck. *b*
2. Hold, feeling the stretch.
3. Return to the starting position.

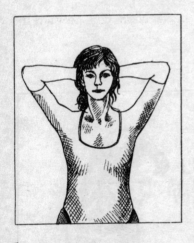

a

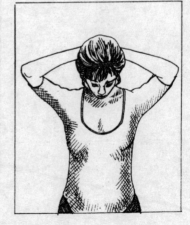

b

Neck Tilt

Instead of a continuous rolling motion, this sideways neck stretch calls to mind the motions of an attentive bird, cocking its head first one way, then the other.

Starting position: Sit or stand comfortably, facing straight ahead.

Steps:

1. Tilt your head to the left, as though trying to touch your ear to your shoulder. Don't try to bring your shoulder up to your ear. *a*
2. When you feel resistance, pause for a few seconds to hold the position.
3. Return to the starting position and relax.
4. Repeat steps 1–3 in the opposite direction, tilting toward the right. *b*

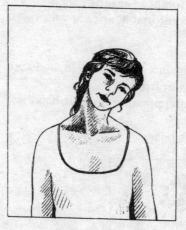

a

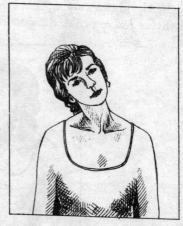

b

To Strengthen the Neck

Bed Head

Your head makes a handy weight for your neck to press and push in this strengthening exercise.

Starting position: Lie on your back in bed or on the floor.

Steps:
1. Press your head straight back into your pillow or mat.
2. Hold for a moment, then release the pressure.
3. Lift your head so that it is just above your pillow or mat, without lifting your shoulders.
4. Hold, feeling the effort in your neck, then release.

Neck Push

This isometric exercise can strengthen your neck by making it work against the pressure of your own arm strength. You can also try doing it by pressing your forehead against a wall!

Starting position: Sit or stand comfortably, arms at your sides.

Steps:
1. Press the palm of one hand against your forehead, and your forehead against the palm of your hand.
2. Hold for a moment, keeping the pressure on your hand and head without moving either one.
3. Relax and return to the starting position.

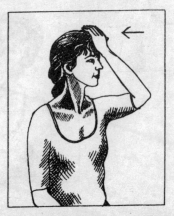

Side Neck Push

The hand-on-head stance called for here may imitate a look of anguish, but the results should bring relief instead.

Starting position: Do this exercise sitting, standing, or even lying down, starting with your arms at your sides.

Steps:

1. Press your left hand against the left side of your head, and simultaneously press your head against your hand.
2. Hold the position, hand and head pushing against each other.
3. Relax and return to the starting position.
4. Repeat steps 1–3, raising your right hand to the right side of your head.

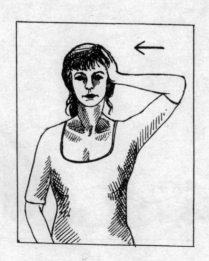

To Stretch the Shoulders and Upper Back

Shoulder Stretch

Try not to raise your shoulders in this exercise, but just let the flowing motion of your arm stretch the neck and shoulder muscles. It may also be worth doing this exercise with both arms simultaneously, as there is less rotation of the upper back and it is likely to be more comfortable.

Starting position: Lie on your back with your knees bent and feet flat, arms at your sides.

Steps:
1. Raise your right arm straight up to a 90-degree angle, and keep moving it through a half-circle until it is extended behind you, palm up.
2. Relax for a moment, and then reverse the movement and return to the starting position.
3. Repeat steps 1 and 2 with your left arm.

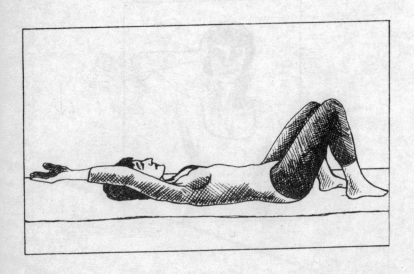

Shoulder Shrug

Even though your shoulders do the work by shrugging, your neck will appear to shrink and grow – and you will feel the positive effects over time.

Starting position: You can do this exercise lying in bed or sitting or standing, with your arms at your sides.

Steps:
1. Slowly and steadily raise your shoulders to a shrug. *a*
2. Hold for a moment, feeling the effect on your neck muscles.
3. Keeping your head still, gently press your shoulders as far down as you can. *b*
4. Hold, feeling the stretch in your neck.

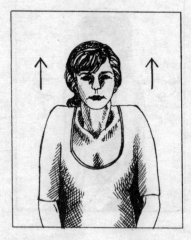

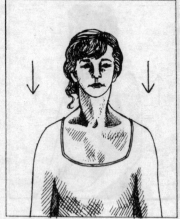

a   *b*

Shoulder Roll

Try to roll your shoulders through a full circle in one fluid motion. Even though each step is numbered separately, keep moving slowly from one to the next without stopping.

Starting position: Sit or stand with your shoulders relaxed.

Steps:
1. Raise your shoulders. *a*
2. Bring your shoulders forward. *b*
3. Push your shoulders down. *c*
4. Pull your shoulders back. *d*
5. Return to the starting position.
6. Circle your shoulders in the opposite direction, reversing the order of steps 1–5.

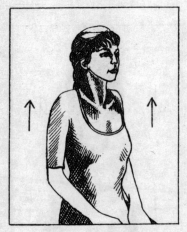

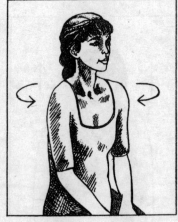

a   *b*

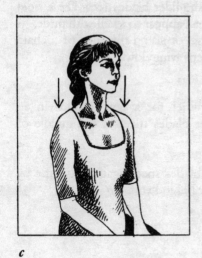

c

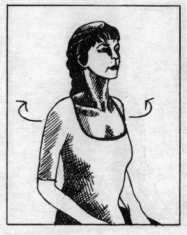

d

Roller Blades

This rolling movement of the shoulder blades feels like a sideways shrug. It will make your chest appear to swell with pride.

Starting position: Stand at ease, or sit on the edge of a chair. You can even do the first two steps lying down.

Steps:
1. Squeeze your shoulders together for a few seconds in an effort to make your shoulder blades meet in the middle of your back. *a*
2. Relax.
3. Try to make your shoulder blades meet again, this time by pushing your elbows together behind you. *b*

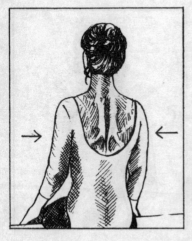
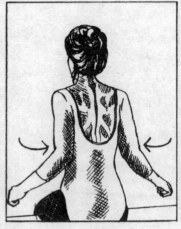

a *b*

Square Shoulder Stretch

Try to keep your neck relaxed as one arm pulls the other to stretch the triceps muscles of your shoulders and upper arms.

Starting position: Sit on a straight-backed chair or stool. Cross your arms in front of you, left over right, so that each hand holds the opposite elbow, raise your arms over your head in this way, and then let your left hand hang free. *a*

Steps:
1. With your right hand, pull your left elbow towards and behind your head. *b*
2. Hold this stretch for several seconds, feeling the stretch in your shoulder and upper arm.
3. Relax and return to the starting position, and switch your grip to hold your right elbow in your left hand.
4. Repeat steps 1–3, using your left hand to pull your right elbow.

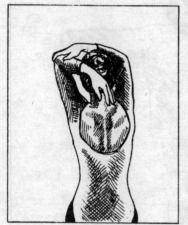 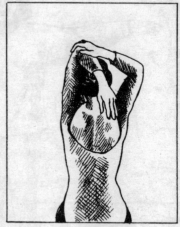

a　　　　　　　　　　*b*

Aeroplane

Try to keep your neck relaxed and your posture aligned as you make these motions of a child imitating an aeroplane.

Starting position: Stand with your arms straight out to the sides at shoulder height, palms down.

Steps:

1. Make several small forward circles with your arms, keeping your elbows straight.
2. Circle your arms in reverse.

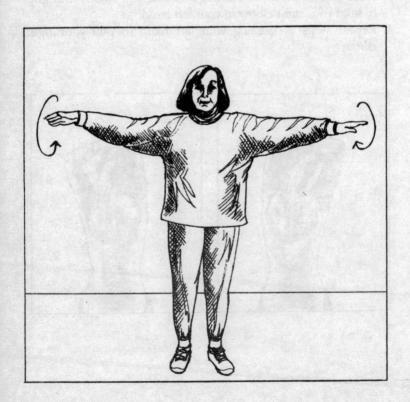

Windmill

Picture your arms as the blades of a windmill as you perform this exercise – but don't try to go as fast!

Starting position: Stand at ease, arms at your sides. Make sure you have sufficient space.

Steps:

1. Keeping your right arm straight, describe several huge circles in the air in a forward motion. *a, b*
2. Without stopping, circle your right arm in the opposite direction, going through a full range of motion.
3. Repeat steps 1–3 with your left arm.

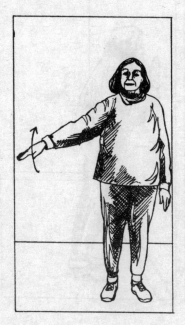

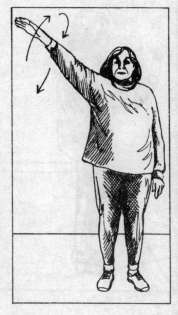

a   *b*

To Strengthen the Shoulders and Upper Back

Push-offs

These standing push-ups are easier than the military kind. They increase in difficulty as you increase the distance between yourself and the wall to as far as 60 cm (2 feet).

Starting position: Stand facing a wall, with your feet apart and about 30 cm (12 inches) away from the wall, with your palms resting on the wall at shoulder height. *a*

Steps:
1. Lean in towards the wall as far as possible, keeping your legs and back straight. *b*
2. Push yourself back to the starting position.

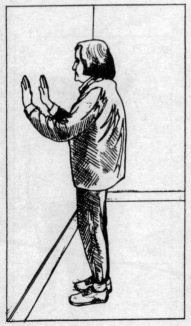 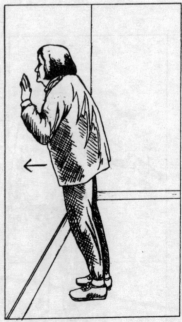

a   *b*

Side Press

Stubbornly pushing against a wall is a sound isometric approach to increasing shoulder strength.

Starting position: Stand near a wall, with the right side of your body about 15 cm (6 inches) away from it.

Steps:
1. Extend your right arm out sideways until your forearm is pressing against the wall. *a*
2. Continue to push for several seconds, feeling the exertion in your shoulder.
3. Relax and return to the starting position.
4. Repeat steps 1–3 twice.
5. Turn, and repeat the exercise with your left arm. *b*

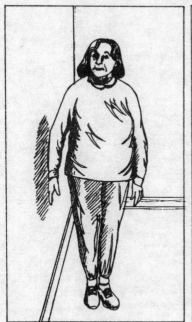 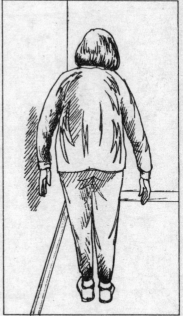

a   *b*

Chapter 24
Exercises for General Fitness

Fitness has become such a popular pursuit that you can barely walk down the street these days without encountering joggers, cyclists and rollerbladers out in force. But if you are walking down the street, you are already engaged in the all-time best activity for building cardiovascular fitness and keeping your back flexible.

This chapter discusses the four most popular fitness exercises for people with back pain – walking, swimming, cycling and dancing.

Walking

Walking is the oldest and best of the weight-bearing exercises for people with back pain. Walking proved helpful in the long run for 98 per cent of the participants in the US survey who made this activity a regular part of their routine. They reported that walking not only increased the flexibility of their backs, but also improved their overall strength and muscle tone. Another important advantage was that walking at least 30 minutes a day, four times a week, greatly reduced stress and tension for these people. Even the twenty-six participants who couldn't lead normal lives because of back pain all improved in the long run by following their practitioners' advice to walk (or swim) regularly.

Hospital studies show that walkers gain the same cardiovascular benefits as runners, and with far fewer injuries. It makes an ideal back exercise because it is low-impact yet high-endurance – that is, once you have built up to taking relatively long walks several times a week. Because most people can walk for a longer time than they can run or play tennis, for example, walking tends to build muscular endurance while it burns calories.

Walking is easy, accessible, effective, enjoyable and free of charge! It can be geared to any level of fitness, and pursued by people of all ages. No exercise could be more convenient than walking. You need no special equipment and no special clothing, other than comfortable shoes. You don't have to travel to the gym or the pool; you just get up and go. For these reasons, you're far less likely to give up your walking regime than any other exercise you might try.

Most people can easily fit walking into their daily activities if they try. You may even find that you can combine your daily activities – your errands, some light shopping – with your walk when you are pressed for time. Walking to work or to appointments is another way to fit exercise into the day's programme. And although walking will quicken your heart rate and get your body into condition, it doesn't usually leave you perspiring so much that you require a shower or a change of clothing when you get where you're going.

If you are already in reasonably good shape, I recommend at least half an hour of brisk walking every other day. You may build up to walking 5–6 km (3–4 miles) in an hour, five to seven days a week. What starts as something you do to improve your back may well turn into the highlight of your day – the time you feel simultaneously relaxed and energized. At that point, you probably won't want to miss your daily walk.

Your walking pace is a measure of your fitness and freedom from pain. Ideally, you should walk at a reasonably quick pace, as if you have somewhere to go. But studies have shown that even a slow pace can benefit your heart and lower your cholesterol level.

Most important, as far as your back is concerned, is to keep your posture aligned, with your abdominals holding your lower back in proper position. And walk with zest – with your hips and legs making great strides as you swing your arms and get the maximum enjoyment out of the activity. At the risk of stating the obvious, remember that the goal of walking is to move forward. Many people add extraneous motions to their walking gait. They may flop from side to side, or bounce up and down as they go. I want you to walk with your posture and purpose in mind. Try to imagine that you are being pulled forward by a string attached to the middle of your chest.

If you are just recuperating from an episode of incapacitating back pain, then you'll want to build up gradually to a fitness level of walking. You can begin by walking as much as you can around your house, as soon as you feel up to it. Even if you stay indoors, wear good shoes as soon as you start spending most of your time up and about. A pair of walking or running shoes, or any comfortable shoes that offer good support, will help you through this recovery period. The best shoes are those you're already used to. If you do need to break in a new pair of shoes, do it gradually, because any sudden change at this point could aggravate your back. (Even after you're up and about, I recommend wearing new shoes just half an hour the first time, then an additional half hour each succeeding day.)

When you venture outside the first few times, try to avoid steep gradients and uneven ground, as walking up or down hills causes more of a strain on the muscles of the lower back. What's more, rocky ground or broken pavements can make it difficult for you to relax and stride comfortably, with your head held high and your gaze out to the world.

Swimming

Swimming is an ideal aerobic exercise for general fitness because it makes the arms and legs work hard to get the heart pumping. Some exercise experts, however, argue that swimming can't match up to walking or running as a weight-bearing exercise. Although it's true that the water provides a virtually stress-free environment, studies have shown that swimmers have thicker, stronger bones than people who perform no exercise at all. Swimming can indeed help you improve your muscle endurance and flexibility.

I didn't hear a single negative comment about swimming in the US survey. I did, however, hear a few cautionary notes about which stroke to choose. A tiring, taxing stroke such as the butterfly, for example, which requires the arms to whirl like windmills while the lower back and legs mimic a leaping dolphin, is clearly too risky for anyone with back problems.

You should also avoid breaststroke unless your back pain is unquestionably a thing of the past. (Even then, you might have difficulty with this stroke.)

Some people with back pain find that the standard overhand crawl or 'freestyle' puts too much of an arch in the lower back. Many prefer the sidestroke, with its froglike kicking motions, to the back-arching flutter-kick of the crawl. I consider the sidestroke to be the easiest on the back, and I recommend that you alternate sides so that you exercise your body evenly. The backstroke – not the back crawl, but the breaststroke flipped on its back – is the next easiest. Keep it simple by keeping your arms close to your sides as you cup your hands to push through the water, instead of reaching way up beyond your shoulder level for power strokes. You may add a frog-kick or a flutter-kick – whichever feels better to you.

You can experiment with different strokes to find the one that suits you best. You may find you like to combine a variety of strokes to add interest to your time in the water. By alternating between difficult and simple strokes, you can pace yourself – getting a good workout while avoiding rapid fatigue.

One advantage of swimming over other fitness activities is that water makes exercise a virtually no-sweat proposition. The reason? Water is four times more efficient than air at dissipating heat. This keeps your body from getting overheated so quickly, and enables you to continue feeling comfortable even though you may be working out very hard in hot weather.

If you have a pool near you and can swim regularly, try to build up to 15 minutes of non-stop swimming, three times a week. You may find that swimming is more beneficial to you than anything else, even walking, depending on your particular condition. (See Chapter 25 for a full discussion of exercises for various back ailments.)

Cycling

A bicycle may be your best friend or your worst enemy, depending on the way it requires you to sit, position your hands, and extend your neck. Fortunately, the racing bike, which requires the rider to assume a near-foetal position and then crane his or her neck up to see straight ahead, has given way in popularity to the upright touring and all-terrain or 'mountain' bike. This trend is a real boon to back sufferers. You will be much more comfortable sitting straight up than hunching over for the sake of reducing air resistance on your body. After all, when your purpose in riding is to gain exercise and fresh air, as opposed to winning a race, sitting up is the position of choice.

Seat comfort is an all-important consideration. Whether you ride as an excuse to get out and about, or restrict your pedalling to an indoor exercise bike, you need to remain seated throughout your workout. Some people experience nothing more annoying than a mild soreness in their buttocks the first few days of getting used to a bicycle seat. Others find that the pain never goes away. This is especially important for people with sciatica pain, which typically runs through the buttocks. Obviously, if you can't get comfortable on a bicycle, then cycling is not for you. But before you give up the advantages of this sport, try experimenting with comfort solutions. You can, for example, add a padded seat cover, or change the seat altogether. Most people find the broad 'saddle' style more comfortable than the small, hard racing seat. You can also gain greater comfort by wearing padded cycling shorts, which are easily available from cycling shops and sports equipment shops.

Since I am recommending cycling as a good fitness activity, I must add that cycling also requires certain safety precautions that have nothing to do with posture or seat selection. Now that the pattern of bicycle-related injuries has been well documented, I urge you to buy and wear a cycling helmet. Head protection is essential on every ride – not only on streets shared with cars, but also on special cycling tracks in parks. If you're a night rider, you'll need reflectors on your bicycle as well as on your clothing and helmet, for safety's sake. It's also a good idea to equip your bicycle with a headlight and tail-light.

Cycling can be enjoyed as an indoor sport with a stationary exercise bike. Many busy people like to work out with an exercise bike, rooted to the floor, because it allows them to pedal away while getting something else done – reading a book or a magazine, say, watching television, or even watching a DVD.

Most of us tend to think of cycling as legwork, and it is, but some stationary bikes include activities for the arms, too. As you pump the pedals with your feet on one of these, you can push and pull handles that will also exercise your upper body.

Dancing

Health experts consider dancing a reasonable alternative to other aerobic activities, including walking, swimming and cycling. As long as you dance on a sprung floor (to lessen the jarring impact), you are likely to find dancing both beneficial and enjoyable. As the most social of all these outlets, dancing provides the combination of good movements and good times with others that puts you in the swing of things and makes you feel good to be alive.

Ballroom dancing and folk dancing may offer just the right activity level for you, as they need not be stressful exercises. If your back is basically strong, causing you only minor aches and pain, you may choose to investigate modern dance, jazz or even ballet instruction.

When you and your partner dance to the music of a long song set, continuing until the music ends, you get great endurance exercise. What's more, the chance to be with other people in an active form of recreation makes dancing virtually boredom-proof. People may abandon their exercise bikes and find excuses to avoid the swimming pool on a chilly day, but dancing retains its appeal over the long term. It's one of the most enjoyable ways to rediscover how much your body can do.

One of the chief benefits of dancing is the relaxed style of movement that comes from mastering steps to music. If you take up dancing, you may well find that as you become accustomed to rhythmically positioning your body in space, you develop dance-like ways of doing other activities. Your motions may become more fluid, so that you improve your walking gait, for example. Instead of striking a rigid pose while you stand at the kitchen counter or sit at your desk, you may bring the good body mechanics of dancing to bear by adding a little motion. Some dancers gently dip and shift their weight from one leg to the other while working standing up, or perform a rock-and-roll stretch of the lower back while typing at the computer keyboard.

Several participants in the US survey learned exercise from dance instructors who taught modern dance and ballet. They went for instruction after a painful episode had ended, not in the throes of back pain. They enjoyed the idea of learning to dance and of practising at least three times a week. Most found they experienced substantial improvement in their posture, abdominal strength and overall flexibility, along with a substantial reduction in back pain.

Some martial arts, such as Tai Chi, offer a non-jarring, dance-like form of aerobic exercise that can be practised daily, by yourself or in a group.

Chapter 25
Exercises for Specific Conditions

When I talk about tailoring a back-exercise programme to your specific needs, I have in mind the specific condition – provided that one can be identified – that is the root cause of your back pain. Many, if not most, back problems elude specific diagnoses agreed on by different kinds of practitioners. Some conditions, however, are easily recognized. And according to the results of the US survey, exercises that take these back problems into account offer the best chance of improvement. Whether or not you can name your condition, you may still be able to categorize your back problem according to the nature of your pain, the type of situation that may aggravate your pain, and the area of your back that hurts most.

Please don't feel at a disadvantage if you can't rattle off a bona fide medical term such as 'herniated disc' or 'scoliosis' that neatly pigeonholes your backache. Hardly anyone knows such things for certain. More than half the US survey respondents had received two or more different diagnoses from two or more practitioners. Most of these discrepancies represented major differences of opinion – not just variations in terminology.

The good news is that even if you never find out exactly what's wrong with your back, you can still get well. After all, you do know your own symptoms, and that knowledge will help you 'categorize' your own pain, so long as serious medical conditions have been ruled out as the cause of your pain.

Following is a list of what we have found to be the seven most common categories of back pain or causes of back pain (for obvious reasons, some of the names sound more specific than others):

- low back pain
- herniated (ruptured or 'slipped') and degenerative disc

- neck pain
- osteoarthritis
- sciatica
- scoliosis
- spondylolisthesis

You may be able to place yourself in one of the above categories, or you may feel that you belong in two or more of them. Indeed, if you have a herniated disc, you may well have sciatica as a result. Low back and neck pain are frequent companions. And osteoarthritis may superimpose itself on one or more existing back problems.

The rest of this chapter will look at these categories one by one, and offer specific exercise suggestions. According to the US survey results, for example, cycling turns out to be an excellent workout for people with scoliosis. If your back pain falls into more than one category, you'll find more than one section of this chapter of value.

Low Back Pain

Back pain is the UK's leading cause of disability, with 1.1 million people disabled by it. The majority of these people suffer from low back pain. Whether you have recently had an acute case of low back pain, or have a chronic painful condition, you can begin to address your needs with the Basic Preparation exercises outlined in Chapter 20. These will help you get back to normal activity.

The part of your exercise routine that brings you the most pleasure will probably be the stretching exercises. By easing the tendency to muscle spasm in your lower back, you will also be helping yourself prevent future pain and disability by faithfully performing your low back stretches.

As you recuperate, try to walk as much as you can. Although you may be tempted at first to spend a lot of time sitting, you'll no doubt find that sitting puts much more strain on your back than lying down or standing up. Keep walking. Try to walk at least 1.6 km (1 mile) a day. Other people may manage to include enough walking while doing their jobs, but this may not be enough to control your low back pain. You will really benefit from daily periods spent in brisk, mind-clearing, arm-swinging, uninterrupted walking.

Herniated (Ruptured or 'Slipped') and Degenerative Disc

Results from the US survey suggest that people with herniated discs need to be especially careful about exercise, since their rate of exercise-related injury is high. Among the US participants, 15 per cent of those who had disc problems incurred injury from exercise, while only 3 per cent of the participants with low back pain found exercise harmful. The point, however, is not to avoid back exercises, but to know which exercises to do and when to do them.

Some specialists and some exercise books offer dangerous exercise advice, such as telling individuals to stretch their hamstrings by bending over and touching their toes. This is a recipe for disaster. Double-leg raises should also be outlawed because of the pressure they put on the discs. The same is true for straight-leg sit-ups.

For you, building strength, especially in your abdominal muscles, takes priority over all stretching exercises. As general fitness exercises, nothing can beat walking and swimming. Try to pursue them both, beginning as soon as possible after your acute pain ebbs. This will help you beat the odds of remaining limited by disability.

The best professional treatment for chronic ruptured-disc pain, as revealed in the US survey, is individualized back-exercise therapy. If you have not been able to perform back exercises because of pain, don't give up yet. Please show the programme in this book to your doctor. It is probably sufficient to put you on the track towards health and well-being, but don't hesitate to seek the personal advice of a physiotherapist or other expert in exercise as rehabilitation.

Neck Pain

Although neck pain is often viewed as a back problem that just happened to land higher up on the spine, the causes and treatments differ substantially. According to the results of the US survey, neck pain was more likely than any other variety of back pain to benefit from chiropractic care.

The survey participants found that no single approach was sufficient to provide long-term help. Chronic neck pain sufferers who did away with disabling pain found the success lay in a combination of exercise, posture adjustment and stress reduction (often achieved through exercise).

Rarely does a person with neck pain require exercise instruction from a professional. Neck-saving manoeuvres can be learned in a matter of minutes. Unfortunately, many people with neck pain miss out on the benefits of exercise simply because they don't think to do it. They may see the value of exercising their arms and legs, but they seem to put their necks in a different category. The truth is, neck exercises offer proven help for pain and stiffness. I encourage you to incorporate the neck exercises outlined in Chapter 23 in your daily routine.

The objective of neck exercise is to promote relaxation, to stretch the neck muscles so as to make them more flexible, and to strengthen them. US survey participants found they tended to perform neck exercises more frequently when they were experiencing some discomfort. In other words, these particular movements seem to provide on-the-spot relief.

Osteoarthritis

Signs of osteoarthritis – pain and stiffness in the joints of the spine, bony growths or spurs that show up on X-rays – seem to multiply with age. Other forms of arthritis, however, including rheumatoid arthritis and ankylosing spondylitis, are found just as often among young adults as among older ones, and follow a completely different course.

Osteoarthritis is often called a 'wear and tear' condition because the cartilage that protects the ends of the bones flakes off, leaving rough edges that prevent the joints from functioning smoothly. One of the reasons that exercise figures so importantly in arthritis treatment is that it helps nourish the joints, to slow or reverse their destruction. Motion squeezes fluids in and out of the joint spaces, facilitating the delivery of nutrients to the cartilage, which has no blood supply of its own, and the removal of waste products.

Rest, which was long touted as the best treatment for arthritis of any kind, has proved to be a poor and even destructive substitute for activity.

Stretching exercises, which are often called 'range of motion' manoeuvres by arthritis specialists, actually preserve the motion of the various joints. Coupled with strengthening exercises, they help protect the joints from injury by building a strong support network in the surrounding muscles, tendons and ligaments. All the exercises in Chapters 24 and 25 are suitable for people with back pain resulting from osteoarthritis.

You may find that exercise improves your function even more than it relieves your pain, though it often serves both purposes equally well.

Walking and swimming were the two fitness exercises that gave the greatest help to US Back Pain Survey participants who suffered from osteoarthritis. (I also conducted a separate Arthritis Survey, to uncover useful information for people with osteoarthritis and rheumatoid arthritis – not solely in the back, but in all the joints of the body.)

Sciatica

Knife-like pain that runs along the sciatic nerve may be linked to disc problems, osteoarthritis, or other, perhaps unidentified, causes. Often compared to a bad toothache of the body, sciatica typically begins in the buttocks, near the spot where the sciatic nerve emerges from the spinal column, then courses through the thigh and calf, and on into the foot.

Participants in US survey who suffered from sciatica were often treated with medication and surgery, but the ones who fared best made progress through prescribed exercise taught to them by physiatrists, physiotherapists and, in some cases, chiropractors.

Some of the best movements for sciatica prove to be Pelvic Tilts (see pp. 359–60), mild stretches of the lower back, and a fitness concentration on swimming or walking. You should proceed with caution, since there can be a risk of exercise-related injury in sciatica.

The exercises in Chapter 22 make up the kind of safe-not-sorry programme that should give you meaningful improvement in a few months' time.

Scoliosis

Unlike other participants in the US survey, people with the spine curvature called scoliosis had better luck exercising without professional input. What's more, they fared better with fitness exercises than with the traditional stretching and strengthening movements. For example, a low back stretch may not achieve for you what it achieves for a person with low back pain. It may even be painful or awkward for you to lie flat on the floor in basic exercise positions, if your curvature makes one side of your back protrude beyond the other. And yet you can benefit enormously from exercises that keep you in motion – especially cycling, swimming and walking.

Participants with scoliosis had nothing but praise for yoga as an exercise technique. Practising yoga with an instructor who selected appropriate positions brought dramatic pain relief and a heightened sense of well-being.

The best scenario for people with scoliosis was to pursue, actively and regularly, a combination of two fitness activities, such as yoga and swimming.

I advise you to try the exercises in Chapters 22 and 23, as I feel they can do no harm. But the more important advice for you is contained in Chapter 24.

Spondylolisthesis

Many people have never even heard of this condition, which involves a forward or backward shift of one or more of the vertebrae, most often the lowest lumbar vertebra. The term 'slipped disc', as mentioned earlier, is a misnomer, as discs do not slip. Unfortunately, vertebrae *can* slip, causing great strain on the back muscles, as well as nerve compression and sciatica.

Only ten of the participants in the US survey had a diagnosis of spondylolisthesis. Seven of them attributed their improved functioning and their pain relief to exercise, and a few specifically mentioned yoga as the form of exercise they favoured. If you have spondylolisthesis, you can use the exercises in Chapter 22 to strengthen your abdominal muscles, as this is one of the most important remedies. Walking and swimming are the safest fitness activities to include in your regime.

Section 9
Mind-Body Work

Mental exercises that promote stress reduction and relaxation can complement any physical exercise programme.

Chapter 26
Yoga

With its traditional emphasis on the integration of spine, mind and spirit, yoga provides an excellent form of backache relief. In fact, the US survey revealed yoga instruction and practice to be among the most successful of all treatments for people who were not incapacitated by their back pain. And those participants who were troubled by osteoarthritis, neck pain and scoliosis found it particularly effective. (The UK survey results were not quite so positive, but 74 per cent of respondents still gained some degree of relief.)

The word yoga means 'unity' or 'harmony'. Yoga is a way of healing the body through exercises that combine postures, movements and breathing techniques.

To the extent that stretching and strengthening your body is helpful – and I believe this beyond a doubt – yoga instruction can be an excellent way to rid yourself of back pain. To the extent that stress contributes to back pain – and most of the survey participants felt that it did – yoga instruction can bring significant relief. The yoga philosophy of never forcing or straining, and of moving in a fluid, meditative manner, makes excellent sense for people with back problems. But yoga philosophy also encompasses the harmony of mind, body and spirit – a concept that is difficult for some back sufferers to grasp, or to take seriously. Although yoga traces its history back to the Hindu culture of India, it is not a religion.

This chapter explains the relative values of self-taught yoga, compared to attending yoga classes or seeking individual instruction. It also includes a step-by-step illustrated guide to modified yoga positions that are safe for people with back problems.

A few of the US survey participants learned yoga entirely on their own, from books and articles. But those who were helped the most got started with professional and personalized instruction. Not all yoga teachers have the experience or the desire to work effectively with people who report a history of back problems. Some of them, however, possess advanced degrees in exercise physiology and may be especially qualified to prescribe exercise. An important determinant of success is the instructor's willingness to modify the therapy to suit your needs.

If yoga instruction is available where you live, drop by the school or studio and speak to an instructor. You may get a chance to see the instructor in action, and determine whether you feel you'll get the kind of intelligent, individual attention that you were hoping to find.

Before I extol yoga any further, however, I must interject a note of caution: Many formal yoga positions are dangerous to attempt during any episode of pain. This is especially true for just-recovering back sufferers.

At least two regular yoga positions could actually cause considerable injury to your back if you tried to perform them while you were in pain, or before you had developed the necessary flexibility. One is the Cobra, which calls for you to lie on your stomach and arch your back by raising your head and chest. The other is the Plough, in which you lie on your back, then raise your straightened legs (ouch!) up and over your head, until you can touch your toes behind your head.

Here's one yoga exercise that you can perform anywhere, as it involves nothing more than deep breathing to help you relax and tone your abdominal muscles:

1. Start by taking a deep breath from your abdomen. (Put your fingers on your belly to convince yourself that it – and not just your chest – is expanding.)
2. Keep inhaling through your nose for 6 seconds.
3. Hold the air inside your lungs for 3 seconds.
4. Exhale through your mouth for 7 seconds. As you do so, let yourself go limp.
5. Repeat this series of steps a few times, alternating the deep breaths with normal breaths (in order to avoid the risk of hyperventilating). Five minutes spent in this kind of deep, relaxed breathing can make you feel both invigorated and relaxed. Try it during your peak work hours, and judge the effect for yourself.

The following series of yoga postures constitutes a safe taste of this form of exercise – provided that you are not in pain when you attempt them. Any or all of these can be combined with the stretching and strengthening exercises in Chapters 22 and 23 to individualize or vary your daily regime.

You may find that you want to attempt the Total Body Relaxation exercise (below) twice a day, for the sheer stress relief it brings. As for the other exercises in this section, I suggest that you begin with three repetitions of each. Once you are comfortable with that number, you can increase it by one repetition every other day until you are performing a total of ten repetitions.

Total Body Relaxation
It may well take you several minutes to spread the feeling of relaxation throughout your body. There's no need to rush. Just enjoy the sensation of willing your body to relax. It will convince you that you can gain control over physical pain, as well as anxiety, stress and fear.

Starting position: Lie on your back with a pillow under your knees, legs slightly apart, and arms at your sides.

Steps:
1. Let your body go limp, so that your neck, arms and legs shift naturally into their most comfortable positions.
2. Think about relaxing your muscles, starting with your feet, ankles and legs.
3. Concentrate on making the individual muscles and joints relax, working your way up your body to your neck and head.

Note: It may help you to tense some of your muscles slightly, before releasing and relaxing them. For example, first make a fist, and then let your hand go limp. Some people find that doing this exercise in the dark is so relaxing that it actually helps them fall asleep!

Sitting Stretch
Reaching over in this sitting posture, you will feel the stretch in your spine all the way down to your coccyx and sitting

bones – and on into the hamstring muscles at the backs of your thighs. Please be careful not to push too far.

Note: This exercise could aggravate symptoms in someone who gets pain on forward bending or sitting. It is definitely not for anyone in any sort of back pain. I cautioned you against this kind of movement in the note with the Hamstring Stretch in Chapter 22. However, you might add it to your regime after you have progressed beyond the pain-free stage and feel ready for more advanced stretching.

Starting position: Sit on the floor with your legs fully extended in front of you, your ankles touching each other. *a*

Steps:
1. Raise your arms in front of you to about shoulder height. *b*
2. Slowly lean your upper body as far forward as you can (*c*), while simultaneously lowering your hands to your knees. *d*
3. When you feel resistance, stop and hold the position for a count of ten.
4. Return to the starting position.
   (See p. 418 for position *d*.)

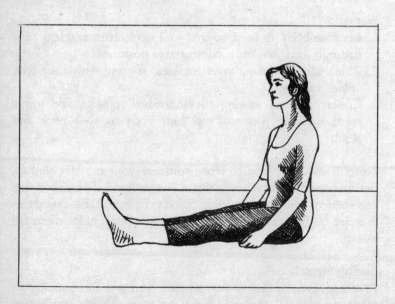

a

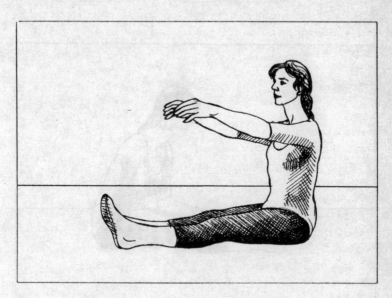

b

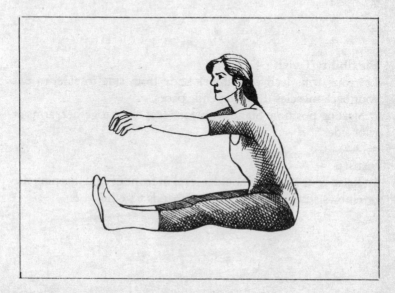

c

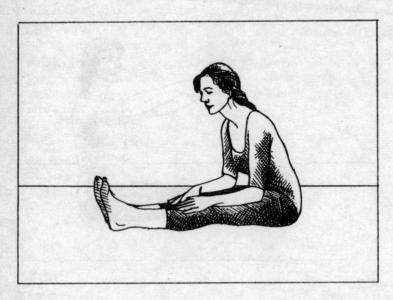

d

Flexibility Twist
Let your arms lead your upper body from side to side, to put
your back muscles through gentle paces.

Starting position: Stand with your feet close together, arms at
your sides. *a*

Steps:
1. Raise your arms to shoulder level in front of you, keeping the
   elbows straight, and touch your hands together. *b*

2. Slowly turn your upper body to the left. *c*
3. When you meet resistance, hold the stretch for 10 seconds. (If you find it hard to keep your balance as you twist your upper body with your feet close together, widen your stance a bit.)
4. Return to the starting position, dropping your arms and relaxing for a few seconds.
5. Repeat steps 1–4, turning to the right this time. *d*

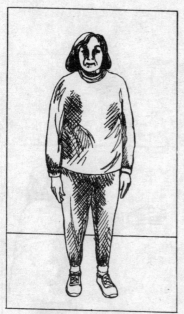

a

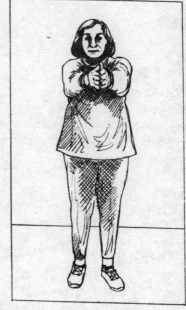

b

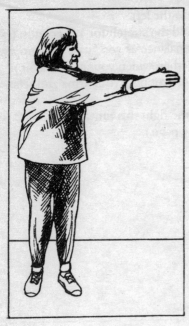

c

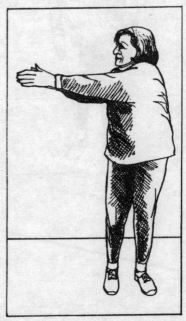

d

Modified Locust

A strategically placed pillow under your abdomen keeps you from arching your back as you raise your legs in this modified locust position.

Note: This exercise may not be suitable for people with cervical spine pain due to the rotation of the neck that is required.

Starting position: Lie face down, arms at your sides, with a pillow tucked under your abdomen for lower back support.

Steps:
1. Keeping your knee locked, raise your left leg about 30 cm (12 inches) off the floor. *a*
2. Hold your leg in this position for a count of six.
   (Turn over the page to see Steps 3–4.)

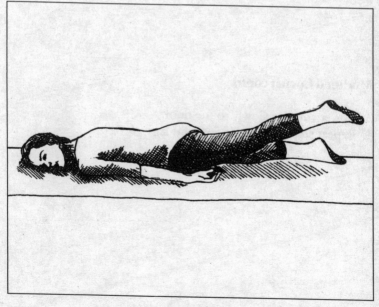

a

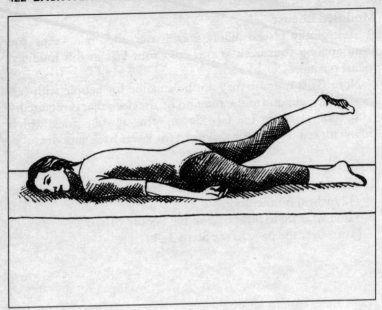

b

Modified Locust contd.

3. Lower your leg slowly to the floor.
4. Repeat steps 1–3 with your right leg. *b*

Chapter 27
Meditation, Imagery and More

Although stress doesn't necessarily cause back pain, there is no doubt that severe back pain causes stress. And stress, in turn, can readily magnify the pain you feel.

Certain kinds of back pain, according to reports from US survey participants, seem more susceptible to aggravation by stress than others. Neck pain, for example, tends to worsen noticeably in times of increased stress. More than 80 per cent of survey participants who suffered from neck pain said their pain grew worse whenever they were under a lot of stress. A possible explanation is that stress and tension make you hunch or stiffen your shoulders, and this strain makes itself felt in the muscles of the neck.

If you have been doing the rounds, seeing different practitioners over a long period of time, you may have heard the term 'stress' used as though it were a diagnosis. When no obvious cause can be found for your pain, someone is bound to suggest that you are suffering from stress. Implicit in this suggestion are several negative messages, including the following:

'There's nothing really wrong with you.'

'You've let stress get the upper hand in your life, and now you're paying the price.'

'I can't do anything to help you.'

If stress is an element in your pain cycle, you deserve some sympathy, not blame. Doctors who understand the connection between pain and stress can help their patients greatly by explaining it – and by encouraging them to learn a few simple stress-reduction techniques that can serve as pain-blockers.

By 'stress reduction' I mean reducing the negative effects of stress – the sensation that your heart is racing away, the knots in your stomach, the rapid breathing, the rising panic, the feeling of spasm in your back or neck. Whether or not you can actually reduce the stress in your life is another matter entirely. The most stressful events or situations may simply be beyond your power to control. Nevertheless, if you can control your reactions to them, you will have accomplished a great deal.

Stress-reduction techniques – including deep breathing, visualization and meditation – can be of great use in helping you feel calmer, reducing your pain, and preparing you for exercise. This chapter explains how to practise a few stress-reduction techniques to best advantage. Think of them as mental exercises, easy and pleasant to perform.

The truth is, any technique that provides a break from stressful activities may turn out to help your back. Even something as simple as taking a 'stretch break' every hour on the hour can be of tremendous benefit. Although I urge you to experiment with the strategies such as deep breathing, meditation, visualization (or imagery) and progressive relaxation, I know of many people who can get their stress and pain levels down by simply taking a walk for 20 minutes.

The US survey participants, as a group, came up with no clear consensus on a favourite method, but individuals expressed strong preferences. Many suppliers of relaxation tapes and stress-reduction gadgets may try to convince you that their approach is the best, but you are the best judge of what technique appeals to you most, and therefore what is most likely to work for you.

Practitioners of yoga know that deep breathing has tremendous powers of relaxation. Just as smiling can sometimes lift your spirits, breathing slowly and deeply can make your whole body feel calmer. Deep breathing figures in virtually every stress-reduction technique, so let's begin with this basic approach.

Deep Breathing

Ordinarily, you don't have to think about breathing. Your body does it automatically. But when the automatic response is panting in response to some stress perceived as a threat, you can make yourself feel better by taking conscious control of the breathing process. Try it. Inhale through your nose for 6 seconds; hold your breath for 1 second; exhale through your mouth for 7 seconds.

Keep your eyes closed. Do you feel yourself getting a bit more relaxed with each exhalation?

Try to become conscious of the breath filling and leaving your lungs. Let your chest expand fully. Relax your shoulders as you inhale, since raising your shoulders does not help to fill the lungs with air. Concentrate instead on widening the girth of your chest, as though it were a balloon being inflated. Put your hand on your abdomen, to feel how it, too, is expanding, as your diaphragm drops down to increase the influx of air into your body.

Stay relaxed as you hold the air in for just a moment or two, and then slowly begin to let it out through your mouth. Exhale so fully that you actually squeeze the air out of your lungs by contracting your chest. Then picture physical tension leaving your body with the expelled breath.

Once you become accustomed to deep breathing, knowing that you can rely on it as an instant aid to relaxation, you may find that you use it periodically throughout the day, any time something unpleasant jars you. You may also use deep breathing at night as a way to relax before falling asleep, and again in the morning, to prepare yourself to meet the day.

Note: Breathing deeply for an extended period can lead to hyperventilation. Remember to alternate deep breathing with regular breathing to avoid this.

Meditation

Heart specialists, such as Dr Herbert Benson of Harvard Medical School, have made meditation a medical treatment. Back sufferers benefit from its stress-reducing effects, too. It was Dr Benson who gave the name 'relaxation response' to the altered state of well-being brought on by meditation. The relaxation response is a physiological state of deep rest while wide awake. It is said to be even more restful and restorative than sleep, because the profound relaxation leaves a lingering sense of calm refreshment. Indeed, a 20-minute period of meditation may exert a positive effect on an entire day.

Many approaches to meditation can be used to good advantage, but I particularly like Dr Benson's approach. The basic outline here is drawn from his book called *Your Maximum Mind*:

- Choose a word or a phrase that will serve as your focus for the meditation exercise. You may choose a pleasant thought, such as 'peace' or the opening words of a prayer, or even a soothing sound that has no particular meaning.
- Sit in a comfortable position. Close your eyes. Relax your muscles.
- Breathe deeply and, with each exhalation, repeat to yourself your focus word or phrase.
- Also use the repetition of your focus word to push away worries or extraneous thoughts that may come into your mind while you are meditating.
- Continue your focused breathing and repetition for 10 to 20 minutes.

It sounds awfully simple, doesn't it? But please don't let the simplicity fool you into thinking that there's nothing much to it. Practice brings total concentration, and total concentration breeds relaxation that works to reduce stress and improve the quality of your life.

If possible, choose a special place for meditation. You might even keep a few items there – photos or memorabilia – that evoke positive feelings. Also try to choose a special time of day when you are least likely to be interrupted. Avoid distractions by taking your phone off the hook, or by asking family and friends not to call you at this time.

Visualization (Imagery)

The power of positive thinking makes it possible for you to soothe yourself with beautiful images that you conjure up and elaborate upon in your mind. These could be landscapes, works of art or wonderful moments in your life. The idea of visualization is to create a safe haven in your mind where you can go to escape from pain or anxiety.

If this sounds far-fetched, try to remember a time when you had the opposite experience – when thinking of a sad event left you feeling depressed, or when planning what you would say in an argument got you so worked up you could barely sit still. The brain and body seem to make little distinction between actual images and imagined ones. This is why you can create the sensation of peaceful relaxation by picturing an idyllic scene where you lie on warm sand, smelling the salt air of the ocean, and hearing the waves pounding on the shore.

Another positive image is to picture a soft glove or gentle hand touching the painful areas of your body with warmth and healing power.

Progressive Relaxation

Relaxing your body, one small part at a time, gets you progressively relaxed until you reach the critical threshold where stress-reduction occurs.

Progressive Relaxation resembles the Total Body Relaxation described in Chapter 26. The idea here is to get relaxed by first tensing the muscles and then releasing them, proceeding in an orderly fashion from one end of the body to the other. It doesn't really matter whether you go from head to toe or begin at your feet and work up.

Here is a plan of action:

* Lie in a comfortable position. Close your eyes.
* Move your body, wriggling your arms and legs, just to settle yourself comfortably.
* Lie still and breathe deeply for a few minutes.
* If you are starting from your head, make some very exaggerated movements with your face – sneer, grin, frown, yawn, raise your eyebrows and then knit them together in a scowl. Then let your face relax.
* Tense your neck by pushing your head down into the floor, then relax.
* One at a time, tighten each arm and raise it, then let it go limp at your side.
* Clench each fist, then let your hands relax.
* Tighten your abdomen and your buttocks, and let them go.
* Spread tension along the length of one leg by straightening the knee and lifting the leg slightly. Then relax that leg and let it slump back into place. Do the same with your other leg.
* Point your toes and arch your foot as sharply as you can, then let it flop free. Do the same with your other foot.
* Lie still and breathe deeply.

You may find that you want to experiment with the different approaches, or mix and match them. What's to stop you, for example, from using a favourite image as your meditation focus?

As you become adept at incorporating these stress-reduction techniques into your daily routines, people may ask you why you're smiling.

Conclusion: Enjoying Life

As you stretch and strengthen your back with the helpful exercises you've learned, you will grow increasingly flexible and resistant to future back injury. This is a great gift that you are giving yourself – one that will enable you to enjoy life more fully.

When I reviewed the comments of survey participants who had overcome the distress and disability that so often results from chronic back pain, I noticed another 'gift' of theirs. It was nothing as tangible as an exercise programme or a set of strategies for completing chores. It was their attitude.

They had promised themselves that they would get well. They had made up their minds to put an end to back pain. And they had put themselves in charge of that task, giving it top priority in their lives. They had stopped asking 'Why me?' They had come to accept their back problem, and that acceptance was the key to finding a solution.

Realizing that they knew more about their own bodies than anyone else possibly could, they listened to the experts without awe. They sought professional care when they needed to, but they did not expect any practitioner to have 'the answer' or to 'cure' them. They acted as partners in their treatment. Even though they were suffering, they did not see themselves as helpless victims waiting to be rescued by someone else.

Exercise can help you develop this attitude of mastery. Exercise is a powerful, effective treatment that you dispense to yourself on a daily basis. In a relatively short time, you can see it working as promised, building your body and your confidence at the same time.

Equally importantly, you need to prioritize your health and well-being, at home and at work, by adopting 'back-friendly' ways of carrying out everyday tasks and activities. Chapters 13 and 14 contain valuable advice on everything from mattresses and chairs to cleaning and gardening. Consult these chapters frequently and ensure that your daily activities are helpful, rather than harmful, for your back.

As you improve your ability to enjoy life by treating your body with exercise and 'back-friendly' ways of living, you will be disproving some long-standing myths about back pain. Maybe you've heard some of these myths, or believed in them yourself:

- *Back pain is inevitable. It's just the price we pay for walking upright.* Pain is not the natural condition of the body. If anything, back pain results from not walking upright enough. Although back pain is extremely common in the USA, where it affects an estimated 80 per cent of all adults, statistics from other countries indicate a much lower incidence. Back pain, therefore, is not an essential part of the human condition, but a reflection of lifestyle trends. Many people in the UK and the USA have adopted an excessively sedentary lifestyle. But that can be changed at will. Exercise, coupled with attention to posture and care in performing daily tasks, will convince your body that there is nothing inevitable about back pain.
- *Back pain is a normal aspect of aging.* Again, pain is neither natural nor normal. Aging does not hurt, unless it is accompanied by illness or neglect of one's health. Analyses of medical records show that back pain is not correlated with advanced age. In fact, the reverse is true: The vast majority of backache sufferers are younger than 45. As you grow older, treating your body well, you have every reason to expect that your back pain will continue to diminish until it disappears altogether.
- *There's nothing really wrong with you.* Even if nothing shows up on the X-rays or other diagnostic tests, even if the doctor cannot imagine why you are in pain, there is something wrong with you if you are in pain.
- *Any exercise programme will help banish back pain.* This is only half true. You know, if you've tried exercise before, that not all routines work for all people. Some non-injurious exercise is better than no exercise, but an individually prescribed programme, or the tailored programme you have now assembled from the ingredients offered here, can do much more for you than an 'off-the-hook' exercise regime. (Indeed, I remind you

that strenuous, arching forms of exercise can aggravate back pain.)

* *Back practitioners routinely offer exercise advice, but back sufferers are too lazy to follow it.* You know from your own experience just how much exercise advice you were offered. Maybe it was an encouraging word, with a few specific suggestions, but more likely you came to the exercise conclusion yourself. You've turned to this book for detailed instructions about assembling and implementing an exercise programme. And now you're going to stick to that programme because you want to improve your own condition. You are taking action, and you will succeed.

Many of the survey participants expressed the opinion that their *approach* to back exercise – and by that they meant their attitude and preparation for exercise – was at least as important as the mechanical components of the exercise therapy itself. Here are some points to remember as you implement your exercise programme over the coming weeks:

* Exercise therapy is more beneficial for your back than anything you can put into or on to your body.
* Although your exercise movements may be slow and gradual now, they will result in dramatic improvements over time. You can expect small but noticeable gains within a few weeks.
* If exercise is something you've never looked forward to before, open your mind to enjoying it now. The time you spend exercising truly is quality time.

As you become used to exercising, you may wonder how you ever got along without it. When you miss a few days of walking or swimming or cycling, you'll miss the relaxation and clear thinking that those activities convey. You'll miss the reassuring physical sensation of tiredness followed by renewed energy. These are the positive additions to your life that exercise has brought. You will be eager to get back to exercising to experience again these pleasant feelings. Exercise, which you once may have viewed as a duty, is now a delight for you – an indulgence of body and mind that you enjoy thoroughly.

To add to your enjoyment of exercise and your new feeling of vitality, try some of the following physical rewards as treats for your body:

- *Massage*. Like exercise, massage offers you another drug-free muscle relaxant that will help your muscles unwind. You can perform self-massage on some areas of your body, but you will probably get the most pleasure out of a full-body massage from a professional – or even from a willing partner. You may need to tell your inexperienced masseur to use a light oil and a fairly light touch, so as to avoid putting too much pressure on your lower back. Also tell your partner to concentrate on your legs, back and neck, massaging towards the heart, and using either a long, gliding motion with the palms, or a circular motion with the fingertips and palms.
- *Good food*. Feeding your body well is part of pampering yourself. Try to eat more fruit, vegetables and wholegrains, and to cut down on junk foods, processed foods, fats, caffeine, sugar and alcohol. Also, avoid constipation (a real hardship for back sufferers) by drinking enough water and including generous portions of fibre in your diet. You may notice a positive change in the appearance of your body, brought on by your commitment to exercise and good posture. Taking care to eat only good foods will help you keep your weight in the ideal range for your height, so that you look even better.
- *Sleep*. Promise yourself the amount of sleep you need to feel comfortable and to maintain good spirits and good posture throughout the day. Try not to think of time spent sleeping as lost or wasted. It isn't. It's crucial time spent restoring your mental and physical energy.
- *Hydrotherapy*. Turn your bath into a relaxing hydrotherapy centre where you can enjoy luxurious warm baths. You may want to purchase a waterproof pillow or a mat that covers the full length of your bath. A less expensive alternative is to pad the bath bottom with a thick bath mat, and roll a towel into a neck support or a lumbar support. Survey participants consider 20 minutes the ideal length for a bath, as longer can make you feel tired. They also prefer warm water to hot, since very hot water can sometimes put muscles in spasm. Experiment to

find the most comfortable position. A safe one is to lean your back against one end of the bath, and bend your knees so you can keep your feet flat on the bottom of the bath. If you feel stiff after maintaining one position for several minutes, prop your feet on the sides of the bath for a change. You can even execute a few exercises in the bath, such as Shoulder Shrugs (see p. 387) and Knee-to-Chest stretches (see pp. 342–4).

• *Join a health club.* Although you can perform all your exercises perfectly well at home, you may still benefit from joining a local health club. If, for example, the club has a swimming pool and a whirlpool or jacuzzi that you can use, these facilities may be worth the price of membership. You can take advantage of the swimming pool for aerobic fitness, and the whirlpool for relaxation and stress reduction. Membership of a health club also puts you in touch with other people who are trying to keep their bodies in the best possible shape, just as you are.

You are about to join the ranks of back sufferers who have endured the pain and managed to get past it. You have decided what you need to do to get well, and you are putting that plan into effect right now.

I salute you in your efforts.

About the Research

The US survey

The individuals in the US Backache Survey volunteered to participate by responding to public notices and advertisements in the following publications: *American Business, Columbia Journalism Review, East-West, Family Weekly, In These Times, Moneysworth, Mother Jones, New Era, New York Magazine, The New York Times, Prevention* and *Saturday Review.* In addition, some participants referred me to other back pain sufferers, who became participants.

Ninety-three of the total 492 participants responded by telephone. Each of these was interviewed for an average of 55 minutes. The remaining participants inquired by mail and were sent a questionnaire. When I received a completed questionnaire, I followed up by telephone whenever necessary to expand or clarify a particular point of information.

Nearly 40 per cent of individuals surveyed were readers of *Family Weekly.* This magazine is distributed in more than 200 medium-sized American cities, and the demographics of its readers closely match those of the general public.

Survey participants represent every stratum of American society, from the wealthy and famous to those who can no longer afford medical treatment. The youngest participant was a 10-year-old girl whose mother helped her fill in the questionnaire. The oldest participant was a 90-year-old woman who had just encountered back pain for the first time and who rid herself of her pain by taking her doctor's advice to walk 1.6 km (1 mile) every day.

At least 55 per cent of the participants were female and 44 per cent were male; 1 per cent chose not to answer the question about sex. The vast majority of individuals were under the age of 50. Persons 18 and younger constituted 1 per cent of the sample; 19 to 29, 28 per cent; 30 to 49, 44 per cent; 50 to 64, 18 per cent; and 65 and older, 7 per cent. These findings concur with available research about the sex and age of back sufferers.

All participants, whether orally or in writing, answered questions contained in a two-page questionnaire. Topics included types of practitioners seen, diagnosis from each practitioner, treatments and advice received, evaluation of each practitioner and treatment, exercise (frequency and source of instruction), emotional stress (its role in back pain and the practitioner's approach to it), tips for back sufferers, and personal data (optional).

Two years passed from the time the first public notice appeared until the results of this survey were tabulated. When the number of participants reached 100, significant trends were already apparent for the most widely seen practitioners – orthopaedic surgeons, chiropractors, general practitioners, physiotherapists and osteopaths. At 200, the reasons behind these trends were clear, and more than twenty-five different kinds of healthcare specialists and thirty-five different kinds of treatments had been reported. However, these could not be adequately evaluated. At 400, I had enough data to appraise virtually every kind of practitioner and treatment available to back pain sufferers.

Why, then, was the final count 492? Because the author had a whim to have participants from every one of the fifty US states.

So, thank you Laura L. of Alaska for allowing me to conclude this research on a happy note.

The UK survey

A total of 2,240 back pain sufferers responded to the UK web-based survey, run by BackCare (registered as the National Back Pain Association), an independent national charity that helps people manage and prevent back pain by providing information, promoting self-help, encouraging debate and funding research into better back health. All the quotations from the UK survey are genuine but in order to preserve the anonymity of our respondents, we have changed people's names. Survey respondents answered the following questions online:

Dear Survey Participant,
Thank you for deciding to take part in the National Back Pain Survey conducted by BackCare in association with Constable and Robinson Publishers.

We will use the information you provide to write a book called *Back Pain: What Really Works*, which is due to be published by Constable and Robinson in February 2006. We ask you to tell us your experiences, opinions about the treatments you have tried and your own tips on how to live with back pain.

Please complete this survey whether you are still suffering from back pain or whether you have now recovered, as all feedback is important to us.

We will treat your personal information with respect and keep it confidential. Your name will not be used in the book or put on any kind of mailing list.

As a token of our thanks for the time you spend completing the form, Constable and Robinson will send a copy of the book FREE to the first 500 people who complete the survey.

Please note that the survey should take between 10 and 15 minutes to complete.

Please answer the questions below:

1. Please tick which of the following describes your back pain: (Please tick any that apply)

   First episode of severe low back pain which came on suddenly and recently
   First episode of mild low back pain which came on suddenly and recently
   Repeat episode of severe low back pain which came on suddenly and recently
   Repeat episode of mild low back pain which came on suddenly and recently
   Long-term low back pain, all the time
   Long-term low back pain, comes and goes
   Pain in legs caused by back (sciatica)
   Pain has gone

Don't know

Other (please state)

....

2. Do you have a medical diagnosis for the cause of your back pain?

(Please tick any that apply)

Ankylosing spondylitis

Arachnoiditis

Arthritis – Osteoarthritis

Arthritis – Rheumatoid arthritis

Fracture

Muscle strain

Osteoporosis (thinning of the bones)

Ruptured/prolapsed/slipped disc

Scoliosis

Spinal Stenosis

Spondylolisthesis

Don't know

Other back diagnosis (please state)

....

3. How long have you suffered from back pain? (Please choose only one option)

One month or less

Between one month and one year

Between one year and five years

Between five years and ten years

Between ten years and fifteen years

Between fifteen years and twenty years

More than twenty years

4. On a scale of 0 to 10, where 0 means pain-free and 10 means intense pain that prevents you from doing anything, please circle the number that describes your condition today. (Please choose only one option)

0   1   2   3   4   5   6   7   8   9   10

5. Which (if any) of the following do you think caused your back pain?
(Please tick any that apply):

Random bad luck
A bone or joint out of place
Wear and tear
Specific medical condition (e.g. Arthritis)
Family history of back trouble
Ageing
Generally unfit
Sudden accident or injury
Longstanding bad posture
Being overweight
Bad lifting technique
Bad sitting posture
Bed that is too hard
Bed that is too soft
Getting out of bed
Getting out of a chair
Picking up something from the floor
Sudden movements (e.g. coughing)
Too much driving
Too much gardening
Too much sport
Stress
Depression
Anxiety
Don't know

6a. Please choose from the practitioners listed below those who have treated you for your back pain. (Please tick any that apply)

Acupuncturist
Alexander Technique Teacher
Aromatherapist
Chiropractor
Dance Instructor

Exercise Trainer
Faith Healer
Feldenkrais Therapist
General Practitioner/GP
Herbalist
Homeopath
Hypnotherapist
Kinesiologist
Massage Therapist
Psychotherapist/Counsellor
Naturopath
Neurologist
Neurosurgeon
Nurse
Nutritionist/Dietician
Obstetrician/Gynaecologist
Occupational Therapist
Orthopaedic Surgeon
Osteopath
Pain Clinic Doctor
Pharmacist
Physiotherapist
Podiatrist/Chiropodist
Reflexologist
Rheumatologist
Rolfer
Shiatsu Therapist
Spinal Surgeon
Sports Medicine Professional
Tai Chi Instructor
Yoga Instructor
Other
....

6b. Now please rate each practitioner using the following scale
(please circle the relevant number).

1 for those practitioners who gave you a great deal of help
that lasted 6 months or more

2 for those practitioners who gave you a little help that lasted 6 months or more

3 for those who gave you only temporary relief

4 for those who didn't help at all

5 for those who made you feel worse

6 for those practitioners you have no experience of

Acupuncturist	1	2	3	4	5	6
Alexander Technique Teacher	1	2	3	4	5	6
Aromatherapist	1	2	3	4	5	6
Chiropractor	1	2	3	4	5	6
Dance Instructor	1	2	3	4	5	6
Exercise Trainer	1	2	3	4	5	6
Faith Healer	1	2	3	4	5	6
Feldenkrais Therapist	1	2	3	4	5	6
General Practitioner/GP	1	2	3	4	5	6
Herbalist	1	2	3	4	5	6
Homeopath	1	2	3	4	5	6
Hypnotherapist	1	2	3	4	5	6
Kinesiologist	1	2	3	4	5	6
Massage Therapist	1	2	3	4	5	6
Naturopath	1	2	3	4	5	6
Neurologist	1	2	3	4	5	6
Neurosurgeon	1	2	3	4	5	6
Nurse	1	2	3	4	5	6
Nutritionist/Dietician	1	2	3	4	5	6
Obstetrician/Gynaecologist	1	2	3	4	5	6
Occupational Therapist	1	2	3	4	5	6
Orthopaedic Surgeon	1	2	3	4	5	6
Osteopath	1	2	3	4	5	6
Pain Clinic Doctor	1	2	3	4	5	6
Pharmacist	1	2	3	4	5	6
Physiotherapist	1	2	3	4	5	6
Podiatrist/chiropodist	1	2	3	4	5	6
Psychotherapist/counsellor	1	2	3	4	5	6
Reflexologist	1	2	3	4	5	6
Rheumatologist	1	2	3	4	5	6
Rolfer	1	2	3	4	5	6
Shiatsu Therapist	1	2	3	4	5	6

Spinal Surgeon	1	2	3	4	5	6
Sports Medicine Professional	1	2	3	4	5	6
Tai Chi Instructor	1	2	3	4	5	6
Yoga Instructor	1	2	3	4	5	6
Other	1	2	3	4	5	6

7a. Do you take prescription drugs or medications for your back pain?

Yes   No

If the answer was YES please tick below any that you take.
(Please tick any that apply)

Antidepressants
Analgesics (painkillers)
Anti-inflammatories
Muscle relaxants/tranquillizers
Other

7b. Do you take non-prescription (over-the-counter) drugs or medications for your back pain?

Yes   No

If the answer was YES please tick below any that you take.
(Please tick any that apply)

Analgesics (painkillers)
Anti-inflammatories
Devil's claw
Glucosamine
Herbal remedies
Homeopathic remedies
Other

7c. Now please rate each drug using the following scale (please circle the relevant number).

1 for those drugs which gave you a great deal of help that lasted 6 months or more
2 for those drugs which gave you a little help that lasted 6 months or more
3 for those drugs which gave you only temporary relief
4 for those drugs which didn't help at all
5 for those drugs which made you feel worse
6 for drugs which you have no experience of

Prescription drugs:

Antidepressants	1	2	3	4	5	6
Analgesics (painkillers)	1	2	3	4	5	6
Anti-inflammatories	1	2	3	4	5	6
Muscle relaxants/tranquillizers	1	2	3	4	5	6

Non-prescription (over-the-counter) drugs:

Analgesics (painkillers)	1	2	3	4	5	6
Anti-inflammatories	1	2	3	4	5	6
Devil's claw	1	2	3	4	5	6
Glucosamine	1	2	3	4	5	6
Herbal remedies	1	2	3	4	5	6
Homeopathic remedies	1	2	3	4	5	6
Other	1	2	3	4	5	6

7d. Have you ever been prescribed medicine for back pain which you have not subsequently taken?

Yes   No

If the answer above is YES, please tick below any that you have been prescribed, but not taken. (Please tick any that apply)

Antidepressants
Analgesics (painkillers)
Anti-inflammatories
Muscle relaxants/tranquillizers
Other

7e. If the answer above was YES, why did you not take it? (Please tick any that apply)

You didn't receive any explanation, from your health professional, of how you should take your medicine, so that it would be most effective

Your back pain stopped before you started taking your medicine

You forgot to take it

You didn't receive any explanation, from your health professional, on how the medicine would help

You don't like taking medicines

Other reason you did not take the drugs (please state)

....

7f. Did you receive any explanation, from your health professional, of how you should take your medicine, so that it would be most effective?

Yes   No

8a. Please tick any of the treatments, listed below, which you have tried for your back pain. (Please tick any that apply)

Acupuncture
Alexander Technique
Aromatherapy
Back exercises
Braces and corsets
Biofeedback
Chymopapain injections
Cold therapy (ice)
Cortisone injections
Counselling
Cycling
Dance
Disc surgery
Epidural
Feldenkrais therapy
Foot orthotics (shoe inserts, lifts, arch supports)
Gravity inversion
Gymnastic ball

Gym circuit
Heat therapy
Hydrotherapy
Implants
Kinesiology
Manipulation (e.g. by chiropractor, osteopath, physiotherapist or GP)
Marijuana
Massage
Meditation
Muscle relaxant injections
Nerve block
Nutrition and vitamins
Physical therapy (e.g. mobilizations, exercises & advice)
Pilates
Reflexology
Relaxation
Rolfing
Sclerotherapy injections
Self-help stress reduction
Swimming
Tai Chi
TENS (Transcutaneous Electrical Nerve Stimulation)
Traction
Trigger point injections
Ultrasound therapy
Walking
Yoga
Other

....

8b. Now please rate each treatment using the following scale (please circle the relevant number).

1 for those treatments which gave you a great deal of help that lasted 6 months or more

2 for those treatments which gave you a little help that lasted 6 months or more

3 for those treatments which gave you only temporary relief
4 for those treatments which didn't help at all
5 for those treatments which made you feel worse
6 for those treatments you have no experience of

Acupuncture	1	2	3	4	5	6
Alexander Technique	1	2	3	4	5	6
Aromatherapy	1	2	3	4	5	6
Back exercises	1	2	3	4	5	6
Braces and corsets	1	2	3	4	5	6
Bio-feedback	1	2	3	4	5	6
Chymopapain injections	1	2	3	4	5	6
Cold therapy (ice)	1	2	3	4	5	6
Cortisone injections	1	2	3	4	5	6
Counselling	1	2	3	4	5	6
Cycling	1	2	3	4	5	6
Dance	1	2	3	4	5	6
Disc surgery	1	2	3	4	5	6
Epidural	1	2	3	4	5	6
Feldenkrais therapy	1	2	3	4	5	6
Foot orthotics (shoe inserts, lifts, arch supports)	1	2	3	4	5	6
Gravity inversion	1	2	3	4	5	6
Gymnastic ball	1	2	3	4	5	6
Gym circuit	1	2	3	4	5	6
Heat therapy	1	2	3	4	5	6
Hydrotherapy	1	2	3	4	5	6
Implants	1	2	3	4	5	6
Kinesiology	1	2	3	4	5	6
Manipulation (e.g. by chiropractor, osteopath, physiotherapist or GP)	1	2	3	4	5	6
Marijuana	1	2	3	4	5	6
Massage	1	2	3	4	5	6
Meditation	1	2	3	4	5	6
Muscle relaxant injections	1	2	3	4	5	6
Nerve block	1	2	3	4	5	6
Nutrition and vitamins	1	2	3	4	5	6
Physical therapy (e.g. mobilizations, exercises & advice)	1	2	3	4	5	6

Pilates	1	2	3	4	5	6
Reflexology	1	2	3	4	5	6
Relaxation	1	2	3	4	5	6
Rolfing	1	2	3	4	5	6
Sclerotherapy injections	1	2	3	4	5	6
Self-help stress reduction	1	2	3	4	5	6
Swimming	1	2	3	4	5	6
Tai Chi	1	2	3	4	5	6
TENS (Transcutaneous Electrical Nerve Stimulation)	1	2	3	4	5	6
Traction	1	2	3	4	5	6
Trigger point injections	1	2	3	4	5	6
Ultrasound therapy	1	2	3	4	5	6
Walking	1	2	3	4	5	6
Yoga	1	2	3	4	5	6
Other	1	2	3	4	5	6

9a. Please tick which of the following forms of self-help you have tried to relieve back pain (Please tick any that apply)

Sleeping on your side with a pillow between your knees
Using a bed board
Using a water bed
Using a special mattress
Using special pillows
Using special seating
Using a lumbar roll
Using a seat insert
Using a corset/body belt
Using massage/vibrating cushions
Taking a hot bath/shower
Applying heat packs/moist heat
Using a hot water bottle
Using a heat pad
Applying cold packs
Stopping/reducing smoking
Losing weight
Other (please
state)...

At the end of the survey, you will have the opportunity to tell us any advice that you might give to another back pain sufferer.

9b. Now please rate each form of self-help using the following scale (please circle the relevant number).

1 for those forms of self-help which gave you a great deal of help that lasted 6 months or more

2 for those forms of self-help which gave you a little help that lasted 6 months or more

3 for those forms that gave you only temporary relief

4 for those forms that didn't help at all

5 for those forms which made you feel worse

6 for those forms of self-help you have no experience of

Sleeping on your side with a pillow between your knees	1	2	3	4	5	6
Using a bed board	1	2	3	4	5	6
Using a water bed	1	2	3	4	5	6
Using a special mattress	1	2	3	4	5	6
Using special pillows	1	2	3	4	5	6
Using special seating	1	2	3	4	5	6
Using a lumbar roll	1	2	3	4	5	6
Using a seat insert	1	2	3	4	5	6
Using a corset/body belt	1	2	3	4	5	6
Using massage/vibrating cushions	1	2	3	4	5	6
Taking a hot bath/shower	1	2	3	4	5	6
Applying heat packs/moist heat	1	2	3	4	5	6
Using a hot water bottle	1	2	3	4	5	6
Using a heat pad	1	2	3	4	5	6
Applying cold packs	1	2	3	4	5	6
Stopping/reducing smoking	1	2	3	4	5	6
Losing weight	1	2	3	4	5	6
Other	1	2	3	4	5	6

10a. Are you currently at work in paid employment or self employed?

Yes   No

10b. If you are NOT working, was your back pain the cause of your stopping work?

Yes   No

10c. If you work, do you believe that working makes you feel: (Please tick only one option)

A lot better
Better
Neither better nor worse
Worse
A lot worse

11. Gender

Male   Female

12. How do you define your ethnic origin? (Please choose only one)

Arab
African
British
Caribbean
Irish
Other European
SE Asian or Chinese
Other Asian
Other

13. Where are you living? (Please tick only one option)

United Kingdom
Other European Community Country
Other European Country
Asia
Australasia
Americas, North

Americas, South
Other

14. What is your age group? (Please tick only one option)

Under 19 years
19–39 years
40–59 years
60 years and over

15. Are you a member of BackCare?

Yes   No

If you would like to be eligible to receive a free copy of the book, please give us your name and address below:
(There will be a free copy for the first 500 people completing the survey.)

Title ....

First Name ....

Last name ....

Address ....
          ....

Town ....

County ....

Postcode ....

Country ....

Thank you for completing our survey

We would also be very interested in what advice you might give another back pain sufferer about any of the following topics:

Getting washed and dressed?
Household tasks?
Driving/travelling?
Working?
Shopping?
Gardening?
Social life (including friends, family, hobbies)?
Keeping positive?

Please write any advice or tips in the space below:

Glossary

abdomen The part of the body between the chest and the legs, containing the stomach, bowels, etc.

Achilles tendon The tendon joining the muscles in the calf to the heel bone.

acupressure See **Shiatsu**.

acupuncture A complementary therapy, designed to relieve pain, in which thin needles are inserted into points along meridian lines designated by ancient practitioners as channels of energy in the body.

Alexander technique A complementary therapy that emphasizes the importance of correct posture and movement in order to ease back and neck problems.

analgesic Medication used to relieve pain.

ankylosing spondylitis A rheumatic condition that mainly affects the spine, in which some of the bones and joints become inflamed and may fuse together. It is also known as 'Bamboo spine'. Entire fusing of the spine is unusual.

anti-inflammatory Medication used to reduce inflammation.

arachnoiditis Chronic inflammation of the arachnoid layer of the meninges (a membrane surrounding the brain and the spinal cord). Often leads to the formation of scar tissue, which may cause long-term back pain.

aromatherapy A complementary therapy that uses essential oils, extracted from plants, which are thought to have specific healing properties. The essential oils can be used in a bath or they can be diluted in a carrier oil and applied in a massage by an aromatherapist.

arthritis Inflammation of the joints. Osteoarthritis is marked by degeneration of the cartilage and bone of the joints. Rheumatoid arthritis is characterized especially by pain, stiffness, inflammation, swelling, and sometimes deformity of joints.

biofeedback A therapy that involves using an electrical device connected to the body via wires and electrodes to monitor one or more vital signs, e.g. heart rate, blood pressure, skin temperature or muscle activity. The machine gives auditory or visual cues as the measures change, and this feedback enables the patient to test new ways of 'thinking relaxed' or altered movement patterns until the monitor indicates that he or she is relaxed.

CAM (complementary and alternative medicine) Complementary and alternative therapies, such as homeopathy, acupuncture, osteopathy and Shiatsu.

cardiovascular Involving the heart and blood vessels.

cartilage A type of soft, elastic tissue in the body, e.g. in the nose and ears, sometimes called gristle.

cervical Of the neck.

chinning bar A bar designed to be secured at an appropriate height so that someone can hang from it by their hands, and then pull themselves up until their chin is level with the bar.

chiropody The medical care and treatment of the human foot.

chiropractic The use of manipulation techniques and advice on exercise and lifestyle to correct spinal problems often diagnosed by means of X-rays. Chiropractic is a profession that specializes in the diagnosis, treatment and management of conditions that are due to problems with joints, ligaments, tendons and nerves, in particular those of the spine. Treatment consists of manipulative techniques designed to improve joint function and relieve pain and muscle spasm. It does not involve the use of any drugs or surgery.

chymopapain injection An injection of a papaya extract, sometimes used to treat sciatic pain caused by a 'slipped' disc.

colitis An inflammation of the colon.

congenital Existing from birth.

cortisone injection A type of steroid injection used to reduce inflammation especially in rheumatoid arthritis.

cryotherapy (or cold therapy) Using ice packs, cold packs and ice massage to ease pain.

CT (computerized tomography) scan or CAT (computer assisted tomography) scan The patient lies inside the CT scanner, and radiation is beamed from several directions to produce a composite image. Unlike X-ray images, a CT scan shows soft tissue as well as bone. But, like standard X-ray procedures, CT scans involve appreciable levels of radiation exposure.

Devil's claw An anti-inflammatory herb, which has become a popular remedy for arthritis.

discectomy An operation to remove the damaged or bulging part of a 'slipped' disc in order to relieve pressure on the nerves in this part of the back.

DMSO (dimethyl sulfoxide) An industrial solvent that is applied to the skin (usually in a diluted form) by some back sufferers in order to gain pain relief. It is illegal to use DMSO in this way.

electrical stimulation therapy A form of therapy most often used by physiotherapists and chiropractors, usually as a supplement to massage, manipulation or trigger point injections. Electrical stimulation devices work by sending an electrical current into muscle areas, causing the muscles to contract and relax.

epidural An injection (usually a mixture of corticosteroid and pain-relieving anaesthetic) into the epidural space, which is just outside the spinal cord.

facet joint A small joint between two vertebrae that allows movement to occur at each level in the spine.

faith healing A method of treating health problems through prayer and faith in God.

Feldenkrais therapy A complementary therapy, developed in the USA by Moishe Feldenkrais, that emphasizes posture, movement and awareness, and attempts to integrate physical, mental and spiritual approaches to well-being.

glucosamine A chemical that occurs naturally in the body and is used to produce the connective tissue for joints. It has become a popular remedy for back pain, especially pain caused by osteoarthritis, in the form of supplements made from shellfish shells.

gravity inversion Hanging upside down or being tilted so that the head is lower than the feet, with the aim of allowing gravity to decompress the vertebrae and stretch the back muscles.

gynaecology A branch of medicine that deal with women's reproductive organs.

hamstring A group of muscles and tendons behind the knee.

herbalism A complementary therapy in which herbal remedies, in the form of tablets, oils, ointments and teas, are used to treat health problems.

herniated disc See 'slipped' disc.

homeopathy A complementary therapy based on the principle that 'like cures like.' For example, a homeopath will treat a fever with a substance that, if taken in normal quantities, would produce a fever. Homeopathic remedies are often diluted many times, until there is no detectable trace of the original substance. This is because homeopaths believe the greater the dilution, the more 'potent' (precise and active) the remedy.

hydrotherapy A form of therapy that uses water, e.g. in whirlpools.

hypnotherapy A complementary therapy in which the practitioner puts the patient into a hypnotic trance in order to help them overcome back pain. Once the patient is in a trance, the hypnotherapist will address their unconscious mind. For instance, people with arthritis may be told that they can turn the pain down like the volume on a radio.

isometric A type of exercise in which muscles contract against a load which is fixed or immovable. In other words, the joints do not move and the muscles work hard in one position.

kelp A type of seaweed, used especially as a source of iodine.

kinesiology A complementary therapy based on the principles and mechanics of muscular movement. Applied kinesiology involves the use of manipulation, massage and exercise.

laminectomy A surgical operation designed to relieve pressure on nerves in either the back or neck by removing a small amount of bone.

ligament A strong band of tissue in the body that connects bones or holds organs in place.

liniment A rub-on balm, e.g. Deep Heat.

lordosis An inward curve, e.g. the hollow in the lower back.

lumbar region The lower back.

MRI (magnetic resonance imaging) scan A scan that is produced using a combination of magnetic force and radio signals. An MRI scanner can 'see' soft tissues (e.g. discs, muscles and ligaments). A computer collects and interprets radio signals from the body, displaying on its screen a composite image of the examined part. The procedure is painless and does not involve any radiation exposure.

musculoskeletal physician An orthodox medical doctor who has done lengthy additional training in the specific diagnosis and treatment of conditions of the spine, muscles and joints. These physicians combine skills and techniques from general practice, rheumatology, orthopaedics, pain management, occupational health, sports medicine, rehabilitation, psychology and psychiatry.

myelogram Taking a myelogram involves placing the patient on a tilting table and injecting a solution opaque to X-rays into the spinal column. Tilting the table disperses the injected dye throughout the spinal column. X-rays are then taken. The dye is supposed to reveal abnormal shapes – such as a ruptured disc or a narrowing of the spine.

naturopathy A complementary therapy based on the idea that body, mind and spirit are interrelated. Naturopaths believe that stress, too little sleep, lack of exercise and fresh air and too many 'toxins' (from processed food and environmental pollution) cause imbalances that can affect the whole person and lead to various health problems.

nerve block injection An injection, often consisting of alcohol or a steroid, designed to numb the nerve centre that is generating the pain.

neurodynamics The dynamics of the nervous system.

neurology Diagnosis and treatment of pathologies involving the nervous system.

neurosurgery Surgery involving the nervous system.

obstetrics A branch of medicine that deals with childbirth and antenatal and postnatal care.

occupational health therapy A form of therapy that offers methods of going about daily activities, with the help of special aids and techniques, that enable people to avoid straining their backs.

orthopaedics A branch of surgery concerned with the prevention or treatment of skeletal abnormalities.

orthotic A shoe insert prescribed for someone whose legs are slightly different lengths.

osteoarthritis See **arthritis**.

osteopathy A complementary therapy in which problems with muscles, ligaments, nerves and joints are treated by using gentle, manual techniques to ease pain, reduce swelling and improve mobility.

pain clinic A clinic specializing in the treatment of all forms of chronic pain.

pelvis The hip and groin area; the bowl-shaped frame of bones at the base of the spine, to which the leg bones are joined.

physiotherapy A profession that specializes in diagnosing and treating problems in the joints and soft tissues. Treatments for back pain aim to relieve pain, promote relaxation and restore movement, and techniques used may include exercise, advice, manipulation, mobilization, massage and electrotherapy (such as TENS and biofeedback).

Pilates A form of exercise that emphasizes correct posture and alignment in order to improve flexibility and mobility.

placebo A pill or treatment with no active ingredients or known medical value, which nevertheless helps some of the patients who receive it.

podiatry A profession that specializes in the assessment, diagnosis and treatment of the lower limbs. Podiatrists are qualified to treat people with arthritis, diabetes, sports injuries, etc. Their biomechanical assessments and foot insoles (orthotics) can be particularly helpful for people with back pain.

prolapsed disc See 'slipped' disc.

prostate A gland, located just below the bladder and found only in men, that produces the liquid component of semen. Prostate cancer is the second most common cancer in men (after lung cancer), though it mainly affects older men.

PSA (prostate specific antigen) A protein that is only secreted by the prostate gland. Rising PSA levels can sometimes indicate prostate cancer.

reflexology A complementary therapy in which pressure is applied to particular areas on the feet or (occasionally) the hands in order to 'rebalance energy in the body' and stimulate natural healing processes.

rheumatoid arthritis See **arthritis**.

rheumatology Diagnosis and treatment of arthritis and related diseases.

Rolfing A vigorous form of massage, developed in the USA and designed to re-align the body and improve posture. Treatment includes instruction on movement and breathing.

ruptured disc See 'slipped' disc.

sacro-lumbar region The base of the spine.

sciatic nerve One of several nerves that come out of the spinal cord in the lower back. There are two sciatic nerves (one for each leg), and each sciatic nerve runs deep inside the buttock and down the back of the leg.

sciatica Pain running down the buttocks, down the back of the thigh, continuing into the calf, and sometimes into the foot, caused by pressure on the sciatic nerve where it emerges from the spinal column.

sclerotherapy A form of treatment that involves injecting a chemical irritant and local anaesthetic into ligaments, usually around a joint thought to be unstable. The body reacts to this irritant by forming scar tissue, which is supposed to help stabilize the back.

scoliosis A lateral (sideways) curvature of the spine.

self-help stress reduction Any one of several different self-help relaxation techniques, including meditation and visualization.

Shiatsu A Japanese massage technique often referred to as 'acupuncture without needles' because it focuses on the same meridian lines, or 'channels of energy' in the body, but uses thumb pressure rather than needles.

'slipped' disc (or herniated/prolapsed/ruptured disc) A condition affecting one of the discs located between the bony segments that make up the spinal column. Part of the soft gel in the centre of the disc bulges through the disc's fibrous outer layer and presses on a nerve as it leaves the spinal cord. The term 'slipped disc' does not really describe the process accurately. Discs do not slip out of place. Instead, they bulge and put pressure on the nerves, which results in leg pain.

soft-tissue back problem A problem involving a strain (torn fibres caused by overstretching), spasms or inflammation of back muscles – or all of the above. Soft-tissue problems can also involve damage to ligaments, tendons or connective tissue.

spina bifida occulta A congenital condition, revealed by X-rays, in which a portion of the spinal column has failed to develop.

spinal cord The cord of nervous tissue that extends from the brain, down the spine, and carries 'messages' to and from the brain.

spinal fusion A surgical operation that permanently joins together two or more spinal vertebrae and prevents movement in that section of the spine.

spinal stenosis A narrowing of the spinal column.

spondylitis Inflammation of the spine.

spondylolisthesis A shift of one of the vertebrae on the segment below. The shift is usually in a forward direction.

spondylolysis A congenital condition involving incompletely formed vertebrae.

subluxation Term used by chiropractors, meaning misalignment.

Swedish massage A relaxing, usually painless form of massage involving smooth, gliding movements.

Tai Chi An ancient Chinese, dance-like martial art that is thought to help increase strength and flexibility.

tendon A tough cord or band of connective tissue that joins a muscle with a bone and transmits the force exerted by the muscle.

traction Form of treatment in which the patient's limbs are suspended for a long period of time, with the aim of pulling joints into alignment. Traction can be done by hand, or by a machine that uses weights to 'stretch' the spine. The idea is that stretching the spine will relieve pressure on discs, and release any trapped nerves and tension in the muscles.

transcutaneous electric nerve stimulation (TENS) machine A small, portable, pain-relieving device, which can be hooked over a belt or concealed under loose clothing. It runs on batteries and sends electrical impulses across the skin via electrodes. These impulses cause a painless buzzing or tingling sensation, and either help prevent pain messages reaching the brain or stimulate the body to make its own natural painkillers (endorphins).

trigger point injection An injection of a painkiller, mixed with saline or cortisone, into an area of soft tissue that seems 'knotted' and radiates pain to other areas of the back, buttocks or legs.

ultrasound therapy A form of therapy that uses sound waves pitched above the range of human hearing. They pass easily through the skin and are thought to produce a micro-massaging effect on the aching joints or muscles underneath.

urology A branch of medicine that deals with the urinary tract.

vertebra One of the bony segments (blocks) that make up the spinal column.

Useful Addresses

The following list of addresses includes some self-help organizations for those in the UK who suffer from back pain, as well as a number of complementary and alternative practitioners' associations from whom you can get a list of registered therapists in your area. This list also contains some Internet sites where it is possible to view and in some cases purchase back-care products online, a potential boon if you do not live near a specialist shop or if your local shop stocks only a limited range of goods. Many house and garden companies, DIY centres and some Internet sites offer useful implements such as long-handled grippers or window washers and long-reach gardening tools.

Organizations

Acupuncture Association of Chartered Physiotherapists (AACP)
AACP Secretariat
Portcullis
Castle Street
Mere
Wiltshire, BA12 6JE
Tel: 01747 861151 (Mondays to Fridays 9a.m.–5p.m.)
Fax: 01747 861717
Email: sec@aacp.uk.com
Internet: www.aacp.uk.com

Aromatherapy Organizations Council (AOC)
PO Box 19834
London SE25 6WF
Tel: 0208 251 7912 (Mondays to Fridays 10a.m.–2p.m.)
Email: info@aoc.uk.net
Internet: www.aocuk.net
The governing body for the aromatherapy profession in the UK. For a list of local practitioners in your area, send an A5 SAE to the above address.

Arthritis Care
18 Stephenson Way
London NW1 2HD
Tel: 0207 380 6500
Fax: 0207 380 6505
Internet:
www.arthritiscare.org.uk
*Arthritis Care is a registered
charity and is the largest voluntary
organization working with people
with arthritis.*

Arthritis Research Campaign
Copeman House
St Mary's Court
St Mary's Gate
Chesterfield
Derbyshire S41 7TD
Tel: 0870 850 500 or
01246 558033
Internet: www.arc.org.uk

**Association of Naturopathic
Practitioners (ANP)**
ANP UK
Secretary General
Coombe Hurst
Coombe Hill Road
East Grinstead
West Sussex RH19 4LZ
Internet:
www.naturopathy-anp.com
*The ANP, an association of
qualified members, seeks to promote
the practice of the healing art of
Naturopathic Medicine in the UK
and Ireland. They have a practi-
tioner referral service for patients
wishing to locate a practitioner.*

Association of Reflexologists
27 Old Gloucester Road
London WC1N 3XX
Tel: 0870 567 3320 (Mondays
to Fridays 9a.m.–5p.m.)
Fax: 01823 336646
Email: info@aor.org.uk
Internet: www.aor.org.uk
*A membership organization for
reflexologists. Provides detailed
information about accredited
members, publications, history of
reflexology, conferences.*

**BackCare – The charity for
healthier backs**
16 Elmtree Road
Teddington
Middlesex TW11 8ST
Tel: 0208 977 5474 (Mondays
to Thursdays 9a.m.–4.30p.m.)
Fax: 0208 943 5318
Email: info@backcare.org.uk
Internet:
www.backcare.org.uk
*BackCare (registered as the
National Back Pain Association) is
an independent national charity that
helps people manage and prevent
back pain by providing information,
promoting self-help, encouraging
debate and funding research into
better back health. BackCare represents people with back pain, a broad
range of health professionals treating back pain, researchers and
employers and is uniquely placed to
act as a conduit for information
exchange and debate.*

British Acupuncture Council
63 Jeddo Road
London W12 9HQ
Tel: 0208 735 0400
Fax: 0208 735 0404
Email:
info@acupuncture.org.uk
Internet:
www.acupuncture.org.uk

**British Association of
Nutritional Therapists
(BANT)**
37 Old Gloucester Street
London WC1N 3XX
Tel: 0870 606 1284 (Mondays
to Fridays 9a.m.–5p.m.)
Email:
theadministrator@bant.org.uk
Internet: www.bant.org.uk
*BANT holds a register of practi-
tioners who are fully qualified in the
science of nutrition as well as clini-
cal practice.*

**British Homeopathic
Association**
Hahnemann House
29 Park Street West
Luton LU1 3BE
Tel: 0870 444 3950
Fax: 0870 444 3960
Internet:
www.trusthomeopathy.org
*A charity founded in 1902 to
promote education and research in
homeopathy.*

**British Institute of
Musculoskeletal Medicine**
34 The Avenue
Watford
Hertfordshire WD17 4AH
Tel: 01923 220999
Fax: 01923 249037
Email: info@bimm.org.uk
Internet: www.bimm.org.uk

**British Massage Therapy
Council**
17 Rymers Lane
Cowley
Oxford OX4 3JU
Tel: 01865 774123 (24-hour
answerphone)
*This is an organization for and rep-
resenting professional massage associations and professional massage
schools, promoting high standards in
the practice of professional massage
therapy, massage training and promoting massage therapy.*

**British Osteopathic
Association**
Langham House West
Mill Street
Luton
Bedfordshire LU1 2NA
Tel: 01582 488455
Fax: 01582 481533
Internet: www.osteopathy.org

British Society for Allergy, Environmental and Nutritional Medicine (BSAENM)
PO Box 7
Knighton
Powys LD7 1WT
Helpline: 0906 302 0010
Tel: 01547 550380
Email: info@bsaenm.org
Internet:
www.jnem.demon.co.uk
BSAENM aims to promote, for the benefit of the public, the study of allergy, environmental and nutritional medicine.

Chartered Society of Physiotherapy
14 Bedford Row
London WC1R 4ED
Tel: 0207 306 6666
Internet: www.csp.org.uk

College of Occupational Therapists
106–114 Borough High Street
Southwark
London SE1 1LB
Tel: 0207 357 6480
Internet: www.cot.org.uk

Complementary Medical Association
The Meridian
142c Greenwich High Road
Greenwich SE10 8NN
Email: info@the-cma.org.uk
Internet: www.the-cma.org.uk

The CMA is a not-for-profit organization that aims to promote ethical, responsible and professional complementary medicine to the public and the medical profession. See the website for details of qualified practitioners and colleges, and extensive information about complementary therapies.

General Council and Register of Naturopaths (GCRN)
Goswell House
2 Goswell Road
Street
Somerset BA16 0JG
Tel: 08707 456 984
Email:
admin@naturopathy.org.uk
Internet:
www.naturopathy.org.uk
The registration body of UK naturopaths who have graduated with a naturopathic diploma (ND) at an accredited college. Aims to establish and maintain standards of education for practitioners and to provide for the inspection of colleges and courses of naturopathy for the protection and benefit of the public. Can search on the website for registered naturopaths.

General Osteopathic Council
176 Tower Bridge Road
London SE1 3LU
Tel: 0207 357 6655
Internet:
www.osteopathy.org.uk

International College of Applied Kinesiology UK
The Administrator
Doneechka Clinic
Southwater
West Sussex RH 13 9EY
Tel: 01403 734321
Email: admin@icak.co.uk
Internet: www.icak.co.uk

International Federation of Reflexologists
76–8 Edridge Road
Croydon
Surrey
CR0 1EF
Tel: 0208 645 9134
Fax: 0208 649 9291
Internet:
www.intfedreflexologists.org
Keeps a register of professional therapists, and a list of accredited schools which all teach to a centrally agreed syllabus. Has a history of reflexology and answers to frequently asked questions.

National Ankylosing Spondylitis Society
PO Box 179
Mayfield
East Sussex TN20 6ZL
Tel: 01435 873527
Fax: 01435 873027
Email: nass@nass.co.uk
Internet: www.nass.co.uk

National Council for Hypnotherapy
PO Box 421
Charwelton
Daventry NN11 1AS
Tel: 0800 952 0545
Internet:
www.hypnotherapists.org.uk
Holds one of the largest registers of independent hypnotherapists in the United Kingdom and strives to maintain the highest standards among its members. Can search for a local hypnotherapist online.

National Federation of Spiritual Healers
Old Manor Farm Studio
Church Street
Sunbury-on-Thames
Middlesex TW16 6RG
Tel: 0845 1232777
Fax: 01932 779648
Email: office@nfsh.org.uk
Internet: www.nfsh.org.uk

National Institute of Medical Herbalists
Elm House
54 Mary Arches Street
Exeter EX4 3BA
Tel: 01392 426022
Email:
nimh@ukexeter.freeserve.co.uk
Internet: www.nimh.org.uk
Professional organization of practitioners of herbal medicine. The Institute maintains high standards

of practice and patient care, and works to promote the benefits of herbal medicine. Website has an online database to find your nearest herbalist, information on training and research, plus links.

National Osteoporosis Society

PO Box 10
Radstock
Bath BA3 3YB
Tel: 01761 471771
Helpline: 0845 4500 230
Internet:
www.nos.org.uk/healthprof.asp

RADAR – The disability network

Head Office
12 City Forum
250 City Road
London EC1V 8AF
Tel: 0207 250 3222
Fax: 0207 250 0212
Minicom: 0207 250 4119
Email: radar@radar.org.uk
Internet: www.radar.org.uk

Research Council for Complementary Medicine

c/o 1 Harley Street
London W1G 9QD
Email: info@rccm.org.uk
Internet: www.rccm.org.uk

Scoliosis Association UK

2 Ivebury Court
323–7 Latimer Road
London W10 6RA
Helpline: 0208 964 1166
Tel: 0208 964 5343
Fax: 0208 964 5343
Email: sauk@sauk.org.uk
Internet: www.sauk.org.uk

Scottish Chiropractic Association

Laigh Hatton Farm
Old Greenock Road
Bishopton
Renfrewshire PA7 5PB
Tel/Fax: 01505 863151
Email:
admin@sca-chiropractic.org
Internet:
www.sca-chiropractic.org

The Shiatsu Society

Eastlands Court
St Peter's Road
Rugby CV21 3QP
Tel: 0845 130 4560 (Mondays to Fridays 9a.m.–5p.m.)
Email: admin@shiatsu.org
Internet: www.shiatsu.org
Set up in 1981 to facilitate communication within the field of shiatsu and to inform the public of the benefits of this form of natural healing. Has formed a network linking individuals, students and teachers to fulfil the role of a professional organization.

**The Society of Chiropodists
and Podiatrists**
1 Fellmonger's Path
Tower Bridge Road
London SE1 3LY
Tel: 0207 234 8620
Internet: www.feetforlife.org

Product Suppliers

The Back Care Warehouse
2a Tower Road
Worthing
West Sussex BN11 1DP
Internet: www.
thebackcarewarehouse.co.uk

Back in Action
11 Whitcomb Street
Trafalgar Square
London WC2H 7HA
Tel: 0207 930 8309
Fax: 0207 925 0250
Internet:
www.backinaction.co.uk

The Back Shop
24 New Cavendish Street
London W1M 7LH
Tel: 0207 935 9148
Internet:
www.thebackshop.co.uk

Fitness Network
129 St John's Hill
London SW11 1TD
Tel: 0207 924 5590
Email:
enquiry@fitnessnetwork.co.uk
Internet:
www. fitnessnetwork.co.uk
*Suppliers of exercise and fitness
products, including gravity inversion
equipment.*

Physio Supplies Limited
The Warehouse
Beck Bank
West Pinchbeck
Spalding
Lincolnshire PE11 3QN
Tel: 08700 545050
Fax: 01775 640044
Internet:
www.physiosupplies.com
*Suppliers of physiotherapy equip-
ment, including massage tables,
Tempur pillows, orthopaedic pillows,
TENS machines, inversion tables,
back supports, lumbar supports and
cushions.*

Further Reading

Back and Neck Pain – The Facts by Loic Burn (Oxford University Press, 2000)

The Back Pain Revolution by Gordon Waddell (Churchill Livingstone, 1998)

The Back Book by Kim Burton et al (The Stationery Office Books, 2002)

The Daily Telegraph Arthritis: The Complete Guide to Relief by Arthur C. Klein (Constable & Robinson Ltd, 2005)

Managing Back Pain (BackCare, 2004)

Living With Back Pain by Helen Parker and Chris J. Main (Manchester University Press, 1990)

Treat Your Own Back by Robin McKenzie (Spinal Publications, 1997)

Overcoming Chronic Pain by Frances Cole, Helen Macdonald, Catherine Carus and Hazel Howden Leach (Constable & Robinson Ltd, 2005)

Index

Page numbers given in italic refer to illustrations